Botulinum Toxin Treatment

Bahman Jabbari

Botulinum Toxin Treatment

What Everyone Should Know

Second Edition

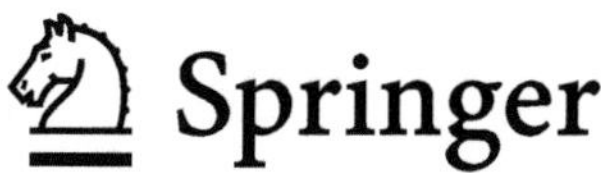 Springer

Bahman Jabbari
Emeritus Professor of Neurology
Yale University School of Medicine
New Haven, CT, USA

ISBN 978-3-031-54473-6   ISBN 978-3-031-54471-2   (eBook)
https://doi.org/10.1007/978-3-031-54471-2

This Springer imprint is published by the registered company Springer Nature Switzerland AG
The registered company address is: Gewerbestrasse 11, 6330 Cham, Switzerland

Paper in this product is recyclable.

Preface

Botulinum toxin therapy is now a major mode of treatment for a variety of medical ailments. The notion that a potent toxin can be used in a safe way to treat so many medical disorders was unimaginable up to 50 years ago. It was through tireless efforts of basic scientists and clinical researchers that the use of this unusual, but effective mode of therapy achieved acceptance in the medical community. Botulinum toxin therapy is now used worldwide in the management of millions of patients. This book describes different approved indications or potential indications of botulinum toxin therapy in a language that would be comprehensible by non-medical individuals. Wherever possible, medical terms are explained in a language understandable to the public.

Since the first edition of this book 5 years ago, a large literature has developed describing the long-term efficacy and safety of toxin therapy in the approved indications such as migraine, bladder disorders and spasticity as well as emergence of more data on potential important indications for this mode of treatment such as efficacy in depression and in certain heart ailments (atrial fibrillation). FDA has approved several toxins (Botox, Dysport and Xeomin) for treatment of spasticity in children with cerebral palsy and other spasticity producing conditions. FDA also approved two new toxins for use in the United States: Jeuveau and Daxxify; Jeuveau has been approved only for cosmetic use, whereas Daxxify was approved for cosmetic use as well as treatment of cervical dystonia—a common movement disorder affecting the neck, often associated with disabling neck pain.

The current edition of the book includes two new chapters, one on the use of botulinum toxin therapy in dentistry and the other on the growing use of toxin therapy in veterinary medicine for canine and equine pains. All chapters of the book are written by Bahman Jabbari M.D. with the exception of Chap. 13 on the cosmetic and aesthetic indications that is provided by Drs Marie Noland and Marissa Dennis. In this edition, the information on safety of botulinum toxin therapy has been considerably expanded with inclusion of new data in Chap. 17. Chapter 19 of this book also provides substantially more information regarding potential indications of botulinum toxin therapy compared to that presented in the first edition of this book.

I would like to express my gratitude to Dr Fattaneh Tavassoli for her editorial assistance and to Drs Tahere Mousavi and Damoun Safarpour for their illustrations. I am also grateful to Merry Stuber and Charlotte Nunes from Springer Nature for their support and to Amrita Unnikrishnan who helped to finalize the printing of this book.

Newport Coast, CA, USA   Bahman Jabbari
April 23, 2024

Contents

Chapter 1
A Toxin that Remedies a Large Number of Medical Problems: How It Happened?

Abstract This chapter provides information on the history of botulinum toxin development into a powerful therapeutic agent. It explains how through tireless efforts of remarkable basic scientists and clinicians one of deadliest toxins in the nature developed into a widely used treatment with high safety profile. Some of the characteristics of different brands of botulinum toxin in the US market are also briefly discussed in this chapter.

Keywords History of Botulinum toxin · Justinus Kerner · FDA approved indications of Botulinum toxins · Botulinum toxin · Botulinum neurotoxin

A group of bacterial toxins called botulinum toxins or botulinum neurotoxins (BoNT) have now become a remedy for a large number of hard to treat medical conditions. They have proven to be the most multipurpose therapeutic agents in modern medicine and possess more clinical applications than any other drug currently in the market [1]. Among these toxins, one type (type A) was first introduced to the medical arena in 1989 under the trade name of oculinum (name changed to Botox 2 years later). It was the only approved toxin in the US for several years. There are now several other type A botulinum toxins and a type B toxin as well, each with their advantages and disadvantages. Four decades of experience with botulinum toxin therapy indicates that these agents can be drugs of first choice for the symptoms of several medical conditions, and when used by trained clinicians, are generally safe. Serious side effects are rare, and in most cases gradually subside if the affected patients are diagnosed early and medically supported.

Botulinum neurotoxin, often abbreviated in the medical literature as BoNT, is produced by a bacterium with the medical name of clostridium botulinum (CB). The bacteria, CB, is present in nature and improper exposure to it can cause a disease called botulism. The term botulinum comes from the Latin word of "botulus" meaning sausage since the earlier (eighteenth and early nineteenth century) outbreaks of botulism in Europe were often linked to consumption of spoiled sausage or ham. The agent can get into the body and cause disease via a variety of routes: food consumption, inhalation, wound contamination and injection. In western countries, botulism is rare due to proper food preparation, wound hygiene, and protective laboratory regulations (to prevent inhalation toxicity). Botulism through therapeutic injections is also rare as the applied units of the toxin for most indications are below 500 units which is far from the lethal dose of 3000 units or more reported in monkeys [2]. Moreover, with modern and advanced life support facilities, even sick patients with respiratory failure, if diagnosed early, often eventually recover as the paralyzing effect of the toxin will not last more than 3–4 months.

The development of a therapeutic utility of botulinum neurotoxin (BoNT) took over a 100 years of clinical observation and laboratory experimentation. For years, physicians in Europe, especially in southern Germany, were familiar with the symptoms of a disease which was caused by consuming rotten sausage "sausage poisoning." After a well- documented outbreak of sausage poisoning in 1793 that affected 13 individuals (6 of whom did not survive), the city of Stuttgart became the major center for investigation of this type of poisoning [3]. At the beginning of the nineteenth century, a leading point of debate was whether the "sausage poisoning" was due to a chemical agent in the sausage or due to a biologic, yet unknown, factor. Several chemical agents were suspected including hydrocyanic acid.

The next major development was the prediction that the agent responsible for "sausage poisoning" could be used for treatment of symptoms of certain medical ailments. The individual who first promoted the idea was a young German physician, 29 years of age at the time, who studied in detail the latest outbreaks of the illness in southern Germany. Justinus Kerner (Fig. 1.1) published two monographs in 1820 and 1822 detailing the clinical aspects of botulism based on case histories of 76 and 155 patients [4]. Kerner's descriptions included almost all manifestations of botulism, as known to us today, including paralysis of the muscles, loss of pupillary reaction to light and diminished sweat and saliva production. After studying all ingredients of the poisoned food, he concluded that something in the fatty portion of the sausage itself and not any other ingredients in the sausage preparation (blood, liver, etc.) was responsible for the sickness. Kerner believed that this "fatty poison" had a biological rather than a chemical origin. He wrote that the toxic agent had to travel through the nervous system to cause paralysis and the other symptoms of the disease. The toxin damaged the nerves and made them like "rusted electrical wires".

Kerner predicted that the "sausage poison" could be used in the future to remedy certain symptoms of some medical disorders, particularly those symptoms arising from hyperexcitability of the nervous system that cause abnormal involuntary movements. He mentioned treatment of the involuntary movement of "chorea" as an example. Chorea is a movement disorder characterized by involuntary twitches which can affect the face or the limbs. Chorea may be hereditary (i.e. Huntington's chorea, often associated with dementia) or it may develop secondary to non-hereditary diseases or drugs. Currently, almost 200 years after Kerner's prediction, medicinal botulinum toxin injections have become the therapy of first choice for several abnormal movement and motor disorders especially dystonias and

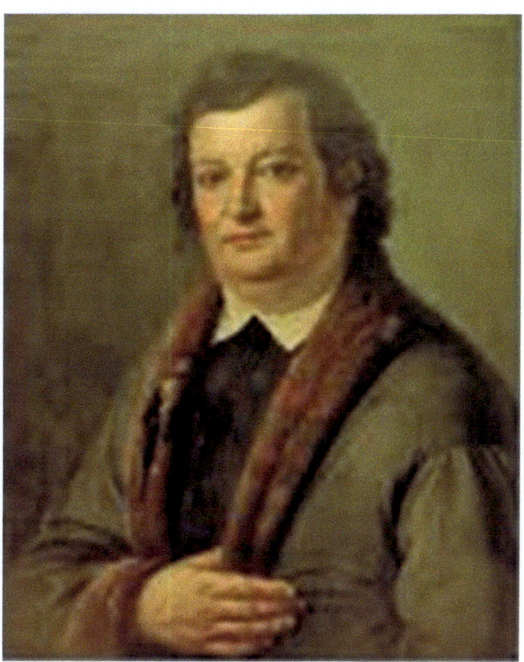

Fig. 1.1 Portrait of Justinus Kerner from Wikimedia (public domain)

spasticity. Interestingly, however, it is least used in management of chorea—the movement disorder that he used as an example.

In 1895, Emile Van Ermengem, a professor of bacteriology at the University of Ghent, Belgium discovered the organism responsible for botulism (Fig. 1.2).

In 1919, Stanford university researcher A. Bruke discovered two different serological strains of BoNT, A and B. In 1924 Ida Bengston a Swedish -American bacteriologist suggested to change the name of bacteria from bacillus botulinum to clostridium botulinum. The word colstrididium is derived from Greek word of kloster meaning spindle.

Further refinement of the botulinum toxin which ultimately facilitated its clinical use, came about during World War II when there was an interest in producing large amounts of the toxin and to find preventive and therapeutic measures in case of exposure and intoxication. Close to the end of World War II, at Fort Detrick Maryland, a US Army research facility, Carl Lamanna and James Duff invented a technique for crystallization and concentration of botulinum toxin [2]. Edward Schantz (Fig. 1.4), purified and produced the first batch of the toxin in 1946. Shantz then moved to the University of Wisconsin where with Eric Johnson further refined botulinum toxin for clinical research.

In 1949, a British investigator, A. Burgen, and his colleagues discovered that botulinum toxin blocks the nerve transmitter substance "acetylcholine" at nerve-muscle junction leading to the toxin's paralytic effect. In 1964, Daniel Drachman at Johns Hopkins University demonstrated that injection of the type A botulinum

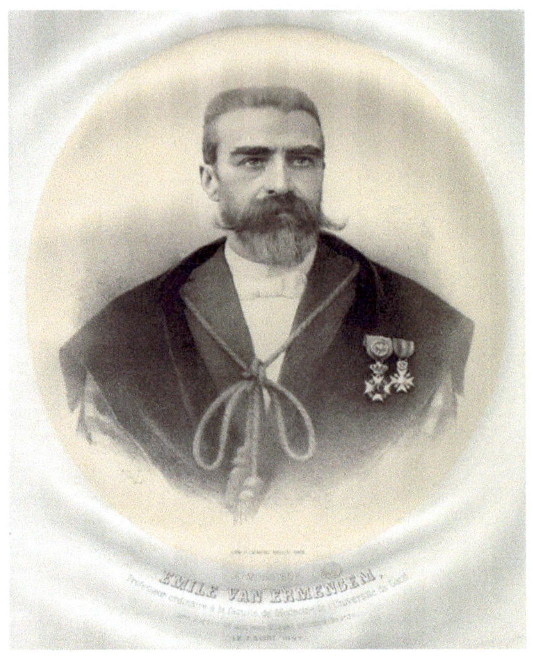

Fig. 1.2 Emile Van Ermengem who discovered the culprit bacteria responsible for botulism. He studied the rotten ham consumed by a group of 34 musicians who all felt sick after an outgoing. He showed that the spoiled ham and the tissue obtained from 3 patients who did not survive, contained a large number of rod–shaped, gram positive bacteria which he named bacillus botulinum (Fig. 1.3)

neurotoxin (BoNT) into the muscles of chick embryos can produce a dose dependent muscle wasting (atrophy) and muscle weakening [5].

The next major step started with the work of Alan Scott and his colleagues in San Francisco, CA. Since early 1960s, Alan Scott, an ophthalmologist, and his colleague Carter Collins were interested in the physiology of eye muscles and correction of strabismus (crossed eyes) in children by a method other than resection of hyperactive muscles around the eye. At the time, their research focused on injection of anaesthetic agents into eye muscles of monkeys under electromyographic guidance. Electromyography records the electrical activity of muscles using a special instrument. Coming across Drachman's work, Dr. Scott started to explore the effects of botulinum toxin injections into the eye muscles of the monkeys. Edward Schantz who was then at University of Wisconsin, provided the purified and injectable toxin for Dr. Scott's experiments. In Scott's laboratory, the toxin was freeze-dried, buffered with albumin and prepared for injection in small aliquots.

In 1973, Dr. Scott published his seminal work on injection of botulinum toxin type A into the external eye muscles of monkeys. The work clearly showed that the toxin injection can selectively weaken a targeted eye muscle and offer an alternative to surgery for strabismus (crossed eyes). His subsequent work on 67 patients with strabismus (under an FDA approved protocol), published in 1980, demonstrated that indeed botulinum toxin injection was effective in correcting human strabismus by decreasing the overactivity of culprit eye muscle(s) and correctly aligning the two eyes [6]. Dr. Scott also showed, in a number of open label, unblinded small studies, that injection of botulinum toxin into face muscles of humans can slow

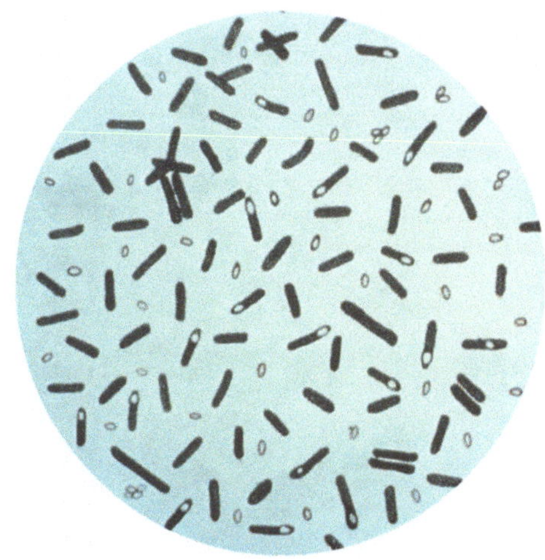

Fig. 1.3 Bacteria responsible for botulism. (Courtesy of Wikipedia)

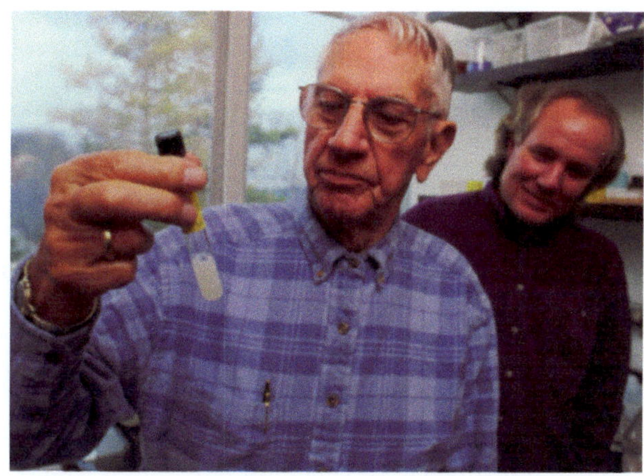

Fig. 1.4 Edward Shantz and Eric Johnson in the laboratory at the University of Wisconsin. (From Dressler & Roggenkeaemper. Reproduced with permission from Springer)

down and even stop involuntary facial movements in conditions like blepharospasm (spasm of the eye lids) and hemifacial spasm (HFS) (involuntary contractions affecting half of the face). These observations ignited substantial interest among Movement Disorder specialists and consequently led to documentation of the efficacy of BoNT therapy for a large number of involuntary movements. Finally, Scott observed that injection of 300 units of Botox for treatment of spasticity (tense muscles with increased tone) in one setting did not cause any side effects. This observation indicated a margin of safety per single injection of botulinum toxin type-A (Botox) in human which was unknown prior to his report [7] (Fig. 1.5).

Dr. Scott's efforts along with the work of Stanley Fahn and Mitchell Brin at Columbia University of New York, Joseph Janckovic at Baylor Medical College and Joseph Tsui at the University of British Columbia led to the approval of botulinum toxin A (then called oculinum, marketed by Allergan- the name was changed

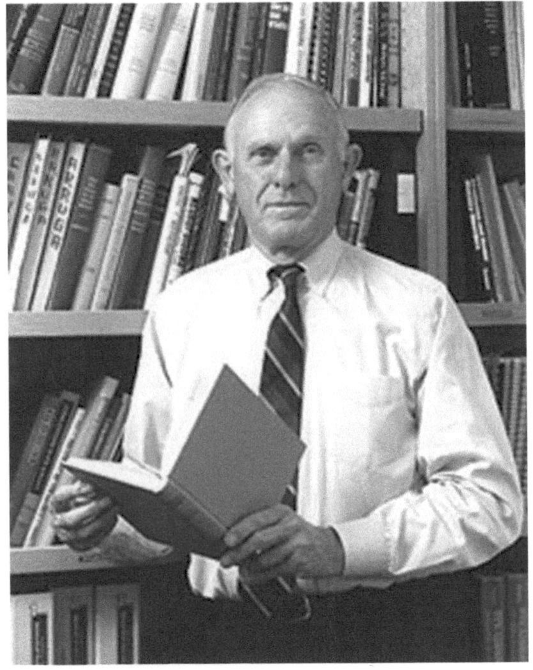

Fig. 1.5 Alan Scott who pioneered the use of botulinum neurotoxin (BoNT) therapy in humans. (From FJ Erbguth in the J Neural Trans. Reproduced by permission from Publisher-Springer)

to Botox 2 years later) for treatment of strabismus, blepharospasm and hemifacial (HFS) in 1989. The path was now open for investigation of the effects of BoNTs in many other movement and motor disorders.

What happened over the next 42 years is one of the most amazing stories in the field of medical treatment. A potent bacterial toxin which was the cause of much fear and apprehension developed into a therapeutic agent with documented or highly suggestive efficacy in alleviating more than 50 different medical symptoms. It was found to be generally safe if used with proper techniques of injection and under appropriate dosing guidelines. Much was learned during these years about the molecular structure of botulinum toxins [8], and their mechanism of action(s) on the nerve-muscle junction (Chap. 2), glandular tissue [9], and even pain pathways [10].

A few years after introduction of Botox, two more BoNT type-As were developed and subsequently marketed in the US under the trade names of Xeomin and Dysport. In Europe, Dirk Dressler, Reiner Benecki, Keith Foster and Andy Picket were leading investigators in defining the characteristics of these two newer forms of BoNTs and their potential for treating medical ailments [11]. A type B toxin was also marketed in the US under the trade name of Myobloc (Neurobloc in Europe). These BoNTs are now all FDA approved for different clinical indications. More recently, more type A toxins have been developed; one of them, Jeuveu received FDA approval in 2019 for aesthetic use and treatment of frown lines. Another type A toxin, Daxxify was approved in 2022 for aesthetic use and then in 2023 for treatment of cervical dystonia. Over time, much was learned about the advantages and disadvantages of these newer toxins (detailed descriptions are provided in Chap. 3 of this book).

Encouraged by earlier promising results of Botox injection, investigators with innovative minds conducted careful, high quality, double blinded clinical trials. The results of these multicenter studies, conducted on a sizeable number of patients led to FDA approval of Botox for management of a variety of medical conditions. In 2002, FDA approved injections of Botox into the face for correction of wrinkles (Chap. 13) and, in 2004, FDA approved Botox for treatment and reduction of excessive sweating (hyperhidrosis) in the arm pit (axilla) (Chap. 14). In 2009, FDA approved Botox injections for treatment of a disabling movement disorder characterized by abnormal neck postures, neck pain and neck shakes (cervical dystonia-Chap. 8). In 2011 and 2013, Botox was approved for two types of bladder dysfunction causing urinary urgency and incontinence (neurogenic and hyperactive bladder (Chap. 10). As clinical research continued, the positive results of two large, multi-center studies (PREEMPT 1 and 2), showed the efficacy of Botox injections into the skin and muscles around the head in subjects with chronic migraine leading to FDA approval of this treatment in 2010 (Chap. 4). During the past 15 years, FDA approved Botox, Xeomin and Dysport for treatment of spasticity. Spasticity (stiff and tense muscles) is a major handicap for patient after stroke, head and spinal cord trauma and multiple sclerosis as well as children affected by cerebral palsy. Injection of botulinum toxin into the affected muscles reduces muscle tone, improves the limb function, and helps ambulation and physiotherapy (Chaps. 6 and 7).

In addition to these FDA approved medical indications, there are more than 20 other medical conditions that, according to the results of small blinded and quality studies, respond to botulinum toxin injections. There are strong suggestions that, BoNT injections into the skin can relieve several types of distressing pains such as pain associated with shingles, painful neuropathy due to diabetes or painful neuropathy secondary to trauma to the limb(s) [12] (Chap. 5). There is also compelling evidence that injection of BoNT into arm and forearm muscles can significantly reduce the hand tremor both in Parkinson disease and in essential tremor (Chap. 8) [13, 14]. This wide range of BoNT applications for treatment of different medical symptoms reflects multiple and diverse mechanisms of the toxin's action which is covered in more detail in the second chapter of this book. It is expected that continued medical research and clinical observations will further expand the indications of botulinum toxin therapy in clinical medicine.

Amid emerging clinical indications for botulinum toxin therapy, basic scientists started to explore specifics of botulinum toxin molecule and its mechanism of action in different medical disorders. In US, at Yale university (New Haven, CT), Professor James Rothman (Fig. 1.6), chairman of the Department of Cell Biology, defined special proteins (called SNARE) that work at synapses (where two nerve cells or a nerve cell and muscle cell connect with each other) and promote the release of a specific chemical at the synapse that conveys the nerve signal from one cell to another. His lab purified SNARE proteins, one of which is blocked by the function of Botox.

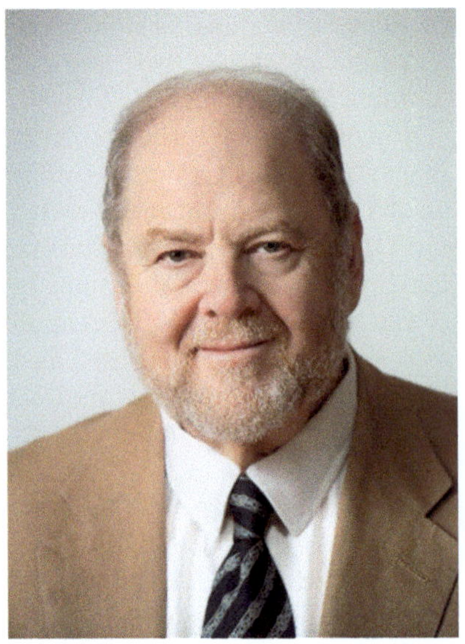

Fig. 1.6 Professor James Rothman, chair of Cell Biology at Yale who won the Nobel Prize in physiology and medicine for his seminal works on the physiology of synapses

Professor De Camilli and his colleagues, also at Yale, identified the protein that is blocked at neuro-muscular junction after Botox injection as SNAP-25 (Chap. 2) [15]. Italian basic scientists Monteccuco, Rossetto, Pirazzini described detailed molecular structure and pharmacology of botulinum toxins as well as the similarity and dissimilarity of this toxin to the tetanus toxin [8, 16]. In Zagreb, Croatia, Zdravko Lackovic, chairman of the Department of Pharmacology and his colleagues, Ivica Matak and Lidjia-Back-Rojecky have shown in a series of elegant experiments compelling evidence for the central action of the botulinum toxins and offered explanations on how the toxin influences pain pathways [17, 18].

Further evidence for the central function of botulinum toxins was provided by Matteo Caleo and his Italian colleagues after finding parts of the toxin in the central nervous system (brain) following injection into the muscle [19]. Gianpietro Schiavo in London, in collaboration with Italian scientists, discovered the enzyme through which botulinum toxins deactivate synapse proteins [20]. Professor Oliver Dolley and his colleagues in Dublin, Ireland have illustrated the mechanisms through which the injected toxin (into muscle) gets through different nerve cells and more recently how the novel recombinant toxin targets sensory cells and alters these cells' functions, an important finding pertaining to the analgesic effects of the toxin [21]. These remarkable achievements in the field of basic science, constantly encourages the clinicians to find new medical indications for botulinum toxins. Table 1.1 demonstrates important time-lines in the history of botulinum toxins from discovery to clinical application.

Table 1.1 Important time-lines of botulinum toxin development for clinical use

Year(s)	Investigator(s)/ FDA approvals	Comment
1820–1822	Justinus Kerner	Described details of botulism; predicted that the toxin could be used in the future as a medical remedy
1895	Emile Van Ermengem	Discovered the bacteria causing botulism
1944–1946	Lamanna and Duffy	Concentrated and crystalized the toxin
1946	Edward Schantz	Purified and produced the toxin in a form suitable for medical research
1949	A. Burgen	Acetylcholine identified as the chemical blocked by BoNT at nerve muscle junction
1953	Daniel Drachman	Intramuscular injection of Schantz's toxin can be quantified and resulted in dose dependent muscle weakness in chicks
1973	Alan Scott	Injection of type A toxin improved strabismus (crossed eyes) in monkeys
1980	Alan Scott	Controlled human study showed efficacy in strabismus. Observations made on potential use for blepharospasm, hemifacial spasm, spasticity
1985–1988	Fahn, Jankovic, Brin, Tsui	Controlled and blinded studies showed efficacy in blepharospasm and cervical dystonia
1989	FDA approval of Type A toxin (oculinum- name later changed to Botox)	Toxin approved for use in blepharospasm, hemifacial spasm and strabismus
1989-present	Other approved indications by FDA	Toxin approved for facial wrinkles, frown lines, cervical dystonia, chronic migraine, bladder dysfunction, upper and lower limb spasticity, excessive sweating of the arm pit and excessive drooling

References

1. Jankovic J. Botulinum toxin: state of the art. Mov Disord. 2017;32(8):1131–8. https://doi.org/10.1002/mds.27072. Epub 2017 Jun 22. PMID: 28639368.
2. Scott AB, Suzuki D. Systemic toxicity of botulinum toxin by intramuscular injection in the monkey. Mov Disord. 1988;3(4):333–5. https://doi.org/10.1002/mds.870030409. PMID: 3211180.
3. Erbguth FJ, Naumann M. Historical aspects of botulinum toxin: Justinus Kerner (1786-1862) and the "sausage poison". Neurology. 1999;53(8):1850–3. https://doi.org/10.1212/wnl.53.8.1850. PMID: 10563638.
4. Erbguth FJ. From poison to remedy: the chequered history of botulinum toxin. J Neural Transm (Vienna). 2008;115(4):559–65. https://doi.org/10.1007/s00702-007-0728-2. Epub 2007 Apr 26. PMID: 17458494.
5. Drachman DB. Atrophy of skeletal muscle in chick embryos treated with botulinum toxin. Science. 1964;145(3633):719–21. https://doi.org/10.1126/science.145.3633.719. PMID: 14163805.

6. Scott AB. Botulinum toxin injection into extraocular muscles as an alternative to strabismus surgery. Ophthalmology. 1980;87(10):1044–9. https://doi.org/10.1016/s0161-6420(80)35127-0. PMID: 7243198.

7. Scott AB. Development of botulinum toxin therapy. Dermatol Clin. 2004;22(2):131–3. https://doi.org/10.1016/s0733-8635(03)00019-6. PMID: 15222571.

8. Pirazzini M, Montecucco C, Rossetto O. Toxicology and pharmacology of botulinum and tetanus neurotoxins: an update. Arch Toxicol. 2022;96(6):1521–39. https://doi.org/10.1007/s00204-022-03271-9. Epub 2022 Mar 25. PMID: 35333944; PMCID: PMC9095541.

9. Lakraj AA, Moghimi N, Jabbari B. Hyperhidrosis: anatomy, pathophysiology and treatment with emphasis on the role of botulinum toxins. Toxins (Basel). 2013;5(4):821–40. https://doi.org/10.3390/toxins5040821. PMID: 23612753; PMCID: PMC3705293.

10. Matak I, Tékus V, Bölcskei K, Lacković Z, Helyes Z. Involvement of substance P in the antinociceptive effect of botulinum toxin type A: evidence from knockout mice. Neuroscience. 2017;358:137–45. https://doi.org/10.1016/j.neuroscience.2017.06.040. Epub 2017 Jul 1. PMID: 28673722.

11. Foster K. Clinical applications of botulinum toxins. New York: Springer; 2014.

12. Jabbari B. Botulinum toxin treatment of pain disorders. 2nd ed. Cham: Springer; 2022.

13. Jankovic J, Schwartz K, Clemence W, Aswad A, Mordaunt J. A randomized, double-blind, placebo-controlled study to evaluate botulinum toxin type A in essential hand tremor. Mov Disord. 1996;11(3):250–6. https://doi.org/10.1002/mds.870110306. PMID: 8723140.

14. Mittal SO, Machado D, Richardson D, Dubey D, Jabbari B. Botulinum toxin in Parkinson disease tremor: a randomized, double-blind, placebo-controlled study with a customized injection approach. Mayo Clin Proc. 2017;92(9):1359–67. https://doi.org/10.1016/j.mayocp.2017.06.010. Epub 2017 Aug 5. PMID: 28789780.

15. Blasi J, Chapman ER, Link E, Binz T, Yamasaki S, De Camilli P, Südhof TC, Niemann H, Jahn R. Botulinum neurotoxin A selectively cleaves the synaptic protein SNAP-25. Nature. 1993;365(6442):160–3. https://doi.org/10.1038/365160a0. PMID: 8103915.

16. Rossetto O, Pirazzini M, Fabris F, Montecucco C. Botulinum neurotoxins: mechanism of action. Handb Exp Pharmacol. 2021;263:35–47. https://doi.org/10.1007/164_2020_355. PMID: 32277300.

17. Filipović B, Matak I, Bach-Rojecky L, Lacković Z. Central action of peripherally applied botulinum toxin type A on pain and dural protein extravasation in rat model of trigeminal neuropathy. PLoS One. 2012;7(1):e29803. https://doi.org/10.1371/journal.pone.0029803. Epub 2012 Jan 4. PMID: 22238656; PMCID: PMC3251614.

18. Matak I, Lacković Z. Botulinum toxin A, brain and pain. Prog Neurobiol. 2014;119-120:39–59. https://doi.org/10.1016/j.pneurobio.2014.06.001. Epub 2014 Jun 7. PMID: 24915026.

19. Caleo M, Spinelli M, Colosimo F, Matak I, Rossetto O, Lackovic Z, Restani L. Transynaptic action of botulinum neurotoxin type a at central cholinergic boutons. J Neurosci. 2018;38(48):10329–37. https://doi.org/10.1523/JNEUROSCI.0294-18.2018. Epub 2018 Oct 12. PMID: 30315128; PMCID: PMC6596210.

20. Schiavo G, Rossetto O, Santucci A, DasGupta BR, Montecucco C. Botulinum neurotoxins are zinc proteins. J Biol Chem. 1992;267(33):23479–83. PMID: 1429690.

21. Dolly JO, Wang J, Zurawski TH, Meng J. Novel therapeutics based on recombinant botulinum neurotoxins to normalize the release of transmitters and pain mediators. FEBS J. 2011;278(23):4454–66. https://doi.org/10.1111/j.1742-4658.2011.08205.x. Epub 2011 Jul 5. PMID: 21645262.

Chapter 2
Structure and Mechanism of Function of Botulinum Neurotoxins: How Does the Toxin Work

Abstract This chapter discusses the molecular structure of botulinum toxin and how the toxin gets into the nerve cells after being injected into the muscle or skin. It describes the sequence of events that occurs inside the muscle or nerve cell that lead to the beneficial effects of the toxin upon the nerve and muscle cells as well as sweat and saliva glands in the body.

Keywords Botulinum toxin · Botulinum neurotoxin · Botulinum toxin molecule · Botulinum toxin mode of action

Introduction

Botulinum toxin or botulinum neurotoxin (BoNT) is a protein produced by certain bacteria named clostridium botulinum (CB). The term clostridium refers to the shape of the bacteria which is spindle/rod shaped, and the term botulinum is derived from the Greek word of "botulus" meaning sausage. The name stems from earlier outbreaks of botulism in Europe (Germany in particular) that were caused by consumption of rotten sausage. The history of early botulism outbreaks, discovery of the responsible agent for botulism, purification and production of the botulinum toxin for medical research as well as early clinical trials with this toxin which led to the discovery of BoNT's effectiveness in treatment of medical disorders are presented in detail in Chap. 1. This chapter explains how this toxin works and how it can be used in different medical conditions.

The results of animal research and early human observations published in 1960s and 1970's, indicating a therapeutic potential for BoNT, encouraged basic scientists to explore the molecular structure of the toxin and its mode of action. Over the past 55 years, the efforts of basic scientists deciphered the exact molecular structure of BoNT and provided a substantial amount of knowledge about how the toxin molecule reaches the nerves and exerts its therapeutic action after peripheral injection (into muscle or skin).

B. Jabbari, *Botulinum Toxin Treatment*,
https://doi.org/10.1007/978-3-031-54471-2_2

Botulinum toxin is structurally a protein with perfect machinery to exert its function through a set of well–defined mechanisms inside the nerve cell. There are 8 distinct types of botulinum toxins (A, B, C, D, E, F, G, X) that are structurally similar with only minor differences. Types A, B, E and F can cause botulism in human, whereas, types C and D cause botulism in domestic animals [1]. The type X toxin has been discovered relatively recently. The type X toxin has low potency and therefore does not seem to be useful for clinical use [2]. Recently, several subtypes of BoNT-A and BoNT-B have been discovered (A1…, B1…) [3–5]. Continued research efforts are underway to define the role of these subtypes. Currently, only types A and B (A1 and B1) are considered suitable for clinical use.

Botulinum toxin molecule (type A) is an approximately 900 KiloDalton (KD) complex which consists of a core toxin (150 KD) and a complex of surrounding proteins (>700 KD). Dalton, the unified atomic mass unit, is a standard unit that quantifies mass on an atomic or molecular scale. The surrounding proteins of the core toxin protect the toxin from being degraded in a hostile environment such as stomach acid after its ingestion. That is why high doses of the toxin presented in infected food resist stomach acid and, after absorption in the gut, cause botulism. However, when the BoNT is injected into a muscle, the tissue enzymes (protease) quickly separate the toxin from the surrounding proteins by a process termed "nicking." The core toxin molecule then reaches its target at nerve endings probably via the blood or lymphatic system [6].

The point where a nerve connects to a muscle is called neuromuscular junction. The point where two nerve cells connect or a nerve cell connects with a muscle cell is called synapse. At both neuromuscular junction (nerve muscle synapse) and at nerve cell to nerve cell synapse, the transfer of nerve impulse to the muscle or to another nerve cell requires presence of a special chemical called neurotransmitter. There are many neurotransmitters in the brain, but the neurotransmitter at neuromuscular junction is called acetylcholine. At neuromuscular junction, there is a membrane on the nerve side (nerve that reaches the muscle) and a membrane on the muscle side with a cleft in between (synaptic cleft). The nerve ending close to the muscle (neuromuscular junction) contain many small vesicles (small pouches) that contain the neurotransmitter acetylcholine (Fig. 2.1). When the nerve's electrical signal reaches the nerve ending, these vesicles rupture and pour their neurotransmitter contents into the cleft between the nerve and muscle membranes. The neurotransmitter (in this case acetylcholine) then attaches itself to the muscle membrane and activates the muscle. The injected botulinum neurotoxin (BoNT), by preventing acetylcholine release, can relax, weaken or even paralyze the muscle (depending on the dose). This is the mechanism by which the injected BoNT into the muscle improves stiffness of the muscles after a stroke, brain trauma or in children with cerebral palsy. The mechanism through which BoNT exerts its effect on nerve-muscle junction is complex and requires some knowledge of the core toxin's molecular structure [7–11].

Each molecule of the toxin consists of two structures, called light chain (designated as L) and heavy chain (designated as H). The molecular weight of light and heavy chains is 50 and 100 KD, respectively. KD stands for kilodalton. Dalton is the

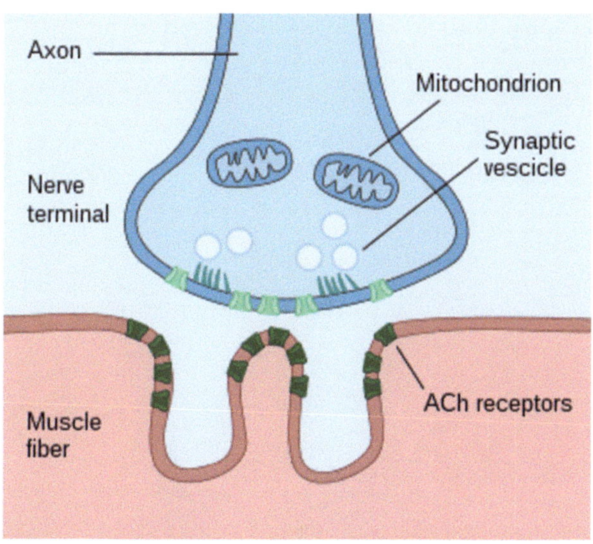

Fig. 2.1 Neuromuscular junction (NMJ): Nerve, nerve terminal, muscle fiber, and the cleft between. Nerve terminal shows vesicles that contain acetylcholine (ACH). Nerve signals reaching the nerve terminal at NMJ cause the rupture of the vesicles and release of acetylcholine into the synaptic cleft. ACH molecules attach to the muscle receptors on the surface of the muscle and activate the muscle. (From Wikipedia reproduced under Creative Commons Attribution-Share Alike 4.0 International license)

unit of atomic weight. The light (L) and heavy (H) chains are connected by a disulfide bond (ss) (Fig. 2.2).

The light chain is the catalytic domain of the toxin and its active moiety after entering the nerve cell. The heavy chain has two parts called HC and HN domains (Fig. 2.2). The HC domain (binding domain) attaches the toxin to the membrane receptors of the nerve cell. There are specific receptors on the nerve cell membrane that the HC domain of the toxin can attach itself to. The receptor for type A toxin is a protein called SV2. For type B toxin, two receptors have been identified. One is a complex sugar called ganglioside and the other is a protein called synaptogamin. After the toxin attaches to the receptor, the receptor undergoes structural modification and ends up working like a channel letting the toxin to go through. After entering the nerve terminal, the disulfide bond of BoNT breaks inside the nerve cell (via action of heavy chain -translocation) and the two chains (light and heavy) of the toxin separate from each other (Fig. 2.3).

The light chain (active moiety of the toxin that has the enzyme protease) is now free to exert its effect and prevent the release of acetylcholine from the synaptic vesicles [12–17]. It does this by attaching itself to specific synapse proteins whose function is to promote the fusion of the vesicle onto the nerve cell membrane. Fusion of the vesicle to cell membrane leads to vesicle rupture and release of acetylcholine into the synaptic cleft. The synapse proteins that promote vesicular fusion and vesicle rupture are called SNARE Proteins.

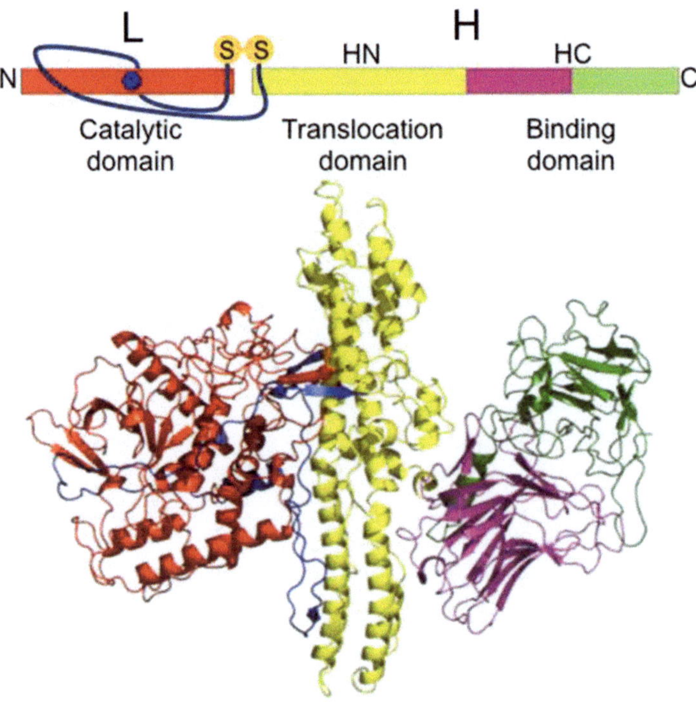

Fig. 2.2 Molecular structure of botulinum toxin. (From Rossetto O and co-workers 2014 reproduced with permission from publisher Nature Portfolio (Springer Nature))

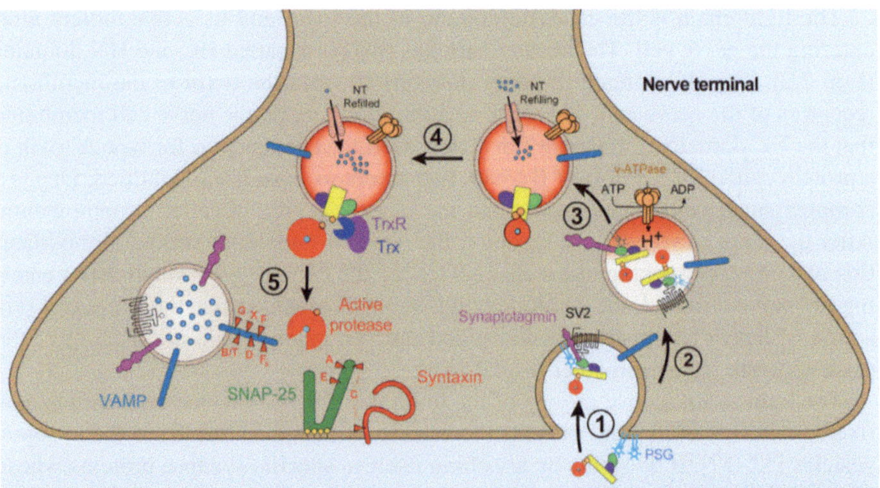

Fig. 2.3 Mechanisms of action of BoNTs. (From Rossetto et al. [10]. Reproduced with permission of publisher (Springer))

Over the past 40–50 years, a group of cell biologists succeeded to determine the mechanisms of vesicle fusion and synaptic machinery including the function of SNAREs [17–20]. Most notable among these scientists are J. Rothman, R. Schekman and TC. Südhof who won the Nobel prize in Medicine & Physiology in 2013 for their work in this area, when inside the nerve terminal and detached from the heavy chain, the light chain of the BoNT attaches itself to a specific SNARE that relates to a specific type of BoNT (for instance type A or B). After attachment to the SNARE protein the light chain of the toxin deactivate the SNARE protein via light chain's enzymatic function (a zinc activated protease). The result is inhibition of release of the neurotransmitter from the vesicle and, in case of nerve-muscle synapse, relaxation, weakness or even paralysis of the muscle depending on the dose of the injected toxin. The SNARE for type A toxins (Botox, Xeomin, Dysport) was first discovered by a group of Yale investigators and named SNAP 25 [21]. It is attached to the membrane of the nerve terminal. For the Type B toxin, the SNARE is attached to the vesicle wall itself and is designated as VAMP/Synaptobrevin (Fig. 2.3). The sequences of botulinum toxin's travel and activation after peripheral injection is presented in Table 2.1.

The binding of the BoNTs (A and B) to the nerve terminal is a long-term binding, that in case of nerve-muscle junction lasts for 3–4 months [22]. This long period of binding is medically desirable. For instance in spastic and tense muscles of patients with stroke or children with cerebral palsy, one injection could maintain the muscle relaxation for the entire period of binding (usually 3–4 months). Over time, the nerve ending starts to sprout and the new endings make contact with different muscle fibers. Finally, when the binding is over, the synapse resumes its full function. This is different from what happens to synapses in certain disease conditions (for instance ALS) where neurodegeneration leads to permanent loss of synapse function.

Table 2.1 Sequence of Botulinum toxin's action after injection into the muscle

1.	After injection into the muscle, protease, an enzyme inside the muscle separates the core toxin from protective proteins around it
2.	The released toxin molecule reaches nerve muscle junction probably via blood or lymphatic system
3.	The heavy chain of the toxin attaches the toxin molecule to certain receptors on the surface of nerve ending (SV2 for Botox)
4.	Receptors open as a channel and let the toxin molecule enter into the nerve terminal
5.	The disulfide bond of the toxin breaks inside of the nerve terminal via function of the heavy chain
6.	Freed light chain of the toxin (active or catalytic moiety) reaches the SNARE proteins and deactivates them via its enzymatic protease function
7.	Deactivation of SNARE protein prevents rupture of synaptic vesicles and release of acetylcholine
8.	Muscle deprived from acetylcholine activation relaxes and slightly weakens, an effect that improves muscle spasms, abnormally high muscle tone (spasticity) and involuntary movements

There is now substantial evidence that BoNT injected into the muscle after reaching the nerve terminal does not stay in the peripheral nerve and part of the molecule of BoNT travels to the central nervous system. The extent of central travel of the toxin is still under investigation. Nevertheless, convincing research evidence exists that a part of toxin molecule reaches the spinal cord and lower part of the brain (brain stem) after injecting the toxin into the muscle [23–25]. It is believed by many researchers, that this central travelling of the toxin may also help modulation of the motor function in a good way. The results would be improvement of motor function for example in spasticity (increased muscle tone) seen in adults with stroke or children with cerebral palsy. Treatment of spasticity with botulinum toxin injection is now approved by FDA for both adults and children and is one of the largest areas of BoNT use in clinical medicine [26–40].

Excessive Sweating and Drooling

Acetylcholine is also the neurotransmitter for the sympathetic nerve endings that supply nerves to sweat and salivary glands. BoNT injections into and under the skin in the areas where these glands are located such as arm pit, palm of the hands or bottom of the feet can significantly reduce sweating and help the affected individuals. Excessive hand sweating can be embarrassing during hand shaking; in case excessive sweating of the arm pit it can cause social discomfort. It many cases excessive sweating is genetic and runs in the family. Excessive drooling is also a nuisance and can be seen in Parkinson's disease or in children with cerebral palsy or individuals (children or adults) with brain damage. The glands that secrete saliva are located close to the angle of the jaw (parotid and submandibular) and are easily accessible from the surface by a thin and small needle. The injected BoNT (A or B) suppresses the excessive salivation within days, an effect that could last for 6 month. Injections are performed with a thin needle and cause minimal discomfort. A sizeable literature indicates efficacy of BoNT therapy for hyperhidrosis and hypersalivation (excessive sweating and excessive salivation) and attests to the safety of this form of treatment [41–52]. The use of BoNT for excessive sweating and excessive secretion of saliva is discussed in detail in Chap. 14 of this book.

Pain

Another important set of chemical neurotransmitters that are affected by peripheral injection (into muscle or skin) of BoNTs is pain neurotransmitters. The pain neurotransmitter(s) is not acetylcholine (in contrast to the muscle and gland) but other transmitters that are present in sensory nerves and in spinal cord or brain. These transmitters convey the unpleasant sensations from periphery to the brain. When they have sufficient intensity they are perceived as pain. Several pain transmitters have been discovered and studies over the past 60–70 years; the most well known among them are glutamate, substance P and Calcitonin Gene Related Peptide (CGRP) [53–57]. Over the past 25 years, animal research have shown that peripheral injection of botulinum neurotoxins A or B can significantly decrease the activity of glutamate, substance P and CGRP in peripheral nerves and in the central nervous system (spinal cord and brain) [58–67].

The animal data demonstrating that peripheral injection of BoNTs can suppress the function of pain transmitters provided grounds for clinical researches to study the role of botulinum toxin therapy in human pain. The first breakthrough came after two large multicenter studies showed efficacy of Botox injections in chronic migraine (see Chap. 4 for detailed information of these studies, recommended sites of injection and applied doses) [68]. Subsequent studies have shown that BoNTs are effective in a number of other pain syndromes as well [69] (Chap. 5).

Over the past 20 years, additional data from animal studies and human observations suggest a "central" mechanism for the action of botulinum toxin molecules in pain disorders. The support for a central (spinal cord and possibly brain) mechanism of action for alleviation of pain after botulinum toxin's injection comes from several lines of research some example of which are described below:

1. In laboratory animals, direct application of BoNT to dura matter (the thin sheet of tissue that covers the brain) alleviated facial pain and reduced the inflammation of the dura caused by experimentally induced facial pain (ligation of a facial nerve) [70].
2. In an animal model of leg pain caused by diabetic neuropathy (nerve damage due to diabetes), injection of BoNT into one leg, not only reduced the pain in that leg but also in the other leg implying an analgesic function through a spinal cord loop (central effect) with participation of spinal cord nerve cells [71].

Much of the seminal works in animal studies of pain are done by Dr. Zdravko Lakovic chairman of department of and Department of Pharmacology and his colleagues in University of Zagreb, Croacia (Fig. 2.4).

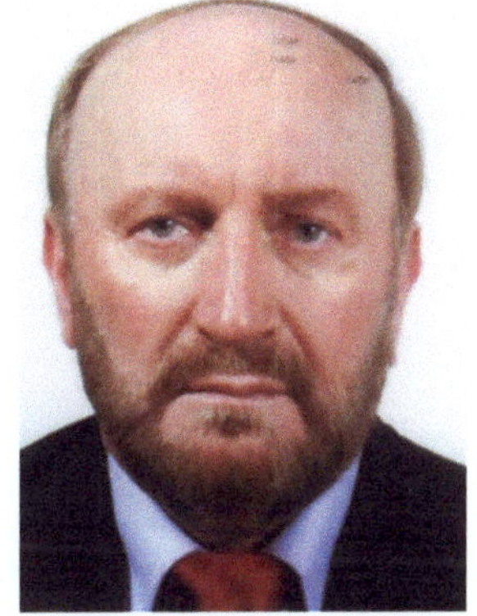

Fig. 2.4 Dr. Zdravko Lacovic whose laboratory provided significant information on how botulinum toxin injection inhibits pain in peripheral and central nervous system(brain and spinal cord). (Photo kindly given to the author by professor Lakovic)

These central mechanisms, however, do not seem to exert any deleterious effect on the spinal cord or brain (in doses approved for clinical use) since millions of patients who receive BoNT injections every year do not complain of any untoward side effects related to central nervous system (seizures, memory loss, specific central motor disorders, etc.).

Recently, scientists have succeeded in making a toxin molecule consisting of combination of two toxins (chimera—for instance for instance E/A toxins), that can specifically target the sensory nerve cells and, hence, specifically treat pain [72–74]. Limited number of studies have shown that in animal models, these toxin chimeras can suppress experimental pain [75]. The effect of these toxin chimeras in human pain is currently under investigation.

The details of botulinum neurotoxins' biology, pharmacology, and toxicology can be found in a recently published comprehensive review [76].

Hyperactive Involuntary Movement Disorders (HIMD)

Botulinum toxins are now widely used for treatment of HIMDs. Most notable examples include cervical dystonia, hemifacial spasm and blepharospasm, three indications that have received early FDA approval for use in the US. Over the past 40 years, experience with botulinum toxin therapy for these movement disorders had been very positive; toxin therapy has now been established as treatment of first choice for these conditions [77, 78]. In the experienced hands using recommended doses, botulinum toxin therapy has proved to be safe and serious side effects are rare and preventable (see Chap. 17 of this book on safety issues).

References

1. Rossetto O. Chapter 1: Botulinum toxins: molecular structures and synaptic physiology. In: Jabbari B, editor. Botulinum toxin treatment in clinical medicine – a disease oriented approach. New York: Springer; 2017. p. 1–12.
2. Martínez-Carranza M, Škerlová J, Lee PG, Zhang J, Burgin D, Elliott M, Philippe J, Donald S, Hornby F, Henriksson L, Masuyer G, Beard M, Dong M, Stenmark P. Structure and activity of botulinum neurotoxin X. bioRxiv [Preprint]. 2023 Jan 11. https://doi.org/10.1101/2023.01.11.523524. PMID: 36712025; PMCID: PMC9882044.
3. Gregory KS, Acharya KR. A comprehensive structural analysis of *Clostridium botulinum* neurotoxin a cell-binding domain from different subtypes. Toxins (Basel). 2023 Jan 18;15(2):92. https://doi.org/10.3390/toxins15020092. PMID: 36828407; PMCID: PMC9966434.
4. Pirazzini M, Montecucco C, Rossetto O. Toxicology and pharmacology of botulinum and tetanus neurotoxins: an update. Arch Toxicol. 2022 June;96(6):1521–39. https://doi.org/10.1007/s00204-022-03271-9. Epub 2022 Mar 25. PMID: 35333944; PMCID: PMC9095541.
5. Davies JR, Liu SM, Acharya KR. Variations in the botulinum neurotoxin binding domain and the potential for novel therapeutics. Toxins (Basel). 2018 Oct 20;10(10):421. https://doi.org/10.3390/toxins10100421. PMID: 30347838; PMCID: PMC6215321.

6. Monteccuco C, Rasso MB. On botulinum neurotoxin variability. MBio. 2015;6:e02131.

7. Clark AW, Bandyopadhyay S, DasGupta BR. The plantar nerves-lumbrical muscles: a useful nerve-muscle preparation for assaying the effects of botulinum neurotoxin. J Neurosci Methods. 1987 Apr;19(4):285–95. https://doi.org/10.1016/0165-0270(87)90071-9. PMID: 3586701.

8. DasGupta BR, Sugiyama H. A common subunit structure in Clostridium botulinum type A, B and E toxins. Biochem Biophys Res Commun. 1972 July 11;48(1):108–12. https://doi.org/10.1016/0006-291x(72)90350-6. PMID: 5041870.

9. Montecucco C, Schiavo G. Mechanism of action of tetanus and botulinum neurotoxins. Mol Microbiol. 1994 July;13(1):1–8. https://doi.org/10.1111/j.1365-2958.1994.tb00396.x. PMID: 7527117.

10. Rossetto O, Pirazzini M, Fabris F, Montecucco C. Botulinum neurotoxins: mechanism of action. Handb Exp Pharmacol. 2021;263:35–47. https://doi.org/10.1007/164_2020_355. PMID: 32277300.

11. Dolly JO, Black J, Williams RS, Melling J. Acceptors for botulinum neurotoxin reside on motor nerve terminals and mediate its internalization. Nature. 1984 Feb 2–8;307(5950):457–60. https://doi.org/10.1038/307457a0. PMID: 6694738.

12. Schiavo G, Rossetto O, Santucci A, DasGupta BR, Montecucco C. Botulinum neurotoxins are zinc proteins. J Biol Chem. 1992 Nov 25;267(33):23479–83. PMID: 1429690.

13. Schiavo G, Poulain B, Benfenati F, DasGupta BR, Montecucco C. Novel targets and catalytic activities of bacterial protein toxins. Trends Microbiol. 1993 Aug;1(5):170–4. https://doi.org/10.1016/0966-842x(93)90086-7. PMID: 8143134.

14. Surana S, Tosolini AP, Meyer IFG, Fellows AD, Novoselov SS, Schiavo G. The travel diaries of tetanus and botulinum neurotoxins. Toxicon. 2018 June 1;147:58–67. https://doi.org/10.1016/j.toxicon.2017.10.008. Epub 2017 Oct 12. PMID: 29031941.

15. Tighe AP, Schiavo G. Botulinum neurotoxins: mechanism of action. Toxicon. 2013 June 1;67:87–93. https://doi.org/10.1016/j.toxicon.2012.11.011. Epub 2012 Nov 29. PMID: 23201505.

16. Lacy DB, Tepp W, Cohen AC, DasGupta BR, Stevens RC. Crystal structure of botulinum neurotoxin type A and implications for toxicity. Nat Struct Biol. 1998;5:898–902.

17. Rothman JE. The principle of membrane fusion in the cell (Nobel lecture). Angew Chem Int Ed Engl. 2014;53(47):12676–94. https://doi.org/10.1002/anie.201402380. Epub2014A.

18. Sherman AD, Hegwood TS, Baruah S, Waziri R. Presynaptic modulation of amino acid release from synaptosomes. Neurochem Res. 1992 Feb;17(2):125–8. https://doi.org/10.1007/BF00966789. PMID: 1371602.

19. Südhof TC. Neurotransmitter release. Handb Exp Pharmacol. 2008;184:1–21. https://doi.org/10.1007/978-3-540-74805-2_1. PMID: 18064409.

20. Südhof TC, Malenka RC. Understanding synapses: past, present, and future. Neuron. 2008 Nov 6;60(3):469–76. https://doi.org/10.1016/j.neuron.2008.10.011. PMID: 18995821; PMCID: PMC3243741.

21. Blasi J, Chapman ER, Link E, Binz T, Yamasaki S, De Camilli P, Südhof TC, Niemann H, Jahn R. Botulinum neurotoxin A selectively cleaves the synaptic protein SNAP-25. Nature. 1993;365(6442):160–3.

22. Kumar R, Dhaliwal HP, Kukreja RV, Singh BR. The botulinum toxin as a therapeutic agent: molecular structure and mechanism of action in motor and sensory systems. Semin Neurol. 2016;36:10–9.

23. Caleo M, Spinelli M, Colosimo F, Matak I, Rossetto O, Lackovic Z, Restani L. Transynaptic action of botulinum neurotoxin type A at central cholinergic boutons. J Neurosci. 2018 Nov 28;38(48):10329–37. https://doi.org/10.1523/JNEUROSCI.0294-18.2018. Epub 2018 Oct 12. PMID: 30315128; PMCID: PMC6596210.

24. Matak I. Evidence for central antispastic effect of botulinum toxin type A. Br J Pharmacol. 2020 Jan;177(1):65–76. https://doi.org/10.1111/bph.14846. Epub 2019 Nov 6. PMID: 31444910; PMCID: PMC6976784.

25. Matak I, Riederer P, Lacković Z. Botulinum toxin's axonal transport from periphery to the spinal cord. Neurochem Int. 2012 July;61(2):236–9. https://doi.org/10.1016/j.neuint.2012.05.001. Epub 2012 May 8. PMID: 22580329.
26. Blumetti FC, Belloti JC, Tamaoki MJ, Pinto JA. Botulinum toxin type A in the treatment of lower limb spasticity in children with cerebral palsy. Cochrane Database Syst Rev. 2019 Oct 8;10(10):CD001408. https://doi.org/10.1002/14651858.CD001408.pub2. PMID: 31591703; PMCID: PMC6779591.
27. Multani I, Manji J, Hastings-Ison T, Khot A, Graham K. Botulinum toxin in the management of children with cerebral palsy. Paediatr Drugs. 2019 Aug;21(4):261–81. https://doi.org/10.1007/s40272-019-00344-8. PMID: 31257556; PMCID: PMC6682585.
28. Datta Gupta A, Visvanathan R, Cameron I, Koblar SA, Howell S, Wilson D. Efficacy of botulinum toxin in modifying spasticity to improve walking and quality of life in post-stroke lower limb spasticity – a randomized double-blind placebo controlled study. BMC Neurol. 2019 May 11;19(1):96. https://doi.org/10.1186/s12883-019-1325-3. PMID: 31078139; PMCID: PMC6511142.
29. Cofré Lizama LE, Khan F, Galea MP. Beyond speed: gait changes after botulinum toxin injections in chronic stroke survivors (a systematic review). Gait Posture. 2019 May;70: 389–96. https://doi.org/10.1016/j.gaitpost.2019.03.035. Epub 2019 Apr 4. PMID: 30974394.
30. Santamato A, Cinone N, Panza F, Letizia S, Santoro L, Lozupone M, Daniele A, Picelli A, Baricich A, Intiso D, Ranieri M. Botulinum toxin type A for the treatment of lower limb spasticity after stroke. Drugs. 2019 Feb;79(2):143–60. https://doi.org/10.1007/s40265-018-1042-z. PMID: 30623347.
31. Baricich A, Picelli A, Santamato A, Carda S, de Sire A, Smania N, Cisari C, Invernizzi M. Safety profile of high-dose botulinum toxin type a in post-stroke spasticity treatment. Clin Drug Investig. 2018 Nov;38(11):991–1000. https://doi.org/10.1007/s40261-018-0701-x. PMID: 30209743.
32. Dong Y, Wu T, Hu X, Wang T. Efficacy and safety of botulinum toxin type A for upper limb spasticity after stroke or traumatic brain injury: a systematic review with meta-analysis and trial sequential analysis. Eur J Phys Rehabil Med. 2017 Apr;53(2):256–67. https://doi.org/10.23736/S1973-9087.16.04329-X. Epub 2016 Nov 11. PMID: 27834471.
33. Pavone V, Testa G, Restivo DA, Cannavò L, Condorelli G, Portinaro NM, Sessa G. Botulinum toxin treatment for limb spasticity in childhood cerebral palsy. Front Pharmacol. 2016 Feb 19;7:29. https://doi.org/10.3389/fphar.2016.00029. PMID: 26924985; PMCID: PMC4759702.
34. Esquenazi A, Albanese A, Chancellor MB, Elovic E, Segal KR, Simpson DM, Smith CP, Ward AB. Evidence-based review and assessment of botulinum neurotoxin for the treatment of adult spasticity in the upper motor neuron syndrome. Toxicon. 2013 June 1;67:115–28. https://doi.org/10.1016/j.toxicon.2012.11.025. Epub 2012 Dec 5. PMID: 23220492.
35. Molenaers G, Van Campenhout A, Fagard K, De Cat J, Desloovere K. The use of botulinum toxin A in children with cerebral palsy, with a focus on the lower limb. J Child Orthop. 2010 June;4(3):183–95. https://doi.org/10.1007/s11832-010-0246-x. Epub 2010 Mar 18. PMID: 21629371; PMCID: PMC2866843.
36. Yılmaz Yalçınkaya E, Karadağ Saygı E, Özyemişci Taşkıran Ö, Çapan N, Kutlay Ş, Sonel Tur B, El Ö, Ünlü Akyüz E, Tekin S, Ofluoğlu D, Zİnnuroğlu M, Akpınar P, Özekli Mısırlıoğlu T, Hüner B, Nur H, Çağlar S, Sezgin M, Tıkız C, Öneş K, İçağasıoğlu A, Aydın R. Consensus recommendations for botulinum toxin injections in the spasticity management of children with cerebral palsy during COVID-19 outbreak. Turk J Med Sci. 2021 Apr 30;51(2):385–92. https://doi.org/10.3906/sag-2009-5. PMID: 33350298; PMCID: PMC8203129.
37. Moccia M, Frau J, Carotenuto A, Butera C, Coghe G, Barbero P, Frontoni M, Groppo E, Giovannelli M, Del Carro U, Inglese C, Frasson E, Castagna A, Buccafusca M, Latino P, Nascimbene C, Romano M, Liotti V, Lanfranchi S, Rapisarda L, Lori S, Esposito M, Maggi L, Petracca M, Lo Fermo S, Altavista MC, Bono F, Eleopra R, Brescia Morra V. Botulinum toxin for the management of spasticity in multiple sclerosis: the Italian botulinum toxin network study. Neurol Sci. 2020 Oct;41(10):2781–92. https://doi.org/10.1007/s10072-020-04392-8. Epub 2020 Apr 12. PMID: 32281038.

38. Li S, Francisco GE. The use of botulinum toxin for treatment of spasticity. Handb Exp Pharmacol. 2021;263:127–46. https://doi.org/10.1007/164_2019_315. Erratum in: Handb Exp Pharmacol. 2021;263:281. PMID: 31820170.

39. Hara T, Momosaki R, Niimi M, Yamada N, Hara H, Abo M. Botulinum toxin therapy combined with rehabilitation for stroke: a systematic review of effect on motor function. Toxins (Basel). 2019 Dec 5;11(12):707. https://doi.org/10.3390/toxins11120707. PMID: 31817426; PMCID: PMC6950173.

40. Jankovic J. Botulinum toxin: state of the art. Mov Disord. 2017 Aug;32(8):1131–8. https://doi.org/10.1002/mds.27072. Epub 2017 June 22. PMID: 28639368.

41. An JS, Hyun Won C, Si Han J, Park HS, Seo KK. Comparison of onabotulinumtoxinA and rimabotulinumtoxinB for the treatment of axillary hyperhidrosis. Dermatologic Surg. 2015 Aug;41(8):960–7. https://doi.org/10.1097/DSS.0000000000000429. PMID: 26218729.

42. Hosp C, Naumann MK, Hamm H. Botulinum toxin treatment of autonomic disorders: focal hyperhidrosis and sialorrhea. Semin Neurol. 2016 Feb;36(1):20–8. https://doi.org/10.1055/s-0035-1571214. Epub 2016 Feb 11. PMID: 26866492.

43. Shayesteh A, Boman J, Janlert U, Brulin C, Nylander E. Primary hyperhidrosis: implications on symptoms, daily life, health and alcohol consumption when treated with botulinum toxin. J Dermatol. 2016 Aug;43(8):928–33. https://doi.org/10.1111/1346-8138.13291. Epub 2016 Feb 15. PMID: 26875781.

44. Vlahovic TC. Plantar hyperhidrosis: an overview. Clin Podiatr Med Surg. 2016 July;33(3):441–51. https://doi.org/10.1016/j.cpm.2016.02.010. Epub 2016 Mar 26. PMID: 27215162.

45. Patakfalvi L, Benohanian A. Treatment of palmar hyperhidrosis with needle-free injection of botulinum toxin A. Arch Dermatol Res. 2014 Jan;306(1):101–2. https://doi.org/10.1007/s00403-013-1425-7. Epub 2013 Nov 7. PMID: 24196236.

46. Orriëns LB, van Hulst K, van der Burg JJW, van den Hoogen FJA, Willemsen MAAP, Erasmus CE. Comparing the evidence for botulinum neurotoxin injections in paediatric anterior drooling: a scoping review. Eur J Pediatr. 2024 Jan;183(1):83–93. https://doi.org/10.1007/s00431-023-05309-1. Epub 2023 Nov 4. PMID: 37924348; PMCID: PMC10858158.

47. Rosell K, Hymnelius K, Swartling C. Botulinum toxin type A and B improve quality of life in patients with axillary and palmar hyperhidrosis. Acta Derm Venereol. 2013 May;93(3):335–9. https://doi.org/10.2340/00015555-1464. PMID: 23053164.

48. Tamadonfar ET, Lew MF. BoNT clinical trial update: Sialorrhea. Toxicon. 2023 Mar 16;226:107087. https://doi.org/10.1016/j.toxicon.2023.107087. Epub ahead of print. PMID: 36931440.

49. Fan T, Frederick R, Abualsoud A, Sheyn A, McLevy-Bazzanella J, Thompson J, Akkus C, Wood J. Treatment of sialorrhea with botulinum toxin injections in pediatric patients less than three years of age. Int J Pediatr Otorhinolaryngol. 2022 July;158:111185. https://doi.org/10.1016/j.ijporl.2022.111185. Epub 2022 May 14. PMID: 35594794.

50. Heikel T, Patel S, Ziai K, Shah SJ, Lighthall JG. Botulinum toxin A in the management of pediatric sialorrhea: a systematic review. Ann Otol Rhinol Laryngol. 2023 Feb;132(2):200–6. https://doi.org/10.1177/00034894221078365. Epub 2022 Feb 18. PMID: 35176902; PMCID: PMC9834812.

51. Hung SA, Liao CL, Lin WP, Hsu JC, Guo YH, Lin YC. Botulinum toxin injections for treatment of drooling in children with cerebral palsy: a systematic review and meta-analysis. Children (Basel). 2021 Nov 25;8(12):1089. https://doi.org/10.3390/children8121089. PMID: 34943284; PMCID: PMC8700360.

52. Yu YC, Chung CC, Tu YK, Hong CT, Chen KH, Tam KW, Kuan YC. Efficacy and safety of botulinum toxin for treating sialorrhea: a systematic review and meta-analysis. Eur J Neurol. 2022 Jan;29(1):69–80. https://doi.org/10.1111/ene.15083. Epub 2021 Sept 12. PMID: 34449931.

53. Gegelashvili G, Bjerrum OJ. Glutamate transport system as a novel therapeutic target in chronic pain: molecular mechanisms and pharmacology. Adv Neurobiol. 2017;16:225–53. https://doi.org/10.1007/978-3-319-55769-4_11. PMID: 28828613.

54. Zieglgänsberger W. Substance P and pain chronicity. Cell Tissue Res. 2019 Jan;375(1):227–41. https://doi.org/10.1007/s00441-018-2922-y. Epub 2018 Oct 3. PMID: 30284083; PMCID: PMC6335504.
55. Robinson P, Rodriguez E, Muñoz M. Substance P-friend or foe. J Clin Med. 2022 June 22;11(13):3609. https://doi.org/10.3390/jcm11133609. PMID: 35806893; PMCID: PMC9267209.
56. Andó RD, Sperlágh B. The role of glutamate release mediated by extrasynaptic P2X7 receptors in animal models of neuropathic pain. Brain Res Bull. 2013 Apr;93:80–5. https://doi.org/10.1016/j.brainresbull.2012.09.016. Epub 2012 Oct 6. PMID: 23047057.
57. Lagerström MC, Rogoz K, Abrahamsen B, Lind AL, Olund C, Smith C, Mendez JA, Wallén-Mackenzie Å, Wood JN, Kullander K. A sensory subpopulation depends on vesicular glutamate transporter 2 for mechanical pain, and together with substance P, inflammatory pain. Proc Natl Acad Sci U S A. 2011 Apr 5;108(14):5789–94. https://doi.org/10.1073/pnas.1013602108. Epub 2011 Mar 17. PMID: 21415372; PMCID: PMC3078395.
58. Matak I, Tékus V, Bölcskei K, Lacković Z, Helyes Z. Involvement of substance P in the antinociceptive effect of botulinum toxin type A: evidence from knockout mice. Neuroscience. 2017 Sept 1;358:137–145. https://doi.org/10.1016/j.neuroscience.2017.06.040. Epub 2017 July 1. PMID: 28673722.
59. Aoki KR. Evidence for antinociceptive activity of botulinum toxin type A in pain management. Headache. 2003 July-Aug;43 Suppl 1:S9–15. https://doi.org/10.1046/j.1526-4610.43.7s.3.x. PMID: 12887389.
60. Hou YP, Zhang YP, Song YF, Zhu CM, Wang YC, Xie GL. Botulinum toxin type A inhibits rat pyloric myoelectrical activity and substance P release in vivo. Can J Physiol Pharmacol. 2007 Feb;85(2):209–14. https://doi.org/10.1139/y07-018. PMID: 17487262.
61. Wang L, Tai NZ, Fan ZH. Effect of botulinum toxin type A on the expression of substance P, calcitonin gene-related peptide, transforming growth factor beta-1 and alpha smooth muscle actin A in wound healing in rats. Zhonghua Zheng Xing Wai Ke Za Zhi. 2009 Jan;25(1):50–3. Chinese. PMID: 19408727.
62. Mustafa G, Anderson EM, Bokrand-Donatelli Y, Neubert JK, Caudle RM. Anti-nociceptive effect of a conjugate of substance P and light chain of botulinum neurotoxin type A. Pain. 2013 Nov;154(11):2547–53. https://doi.org/10.1016/j.pain.2013.07.041. Epub 2013 Aug 8. PMID: 23933181; PMCID: PMC3808523.
63. Marino MJ, Terashima T, Steinauer JJ, Eddinger KA, Yaksh TL, Xu Q. Botulinum toxin B in the sensory afferent: transmitter release, spinal activation, and pain behavior. Pain. 2014 Apr;155(4):674–84. https://doi.org/10.1016/j.pain.2013.12.009. Epub 2013 Dec 11. PMID: 24333775; PMCID: PMC3960322.
64. Kim DW, Lee SK, Ahnn J. Botulinum toxin as a pain killer: players and actions in antinociception. Toxins (Basel). 2015 June 30;7(7):2435–53. https://doi.org/10.3390/toxins7072435. PMID: 26134255; PMCID: PMC4516922.
65. Sanchez-Prieto J, Sihra TS, Evans D, Ashton A, Dolly JO, Nicholls DG. Botulinum toxin A blocks glutamate exocytosis from Guinea-pig cerebral cortical synaptosomes. Eur J Biochem. 1987 June 15;165(3):675–81. https://doi.org/10.1111/j.1432-1033.1987.tb11494.x. PMID: 2439334.
66. McMahon HT, Foran P, Dolly JO, Verhage M, Wiegant VM, Nicholls DG. Tetanus toxin and botulinum toxins type A and B inhibit glutamate, gamma-aminobutyric acid, aspartate, and met-enkephalin release from synaptosomes. Clues to the locus of action. J Biol Chem. 1992 Oct 25;267(30):21338–43. PMID: 1356988.
67. Bittencourt da Silva L, Karshenas A, Bach FW, Rasmussen S, Arendt-Nielsen L, Gazerani P. Blockade of glutamate release by botulinum neurotoxin type A in humans: a dermal microdialysis study. Pain Res Manag. 2014 May–June;19(3):126–32. https://doi.org/10.1155/2014/410415. PMID: 24851237; PMCID: PMC4158957.

68. Aurora SK, Winner P, Freeman MC, Spierings EL, Heiring JO, DeGryse RE, VanDenburgh AM, Nolan ME, Turkel CC. OnabotulinumtoxinA for treatment of chronic migraine: pooled analyses of the 56-week PREEMPT clinical program. Headache. 2011;51:1358–73.
69. Jabbari B. Botulinum toxin treatment of pain disorders. 2nd ed. New York: Springer; 2022.
70. Lacković Z, Filipović B, Matak I, et al. Activity of botulinum toxin type A in cranial dura: implications for treatment of migraine and other headaches. Br J Pharmacol. 2016;173:279–91.
71. Bach-Rojecky L, Salković-Petrisić M, Lacković Z. Botulinum toxin type A reduces pain supersensitivity in experimental diabetic neuropathy: bilateral effect after unilateral injection. Eur J Pharmacol. 2010;633:10–4.
72. Wang J, Casals-Diaz L, Zurawski T, et al. A novel therapeutic with two SNAP-25 inactivating proteases shows long-lasting anti-hyperalgesic activity in a rat model of neuropathic pain. Neuropharmacology. 2017;118:223–32.
73. Dolly JO, Wang J, Zurawski TH, Meng J. Novel therapeutics based on recombinant botulinum neurotoxins to normalize the release of transmitters and pain mediators. FEBS J. 2011 Dec;278(23):4454–66. https://doi.org/10.1111/j.1742-4658.2011.08205.x. Epub 2011 July 5. PMID: 21645262.
74. Wang J, Zurawski TH, Meng J, Lawrence GW, Aoki KR, Wheeler L, Dolly JO. Novel chimeras of botulinum and tetanus neurotoxins yield insights into their distinct sites of neuroparalysis. FASEB J. 2012 Dec;26(12):5035–48. https://doi.org/10.1096/fj.12-210112. Epub 2012 Aug 31. PMID: 22942075.
75. Antoniazzi C, Belinskaia M, Zurawski T, Kaza SK, Dolly JO, Lawrence GW. Botulinum neurotoxin chimeras suppress stimulation by capsaicin of rat trigeminal sensory neurons in vivo and in vitro. Toxins (Basel). 2022 Feb 4;14(2):116. https://doi.org/10.3390/toxins14020116. PMID: 35202143; PMCID: PMC8878885.
76. Pirrazzini M, Rossetto O, Elopra R, Montecucco C. Botulinum neurotoxins: biology, pharmacology, and toxicology. Pharmacol Rev. 2017;69:200–35.
77. Dressler D, Adib Saberi F, Rosales RL. Botulinum toxin therapy of dystonia. J Neural Transm (Vienna). 2021 Apr;128(4):531–7. https://doi.org/10.1007/s00702-020-02266-z. Epub 2020 Oct 30. PMID: 33125571; PMCID: PMC8099791.
78. Brin MF, Blitzer A. The pluripotential evolution and journey of Botox (onabotulinumtoxinA). Medicine (Baltimore). 2023 July 1;102(S1):e32373. https://doi.org/10.1097/MD.0000000000032373. PMID: 37499079; PMCID: PMC10374190.

Chapter 3
Beyond Botox: Other Neurotoxins—What Are Similarities and Differences?

Abstract This chapter describes the pharmacological and clinical characteristics of six botulinum toxins—Botox, Xeomin, Dysport, Myobloc, Jeuveau and Dixxify—currently approved by FDA for use in the US. Two other unapproved, but widely used, botulinum toxins in Asia, Prosigne and Meditox are also briefly discussed. In addition, a brief account on the structure of clinical trials and definition of study phases, I, II, III, IV as it pertains to clinical investigations in the field of toxicology is also provided. The classification of clinical studies based on their quality—class I to IV and their level of study efficacy—A, B, C, U—are described using the guidelines provided by the Assessment and Therapeutics Subcommittee of the American Academy of Neurology.

Keywords Botulinum toxin · Botulinum neurotoxin · Botox · Xeomin · Dysport · Myobloc · Jeuveau · Dixxify

Introduction

The history of botulinum neurotoxin (BoNT) and how it developed and evolved from a lethal toxin to a widely used and relatively safe medical agent has been discussed in Chap. 1 of this book. In Chap. 2, the molecular structure and mechanisms of function of botulinum toxins were discussed. This chapter, defines the qualities and characteristics of six FDA approved botulinum toxins currently used in the US. These are Botox, Xeomin, Dysport, Myobloc, Jeuveau and Daxxify. Figure 3.1 shows some of the marketed vials of four commonly used FDA approved botulinum toxins. These four toxins have been approved by FDA for several years and for more than one indication. Jeuveau and Daxxify recently approval by FDA only for cosmetic use in 2019 and 2022, respectively. In 2023, FDA approved Daxxify for treatment of cervical dystonia (for definition see Chap. 8), additionally.

B. Jabbari, *Botulinum Toxin Treatment*,
https://doi.org/10.1007/978-3-031-54471-2_3

25

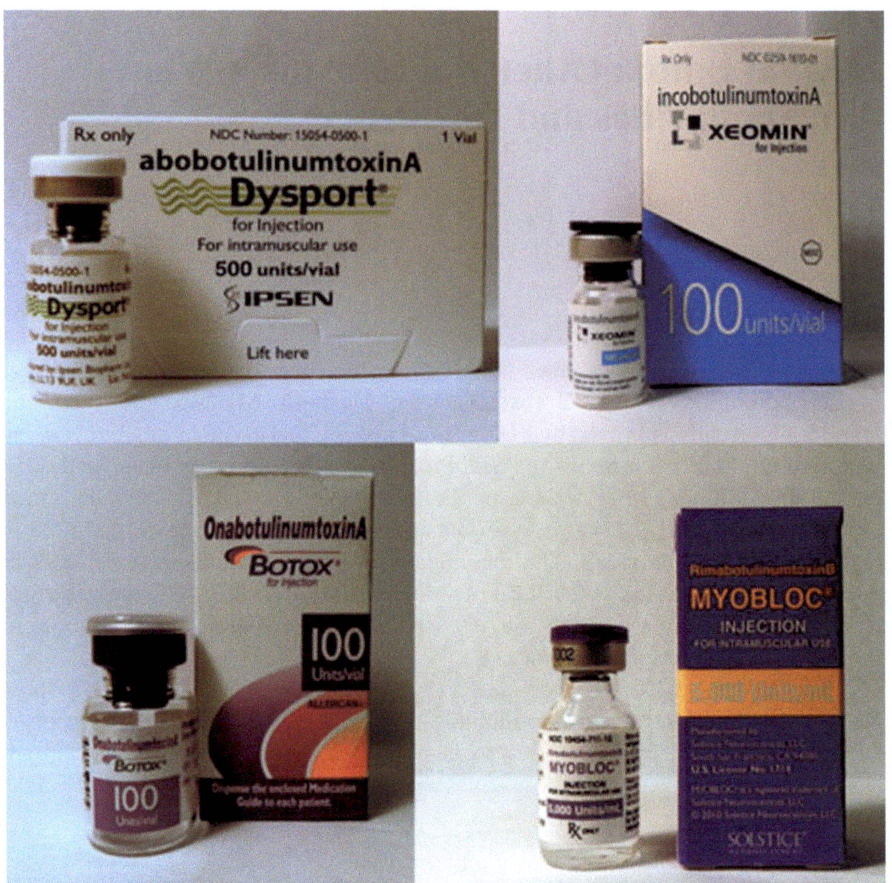

Fig. 3.1 FDA approved, commonly used botulinum toxins: type A (Botox, Xeomin, Dysport) and type B (Myobloc). (From Chen and Dashtipour 2013 [1]. Courtesy of Wiley & Sons Publisher)

Of 9 subgroups of botulinum toxins (A, B, C, D, E, F, D, G, X) (see Chap. 2), only types A and B are used for treatment in clinical medicine. This is due to the prolonged action of types A and B providing suitability for medical use. Botox, Xeomin, Dysport and Jeuveau and Daxxify are type A; Myobloc is a type B toxin. In medical communications and research manuscripts, usually the trade names, as cited above, are avoided, and the proprietary names (designed by FDA) are used instead (Table 3.1). Currently, two other type A toxins are used widely in Asia, but they are not approved by FDA for use in the US (Table 3.1).

There is a difference between these toxins in term of preparation, dilution, refrigeration, unit potency and immunogenicity. Some of these differences are summarized in Table 3.2.

Table 3.1 The eight commonly used botulinum toxins: trade name, proprietary name, manufacturer, FDA approval

Trade name	Propriety name	Abbreviation	Manufacturer	FDA approval
Botox	Onabotulinum toxin A	Ona-A	Allrgan-Inc., Dublin, Ireland	Yes
Xeomin	Incobotulinum toxin A	Inco-A	Merz Pharma, Frankfurt, Germany	Yes
Dysport	Abobotulinum toxinA	AboA	Ipsen Pharmaceuticals, UK	Yes
Myobloc[a]	Rimabotulinum toxinB	RimaB	US Woldwide Med, Solstice	Yes
Jeuveu	Probobotulinumtoxin A	ProboA	Evolus Inc., Santa Barbars, CA	Yes
Daxxify	Daxibotulinumtoxin A	DaxiA	Revance Therapeutics, Nashville, TN	Yes
Prosgine (Inotox)	–	–	Lanzhou Institute, China	No
Meditoxin (Neuronox)	–	–	Medytox, South Korea	No

[a]Marketed as neurobloc in Europe

Table 3.2 Trade name, preparation, need for refrigeration, unit equivalency and vial size of botulinum toxins

Trade name	Dilution with saline	Refrigeration	Approximate unit equivalency	Units/vial
Botox	Yes	2–8 degrees©	1	50,100,300
Xeomin	Yes	No need for refrigeration	1	50,100,200
Dysport	Yes	2–8 degrees©	2.5–3	300.500.1000
Myobloc[a]	No	2–8 degrees©	40–50	2500, 5000,10,000
Prosigne	Yes	2–8 degrees©	1–1.5	50,100
Meditoxin(neuronox)	Yes	2–8 degrees c	1	50

[a]Myobloc comes prepared and does not need reconstruction

Botox (Allergan Inc., Irvine California)

Botox is the first botulinum toxin marketed for clinical use. It was initially introduced in 1989 under the trade name of oculinum (related to the eye) since at that time, the focus was on eye related indications such as strabismus (crossed eyes) and abnormal contractions of the eyelids (blepharospasm) and hemifacial spasm (HFS—involuntary twitches of half of the face). Two years later, noticing the wide potential application of this toxin in the medical field, the name was changed to Botox. Botox is the most widely used of botulinum toxins and currently has over 80% of the US market. Botox is a type A botulinum toxin similar to the other two of its competitors, Xeomin and Dysport. Out of 9 different serotypes of the BoNTs, only types A and B have medical applications. Part of this is due to the long duration of action of these two types of BoNTs (A and B); a single intramuscular or subcutaneous (underskin) injection, provide 3–6 months duration of action (depending on the clinical condition).

Botox is provided in small vials (Fig. 3.1) that contain 50 (for cosmetic use), 100 and 300 units of botulinum toxin. The unit of the toxin is based on toxin's lethality in mice.

Botox is heat sensitive. The original vial of Botox as well as prepared Botox (mixed with normal saline-salt water, before injection) needs to be kept in the refrigerator. The manufacturer recommends the prepared solution to be used within 4–6 h after reconstruction. There are studies, however, that claim reconstructed Botox solution can maintain its potency for up to 6 weeks if kept in the refrigerator. Patients who buy Botox from the pharmacy and plan to take it to the physician's office for injection need to be particularly diligent about the issue of Botox's heat sensitivity. The Botox content of the vial will lose its potency if left at room temperature for more than a few hours. If a patient buys a Botox vial today from the pharmacy and plans to go to the treating physician's office the next day, the Botox vial should be refrigerated.

The effect of Botox starts between 24 and 72 h after injection into the muscle. Like other botulinum toxins in the market, the effect of Botox for most indications, lasts on average about 3–4 months. It needs to be reinjected to maintain a long-term efficacy. Injections are done by a small and thin needle (gauge 27.5 or 30) and, in experienced hands cause little discomfort. For some indications such as drooling and excessive sweating as well as bladder dysfunction (see Chaps. 10 and 14), the duration of action may be as long as 6 months.

Most FDA approved botulinum toxin preparations (Botox, Xeomin, Dysport, Myobloc, Jeuveau) have some foreign protein (human albumin) in them that may produce antibodies. Injection of botulinum toxins, especially in large amounts (such as used for relaxing large spastic limbs after stroke or brain/spinal cord injury), can facilitate formation of antibodies and, as a result make the patient unresponsive to the effects of subsequent Botox injection(s). This was an issue with earlier preparations of Botox (up to 1997) when approximately 10% of the patients receiving repeated injection developed antibodies and became unresponsive. However, great improvements have been made in this regard over the past 25 years to improve Botox's sustained efficacy. Current Botox vials contain only 0.5 ng of human albumin with a protein load of 5 ng/100 units. This is substantially reduced from 25 ng/100 units which was present in the Botox formulations prior to 1997. The low protein load of the current Botox preparations has reduced Botox's antibody formation to less than 1.2% and the development of non-responsiveness down to 1% or less after repeated applications [2]. The antibody formation after application of a substance is referred to as antigenicity in medical terminology. The albumin content of each of the five FDA approved botulinum toxin preparations and the level of their antigenicity are illustrated in Table 3.3.

Table 3.3 Albumin content of FDA approved marketed botulinum toxins and their level of antigenicity

Toxin name	Botox	Xeomin	Dysport	Jeuveau	Myobloc
Albumin content	5 ng/100 units	0.44 ng/100 units	4.35 ng/500 units	0.5 mg/100 units	55/2500
Level of antigenicity	Low	Very low due to low albumin content	Low	Low	Low

Modified from Benecke in Biodrugs. Springer 2012 [3]

It is important to remember that the units of these different toxins have different strengths. When a patient goes to a different doctor, if a different toxin is going to be used, a proper unit conversion is necessary. Botox and Xeomin units are approximately comparable (1:1) but both are very different from Dysport or Myobloc as illustrated in Table 3.2.

Xeomin (Merz Pharmaceuticals, Frankfurt, Germany) [4]

This is another type A botulinum toxin with activities very similar to Botox. The units of Xeomin are close to Botox in potency and, in comparative clinical trials, researchers often use a 1:1 Xeomin/Botox ratio. It should be remembered that the units of different botulinum toxins are never truly comparable and the given equivalents are at best an approximation.

Xeomin's structure is very similar to the South Korean toxin, Meditoxin/Neurotox produced in year 2000 by the Korean Medytox pharmaceutical. Merz, a German pharmaceutical company, produces and distributes Xeomin in US. Although Xeomin still does not have FDA approval for some major clinical indications (migraine, bladder dysfunction), but like Botox it possesses efficacy in treatment of two very common medical indications namely, spasticity (abnormally increased muscle tone) and dystonias (involuntary movements and postures of the neck and face). It is also approved by FDA for treatment of excessive sweating and excessive drooling. Xeomin is provided in vials containing 50 and 100 units (Fig. 3.1, Table 3.3).

Xeomin has three advantages over Botox and other toxins:

1. It does not have to be refrigerated—a feature that is often helpful both to patients and medical providers.
2. It has a negligible amount of albumin (protein load of 0.44 ng/100unit), hence possesses very low antigenicity, hence, rarely leading to harmful antibody formation. This means that the incidence of unresponsiveness even with large doses and repeated injections is extremely low with xeomin (Table 3.3). In practice, however, this is a minor advantage over Botox since, as mentioned above, the new formulations of Botox have low incidence of unresponsiveness after chronic use even with large doses.

3. Reconstituted Xeomin does not show reduction of potency throughout 52 weeks (when kept in refrigerator) and, hence, may make it economically more favorable than other toxins [5].

Dysport (Ipsen Limited, Paris France) [6]

Dysport, a type A toxin similar to Botox, can be used for many neurological conditions (cervical dystonia, blepharospasm, hemifacial spasm, upper and lower limb muscle spasticity). Like Botox and Xeomin, it is approved by FDA for cervical dystonia, spasticity [7] and treatment of excessive sweating. It is the first botulinum toxin approved by FDA for treatment of lower limb spasticity in children based on high quality clinical trials (Table 3.4) [8]. Units of Dysport are different from that of Botox and Xeomin. Each 2.5–3 units of Dysport are approximately equivalent to 1 unit of the other two toxins. Dysport is provided in vials containing 300, 500 and 1000 units (Table 3.2).

Jeuveau and Daxxify [7, 8]

These two type A botulinum toxins were approved by FDA only for treatment of wrinkles and frown lines in 2019 and 2022, respectively. More recently (2023), Daxxify has also benn approved by FDA for treatment of cervical dystonia.

Jeuveau comes in single vials containing 100 units. Its effect on wrinkles is similar to that of Botox. Some studies have suggested that its effect on improving wrinkles lasts longer than Botox. Like Botox, it needs to be mixed with saline (salt water) before injection. Unlike Botox, Jeuveau does not have FDA approval for any other indication.

Daxxify works faster than Botox—on average, within 2 days versus 3–5 days for Botox. Daxxify lasts longer than Botox (6 months versus 3–4 months). It is however, almost twice more expensive than Botox. The cosmetic use of botulinum toxins are discussed in Chap. 13 of this book.

Myobloc (Neurobloc in Europe: WorldMed/Solstice Neurosciences, Louisville, Kentucky) [9]

Myobloc is the only type B toxin available for clinical use in US. It is approved for two indications: cervical dystonia which is involuntary movement/postures and stiffness of neck muscles, often associated with pain and for excessive salivation or sweating (autonomic disorder). In cervical dystonia, there is some literature

Table 3.4 Clinical indications (approved by FDA) for different botulinum toxins marketed in the USA

Trade name	Proprietary name given by FDA	Manufacturer	Medical condition	Year of FDA approval
Botox	OnabotulinumtoxinA	Allergan/Abvie Irvine, Ca	Blepharospasm	1989
			Hemifacial spasm	1989
			Strabismus (crossed eyes)	1989
			Cervical dystonia	2000
			Armpit sweating	2004
			Chronic migraine	2010
			Upper limb spasticity	2010
			Bladder (NDO)[a]	2011
			Bladder (OAB)[a]	2013
			Lower limb spasticity (adult)	2014
			Esthetics(forehead wrinkles)	2017
			Upper limb spasticity (child)	2019
Xeomin	incobotulinumtoxinA	Merz Pharma Frankfurt, Germany	Cervical dystonia	2010
			Blepharospasm	2010
			Excessive sweating	2010
			Esthetics (glabellar lines)	2011
			Upper limb spasticity(adult)	2015
			Excessive drooling	2018
Dysport	AbobotulinumtoxinA	Ipsen Pharma-UK	Cervical dystonia	2009
			Esthetics (glabellar lines)	2009
			Upper limb spasticity (adult)	2015
			Lower limb spasticity (child)	2016
			Lower limb spasticity adult	2017
Jeuveau	Probobotulinum toxinA	Evolus, Inc. Santa Barbara, CA	Esthetics (wrinkles)	2019
Daxxify	DaxibotulinumtoxinA	Revance Nashville, TN	Esthetics	2022
			Cervical dystonia	2023
Myobloc	RimabotulinumtoxinB	Solstice Neuroscience	Cervical dystonia	2009
			Excessive drooling	2010

[a]*NDO* neurogenic detrusor over-activity. Detrusser is the main muscle of the bladder wall. *OAB* overactive bladder (see Chap. 10)

suggesting that Myobloc works better than other toxins for associated neck pain and for this indication, the higher doses of Myobloc are more effective than lower doses [10, 11]. It is used, off-label, for treatment of spasticity and muscle spasms as well as excessive drooling based on clinical trials demonstrating its efficacy. Myobloc is provided as a "ready to use" solution and does not require reconstruction (mixing the toxin with saline). The units of Myobloc are very different from the units of other botulinum toxins. Myobloc vials contain 2500, 5000 and 10,000 units. Each 40–50 units of myobloc approximates 1 unit of Botox or Xeomin and 2.5–3 units of Dysport.

The times lines of FDA approval for each indication of botulinum toxins is presented in Table 3.4.

Preparation/Injection

All botulinum toxins are administered through intramuscular or intradermal (into the skin) injection. Before injection, Botox, Xeomin and Dysport need to be prepared for injection. These toxins are provided in the vial as a white powder and need reconstitution with salt water (saline) before injection. For most indications, the dilution is with 1–2 cc of normal saline (0.9% sodium salt solution commonly used in clinical practice). When injecting large muscles, mostly for spasticity (abnormally increased muscle tone such as seen after stroke), some injectors prefer to dilute with 4 or even 8 cc of normal saline to enhance diffusion of the toxin within the muscle. After inserting sterile saline into the vial, in case of Botox, the vial is gently shaken 3–4 times to accelerate the mixing process. For Xeomin, it is recommended to invert the vial several times. For most indications, a 1 cc thin syringe with 10 divisions is used to draw the solution. Because of the small size of the syringe drawing the reconstituted solution from the vial into injecting syringe is often problematic. The drawing process is tight and some of the solution is lost in the process. Adding a couple of cc's of air into the vial before drawing the solution into a 1 cc syringe will help. This will allow smooth drawing of the solution into the small syringe and full recovery of the solution from the vial.

For most indications of botulinum toxin therapy (with Botox or others), injecting muscles and skin around the head (in case of migraine), spasticity and dystonias (neck, limbs), injection are done with a small and thin needle to avoid pain and discomfort. A 27.5 gauge needle, ¾ inch long, is commonly used in clinical practice for these injections. For injections into the face for blepharospasm (spasm of eyelids) and hemifacial spasm (spasm of half of the face) as well as injecting into sweat gland and salivary glands, a smaller, 30-gauge needle is preferable. For most indications, injections are performed quickly and do not need prior numbing of the skin. For management of excessive sweating (palm, sole of the feet, arm pit) which requires multiple injections—20 to 30 injections under into or under the skin in a grid—like fashion—the skin is usually numbed with an anaesthetic cream first (for example Emla cream), about 1–2 h before injections. The skin is then cleaned and can be further numbed by an anaesthetic spray during the injections.

Specific side effects after treatment for each medical indication are discussed in different chapters of this book. The safety issues with botulinum toxins, in general, and for specific indications are discussed in Chap. 17.

Non-FDA Approved Botulinum Toxins Used in Far East Asia

Prosigne [12]

Prosigne is a type A toxin which was developed by Chinese scientists at the Lanzhou Institute. The toxin has properties similar to other type A toxins and targets the same set of proteins in nerve-muscle junction to prevent release of neurotransmitters from vesicles located inside the nerve terminal (see Chap. 2). The external expedients of Prosigne per vial, unlike all other type A toxins which is albumin is porcine gelatin 5 mg, dextran 25 mg and sucrose 25 mg with a protein load of 4–5 ng/100 units. It is generally believed that Prosigne's potency is close to that of Botox. In one report, a similar potency has been described (Botox/Prosigne 1:1 ratio) [12] while another report [13] used 1:1.5 ratio, with Botox being more potent. Although Prosigne has been shown to be effective in several indications similar to Botox including some pain indications, it is not approved by FDA for use in the US.

Meditoxin/Neuronox

Meditoxin (Neuronox) is a type A toxin manufactured by Medytox company in South Korea; it is widely used in Asian countries. The toxin has almost an identical structure to Xeomin and possesses a very low protein load. Neuronox comes in 50,100 unit vials with a potency similar to Botox. The external expedient in meditoxin is a plant protein unlike that of Botox which is serum albumin. A liquid formulation of Meditoxin has been developed which does not need reconstitution and can be kept at room temperature.

Meditoxin has been studied recently in several high quality investigations for possible approval by FDA. A phase III study (see definition of study phase later in this chapter) was completed on 7-4-2017 for blepharospasm (involuntary eyelid closure and spasms). Another phase III study was completed in 7-6-2017 on cervical dystonia, a medical condition characterized by involuntary neck movements and postures often associated with neck pain. Another phase III study for wrinkles with Meditoxin was initiated on 4-17-2017. However, recently, Meditox use and distribution has been the subject of critical investigations. In 2020, the Thai government suspended the sale of Meditoxin and recalled all the Meditoxin products distributed in the market based on alleged use of unauthorized ingredients and faked test results. In US, on December 2022, one distributor that falsely claimed FDA approval for Meditoxin was fined $10,000 in a Florida Court.

Definition of Clinical Trials

Before a drug gets approved by FDA for human use, it needs to go through three phases of clinical trials. Phase I clinical trial investigates if the drug is safe for human use. This is done usually on a small number of patients (n = 10–30) assessing the effect of different dosages of the drug and recording carefully tolerability and side effects. It is not the test of efficacy of the drug, although some observations on the patients' response to the drug can be made. No placebo (sham drug) is involved in a phase I clinical trial.

In a phase II clinical trial, larger number of patients are tested (usually between 25–100) looking at the efficacy of the drug for a specific indication based on different doses that have been found to be safe in the phase I trial. The patients' response to the drug is carefully tested by using different rating scales. This is usually a blinded and placebo controlled study i.e. the effect of the drug is blindly compared with a placebo (usually salt water injection in comparison with botulinum toxin). Double blinding means that the design of the study is as such that neither the patient nor the physician know the type of injection (toxin or placebo).

A phase III clinical trial is usually a multicenter trial involving a large number (hundreds or thousands) of patients. Phase III clinical trials use a placebo arm and the response of the patients' symptoms to the therapeutic agent (for instance botulinum toxin) is measured against that of a placebo. The results are presented after careful statistical assessment. Phase III clinical trials are longer than phase I and II, often lasting for months.

A phase IV clinical trial is done after FDA approval in order to investigate the clinical efficacy, quality of life and cost effectiveness in greater detail. These studies may involve several thousands of patients and are often conducted over several years.

The FDA approval for any drug (including botulinum toxins) for use in the US is based on availability of high quality, phase III trials. In most cases, FDA requires two phase III, class I (very high quality) studies that have proven the efficacy of the therapeutic agent for a given indication. For some indications, however, FDA has approved a drug for US use based on only one large, multicenter and exceptionally well done, Class I, phase III trial.

Study Class and Efficacy Evaluation

In this book, the definition of study class and efficacy are based on the criteria previously published by the American Academy of Neurology (AAN) [14, 15]. Clinical trials are classified into Class I, II, III and IV based on the quality of the study.

A class I study (highest quality) is a randomized, controlled clinical trial of the intervention of interest with masked or objective assessment in a representative population [14, 15]. The study is double blind i.e. the rating physician and the patient do not know what the given pill or injection was (drug or a placebo—a sham substance). Usually another physician not involved in the rating (assessment of symptom improvement) or a nurse conceals the information in a computer. Also, there should not be any substantial differences between the two study groups (toxin or placebo) in regard to relevant characteristics (sex, age, duration of illness, etc.).

The following also need to be clearly defined:

(a) How the allocation to drug group versus placebo group is concealed from the patient or rating physician
(b) Primary outcome(s)
(c) Exclusion and inclusion criteria
(d) Adequate accounting for dropouts. The dropout should not exceed 20% of the studied population

A class II study is a randomized, double blind study which lacks one of the 4 additional criteria (a–d) mentioned above or a prospective cohort which meets b, c or, d criteria. A class III study is all other controlled trials (including well-defined natural history controls or patients serving as their own control) in a representative population where outcomes are independently assessed or independently derived by objective outcome measurements. Class IV studies are all other studies not meeting Class I, II and III criteria. These studies are often retrospective reviews of a small cohort.

Based on the availability of high quality studies, the efficacy of a drug is classified as A, B, C and U. An A level of efficacy means that the efficacy is established or refuted based on two class I studies. For instance, the efficacy of Botox treatment is established in chronic migraine based on two class I studies (Chap. 4). A level B efficacy means probable efficacy (or lack of it) based on one class I or two class II studies. For example the efficacy of Botulinum toxin in nerve damage due to diabetes (diabetic neuropathy) has been assigned a B level based on two class II studies (Chap. 5). Level C efficacy denotes possible efficacy or possible lack of efficacy based on one class II study. The U efficacy level means that the reported high quality studies (class I and II) have described contradictory results or that there are no high quality studies reported for that indication. An example that has been assigned a U level of efficacy would be the use of botulinum toxin therapy in a condition called myofascial spasm. Throughout this book, wherever study class and efficacy level is quoted, it refers to the above-described classes and levels as defined by AAN guidelines.

References

1. Chen JJ, Dashtipour K. Abo-, inco-, ona-, and rima-botulinum toxins in clinical therapy: a primer. Pharmacotherapy. 2013;33:304–18.
2. Brin MF, Comella CL, Jankovic J, Lai F, Naumann M. CD-017 BoNTA study group. Long-term treatment with botulinum toxin type A in cervical dystonia has low immunogenicity by mouse protection assay. Mov Disord. 2008;23:1353–60.
3. Benecke R. Clinical relevance of botulinum toxin immunogenicity. BioDrugs. 2012 Apr 1;26(2):e1–9. https://doi.org/10.2165/11599840-000000000-00000. PMID: 22385408; PMCID: PMC3683397.

4. Dressler D. Five-year experience with incobotulinumtoxinA (Xeomin®): the first botulinum toxin drug free of complexing proteins. Eur J Neurol. 2012;19:385–9.
5. Dressler D, Bigalke H, Frevert J. The immunology of botulinum toxin therapy: a brief summary. Toxicology. 2022 Nov;481:153341. https://doi.org/10.1016/j.tox.2022.153341. Epub 2022 Sep 30. PMID: 36191878.
6. Monheit GD, Pickett A. AbobotulinumtoxinA: a 25-year history. Aesthet Surg J. 2017 May 1;37(suppl_1):S4–11. https://doi.org/10.1093/asj/sjw284. PMID: 28388718; PMCID: PMC5434488.
7. Gadarowski MB, Ghamrawi RI, Taylor SL, Feldman SR. PrabotulinumtoxinA-xvfs for the treatment of moderate-to-severe glabellar lines. Ann Pharmacother 2021 Mar;55(3):354–61. https://doi.org/10.1177/1060028020943527. Epub 2020 Jul 22. PMID: 32698599.
8. Hanna E, Pon K. Updates on botulinum neurotoxins in dermatology. Am J Clin Dermatol 2020 Apr;21(2):157–62. https://doi.org/10.1007/s40257-019-00482-2. PMID: 31782076.
9. Callaway JE. Botulinum toxin type B (myobloc): pharmacology and biochemistry. Clin Dermatol 2004. Jan–Feb;22(1):23–8. https://doi.org/10.1016/j.clindermatol.2003.12.027. PMID: 15158541.
10. Lew MF, Chinnapongse R, Zhang Y, Corliss M. RimabotulinumtoxinB effects on pain associated with cervical dystonia: results of placebo and comparator-controlled studies. Int J Neurosci. 2010;120:298–300.
11. Kaji R, Shimizu H, Takase T, Osawa M, Yanagisawa N. A double-blind comparative study to evaluate the efficacy and safety of NerBloc® (rimabotulinumtoxinB) administered in a single dose to patients with cervical dystonia. Brain Nerve. 2013;65:203–11.
12. Quagliato EM, Carelli EF, Viana MA. A prospective, randomized, double-blind study comparing the efficacy and safety of type a botulinum toxins botox and prosigne in the treatment of cervical dystonia. Clin Neuropharmacol. 2010;33:22–6.
13. Rieder CR, Schestatsky P, Socal MP, et al. A double-blind, randomized, crossover study of prosigne versus Botox in patients with blepharospasm and hemifacial spasm. Clin Neuropharmacol. 2007;30:39–42.
14. French J, Gronseth G. Lost in a jungle of evidence: we need a compass. Neurology. 2008;71:1634–8.
15. Gronseth G, French J. Practice parameters and technology assessments: what they are, what they are not, and why you should care. Neurology. 2008;71:1639–43.

Chapter 4
Botox: A Miracle Drug for Chronic Migraine

Abstract Headache is a common human ailment. Migraine is a recurrent and distressing headache that often impairs the quality of life. Uncontrolled and chronic migraine is a huge financial burden to the individual and to the country's economy. The data from high quality studies have shown efficacy of botulinum toxin injections in chronic migraine. Based on these data, in 2010, Botox was approved for chronic migraine in Europe and by FDA for use in the US. This chapter discusses the role of botulinum therapy in primary headaches, migraine and tension headache. It also provides information on the limited data published on secondary headaches such as those occurring after head injury. Information on different techniques of botulinum toxin injection for treatment of chronic migraine is also provided. The results of botulinum therapy for migraine are compared with the results of pharmacological therapy in migraine including the newer drugs introduced to the market over the past 10 years.

Keywords Botulinum toxin · Botulinum neurotoxin · Migraine · Chronic migraine · Tension headaches

Introduction

Headache is a common ailment. On average, 50% of the population experiences one headache per month and a quarter of the population acknowledge having one headache per week. Headache disorders are not only among the most prevalent, they are also among the most disabling disorders worldwide [1]. The international society for classification of headaches, categorizes headaches into primary and secondary headaches [2]. Primary headaches are those that occur in individuals with no evidence of brain disease or no abnormalities on brain imaging (CT, MRI) or laboratory testing. Secondary headaches arise as a result of brain pathology or systemic disorders. Although secondary headaches reflect a more serious condition (tumor, inflammation, bleeding, etc.), at times, primary headaches can be also as severe and as disabling.

The major primary headache disorders consist of migraine, tension headaches and cluster headaches. Over the past 25 years, the effects of botulinum neurotoxin therapy on primary headaches has been studied extensively, especially with type A toxin, Botox (see Chap. 3 for different types of botulinum toxins in the market). These studies have shown the efficacy of Botox in treatment of chronic migraine, an indication for which approval was received in summer of 2010 in Europe and Canada; it received approval by FDA for use in US, later that year. It is now considered a major treatment modality for treatment of chronic migraine.

Migraine and Chronic Migraine

The word migraine is derived from the French word migraine (pronounced migren) which itself originates from the Greek word hemikrania (pain involving half of the head—Galen 200 AD). Although in many patients with migraine, pain of migraine involves mainly one side of the head, a sizeable number of migraine victims complain of bilateral headaches. Migraine is much more common among women than men with a reported prevalence of 17% among women and 6% in men [3]. The exact cause of this huge gender difference in migraine is not clear but, undoubtedly, hormonal issues play a major role as migraine frequency often diminishes during pregnancy and after menopause following the drop in estrogen levels. Migraine's impact on the quality of life is substantial. Migraine is currently rated as the seventh cause of medical disability [4]. In terms of years lived with disability [YLD], headaches are the third most common cause of (YLD); 88% of YLD in headache field is due to migraine [5]. Migraine headaches usually begin during the second and third decades of life and decrease substantially after age 40 [6]. Migraine is considered a genetic disease since over 50% of the patients report a family history of migraine.

The pathophysiology of migraine is still not fully understood. The old concept that a sequence of constrictions of brain vessels followed by dilatation causes migraine is no longer tenable. According to current thinking, before onset of pain, an electrical wave starts and travels over the cortex resulting in depression of brain activity and release of potassium, calcitonin gene related peptide (CGRP) and other substances. These substances lead to inflammation of brain coverings which then conveys signals to the pain sensitive trigeminal system inside and outside of the brain. This system innervates the skull, scalp and blood vessels; irritation and sensitization of this system results in pain. A genetically related mechanism triggers the initial event of this cascade in migraine which is yet to be explained.

Clinically, migraine headaches are often of moderate to severe intensity and, on the average, last from 4 to 72 h. Migraine attacks may be one sided, but changing sides is not unusual. During the attacks, patients often complain of nausea and report unusual sensitivity to light or sound. Most affected patients prefer to go to a quiet room, close their eyes and avoid noisy environments.

In 20% of the patients, a migraine attack begins with an "aura." Aura means "breeze" in Greek and, in migraine, denotes a transient objective sensation before the onset of headache. The most common type of aura in migraine is a visual aura. Patients describe seeing lights in part of their visual field. These light auras are usually on one side of the patients' visual fields (sometimes affecting half of the field in both eyes) while taking many shapes and forms. They can present in the form of flickering or zigzag lights also called scintillations. These lights often start in a small part of the visual field and then evolve into larger areas. The enlarging lights in the field of vision (positive aura) sometimes end to momentary loss of vision in the same area (scotoma). In some patients, the scotomas or negative auras can occur without positive auras. Another common aura in migraine is a sensory aura which presents with experiencing unusual sensations over the face or parts of body. These sensations are usually in form of tingling, numbness or transient loss of sensation, affecting one side. Such experiences in older individuals need to be differentiated from initial symptoms of an impending stroke which is totally different from migraine. Other auras, such as experiencing intense smell or taste or having episodes of vertigo, are less common.

Patients may explain their first migraine as the most severe headache of their life with a very sudden onset. Such headaches (thunderclap headache) need to be investigated by computed tomography (CT scan) or magnetic resonance imaging (MRI) to ensure that they do not represent bleeding inside the head as a consequence of a ruptured aneurysm that requires immediate and urgent care due to its potentially life threatening nature (re-bleed). Aneurysm is an abnormal bulging, weakened wall of a blood vessel, usually an artery, that has a tendency to rupture.

Based on the frequency of headaches, migraine is classified as episodic or chronic migraine. The term episodic migraine defines a form of migraine with headache days of less than 15 per month, while definition of chronic migraine requires 15 or more headache days per month, with at least 8 of them being of migraine type (as described above).

Treatment of migraine includes abortive and prophylactic (preventive) measures. Abortive medications suppress the acute pain, whereas prophylactic medications prevent recurrence of severe headaches. Abortive treatments are short term and usually limited to the day of the migraine attack. Prophylactic treatments require taking daily medications. Migraine is an underdiagnosed disease and it is generally believed that preventive treatment in migraine is underutilized.

Treatment of Acute Attacks

Different categories of medications are available for inducing significant relief of acute migraine attacks within 2 h, usually in over 50% of the patients. These abortive drugs consist of Triptans, the Ergot derivative DHE, antiemetic (against vomiting) agents (metoclopramide, chlorpromazine), ketorolac, lasmiditan and small molecule CGRP (see above) inhibitors called Gepants.

Triptans (sumatriptan, eletriptan and other triptans) [7] are available in oral, injectable and nasal spray forms; generally abort the acute migraine attacks in a couple of hours. They are not, however, indicated in patients with history of stroke and heart disease. Subcutaneous (under the skin) injection of or nasal spray form of DHE has similar effects; to abort severe attacks intravenous DHE combined with metochlopromide (to reduce nausea) is often used. Ketoralac is in the category of non-steroidal (not a steroid) anti-inflammatory (working against inflammation) drugs which can be used for aborting acute migraine attacks. Ketorolac for migraine can be injected into the muscle (60 mg) or into the veins (15–30 mg). Lasmiditan (approved by FDA for use in the US in 2019) by reducing the activity of the trigeminal system (the part of the nervous system that supplies nerves for the face and scalp), aborts acute migraine attacks. Since it does not affect the vascular system, it can be used in patients with the history of heart disease or stroke [8]. Sleepiness is a side effect and driving should be avoided after taking lamisidin.

Recently, gepants have been introduced to the market for treatment of migraine. Among the three FDA approved gepants, ubrogepant (Ubrelvy) was the first gepant approved in 2019. It is now often used for treatment of acute migraine. A single 50 or 100 mg pill is able to abort the acute migraine attack, in a few hours. It is usually well tolerated with occasional side effects of dry mouth and sleepiness [9]. Long-term treatment data are now available and attest to the safety of this drug [10].

Transcranial magnetic stimulator is an FDA approved device that provides a magnetic pulse to the brain surface through the skull. In acute migraine, it has been shown to make 17% of the patients free of headache within 2 h [6]. This percentage, however, is considerably lower than 30% or higher improvement rates achieved by gepants or lasmiditan.

Preventive Treatment of Migraine

Several categories of medication are used for prevention of acute attacks of migraine. These include tricyclic antidepressants (amitryptiline and nortryptiline), betablockers (propranolol, nadolol, metoprolol, timolol) that also used for treatment of tremor, and drugs commonly used for treatment of seizures (anticonvulsant agents -topiramate, divalproex sodium). More recently, so-called monoclonal antibodies that block the function of CGRP (calcitonin gene related peptide) have been added to this list. As described earlier in this chapter, CGRP is a major pain transmitter and modulator that, based on laboratory tests, plays a major role in the pathophysiology of migraine. In high quality, blinded, phase 3 studies (see definition in Chap. 3), this group of drugs has been found to be extremely effective in prevention of migraine [11]. The mode of application for CGRP inhibitors can be either in the form of subcutaneous or intravenous injections, used once every 1–3 months. Table 4.1 shows different types of CGRP inhibitors (monoclonal antibodies) currently approved by FDA for treatment of migraine.

Table 4.1 CGRP inhibitors approved by FDA for treatment of migraine

Generic name	Trade name	Molecular size	Mode of application	Date of approval by FDA
Erenumab	Emimovig	Large	Pill	2018
Fremanezumab	Ajovy	Large	Pill	2018
Galcanezumab	Emgality	Large	Pill	2018
Epitinezumab	Vyepti	Large	Pill	2020
Ubrogepant	Ubrely	Small	Pill	2019
Rimegepant sulfate	NurtecODT	Small	Pill	2020
Atogepant	Qualipta	Small	Pill	2022
Zavegepant	Zavzpret	Small	Nasal spray	2023

Modified from Jabbari, B: in Botulinum Treatment of Pain Disorders, Second edition, 2022-Springer [12]

The pharmacological treatment of migraine has improved significantly with introduction of CGRP inhibitors. Prior to CGRP era, all medications used for prevention of acute migraine attacks had a low to medium rate of efficacy especially in chronic migraine when the attacks occur 15 or more days per month. Moreover, the side effects of these medications such as hypotension (low blood pressure) and sexual dysfunction (in case of betablockers), unusual sensory experiences, cognitive decline, depression, weight loss (topiramate), tremor and hair loss (divalproex), dry mouth, urinary retention and weight gain (tricyclic antidepressant and divalproex) concerned many patients. Over the counter medications such as co-enzyme Q, magnesium, vitamin B1 and melatonin or acupuncture have questionable preventive effect. Exercise, yoga, and meditation help some patients through relaxation. Furthermore, drugs that are used for aborting the acute migraine attacks are, themselves, sometimes hard to tolerate due to undesirable side effects. For instance, triptans and DHE are contraindicated in patients with coronary artery disease and can cause dizziness, nausea and light headedness, while antiemetic medications cause sedation and acute abnormal movements (dystonia: twisting of the limbs and akathisia: excessive restlessness).

CGRP inhibitors are generally well tolerated and have less side effects than the above-mentioned traditional drugs used for prevention of migraine [7]. Because of their expense, however, it is recommended to be used after traditional treatment of migraine fails [7]. Erunumab (Table 4.1), the most widely used CGRP inhibitor, can cause constipation and increase blood pressure. Since CGRPs have a potential to constrict blood vessels, The European Headache Federation guidelines suggests not to use CGRP inhibitors in patients with heart disease or stroke [13]. There is also the issue of losing the original efficacy over time with the use of CGRP inhibitors that needs to be further investigated [14]. For these reasons, a mode of preventive treatment which is effective and has a low side effect profile while providing sustained action, deserves exploration for prevention of frequent migraine attacks.

Botulinum Toxin Treatment of Migraine

During final years of the twentieth century, several reports indicated that Botox injection into forehead muscles can improve forehead wrinkles. To the surprise of clinicians that treated patients for wrinkles, some patients who received forehead injections reported a reduction in intensity and frequency of their migraine headaches. Following these observations, a headache specialist and researcher, Stephen Silberstein and his co-workers conducted the first randomized, double-blind, placebo-controlled clinical trial (see Chap. 3 for definition of clinical trials) of Botox in patients with migraine [15]. In that study, published in the year 2000, 123 patients with migraine were stratified into three groups receiving either Botox (75 units), Botox (25 units) or placebo (normal saline) into the forehead muscles. Although the study did not show a statistically significant improvement of the primary outcome measure—increased pain free days/month, it showed that injection of Botox into forehead muscles reduces the intensity of migraine attacks and the number of pain days/month. Between the year 2000 and 2010, several high quality studies [16–29] demonstrated that, in human, botulinum toxin injection can improve pain in several ailments, hence, encouraging further research in migraine. Furthermore, animal studies have shown that injection of botulinum toxins (A or B) into muscles and under the skin can inhibit the function of pain transmitters both in peripheral and in central nervous system [30–34].

It took 10 years after Silberstein's publication and several failed reports for use of Botox in large population of patients with migraine (mostly episodic migraine— migraine attacks of less than 15 times a month) [35] that convincing data about the role of Botox in migraine appeared in the literature.

In 2010, publication of two large PREEMPT studies demonstrated that injection of Botox into the pericranial (around the head) muscles, with a certain injection paradigm and dose, can significantly reduce the number of pain days in patients with chronic migraine. The total dose and number of injected sites in PREEMPT studies was substantially higher than that of prior studies.

PREEMPT Studies

The two PREEMPT [36, 37] studies were multi-center and investigated the efficacy of Botox in chronic migraine (15 or more pain days per month) on a total of 1384 patients. The PREEMPT studies were double blind, meaning that the patients did not know what they were receiving, also physicians and raters of the response were blinded to the type of the injections. Both studies had an open label arm (unblinded). The blinded arm of the studies lasted for 24 weeks with placebo or Botox injection every 12 weeks. Patients were evaluated with weekly visits during which they had several ratings of pain, sleep, and quality of life throughout the duration of the study. The open, unblinded arm which began after completion of the blinded arm, lasted

32 weeks during which the patients received Botox only and were evaluated the same way for their response. Evaluation of the pooled data from the two PREEMPT studies showed that a single injection of Botox produced not only reduction of pain days and migraine episodes per month, but it also reduced the pain intensity of each episode [38]. All findings had a high level of statistical significance (P < 0.0001). Since then, Botox has been used for treatment of chronic migraine on millions of patients worldwide. The positive results of PREEMPT studies raised several practical questions:

- Can the positive effect of Botox treatment in chronic migraine be sustained over a long period of time (years) with repeat injections?
- A sizeable number of patients with chronic migraine also have superimposed medication overuse headaches may complicate treatment. Does this population of patients with chronic migraine also respond to Botox therapy?
- Generally, patients with chronic migraine have a poor quality of life. Do the positive effects of Botox therapy in chronic migraine lead to improvement of quality of life?
- Is long-term treatment of chronic migraine with Botox safe? Are there any serious side effects with long-term use?

Aurora and co-workers [39] studied the sustenance of Botox effect on 1005 patients with chronic migraine who received Botox injections into pericranial (around the head) muscles every 3 months for 5 cycles (every 3–4 months) of treatment. Patients continued to enjoy pain relief during all 5 cycles of treatment (56 weeks) and also showed a substantial improvement in their quality of life as measured by migraine-specific quality of life questionnaire scores. Another group of investigators demonstrated that quality of life improved significantly both in the blinded and open label phase of the PREEMPT study in the Botox group (607 patients) compared to the placebo group (629 patients) [40]. Silberstein and co-workers [41], studied another cohort of the PREEMPT population. Of 688 patients who received Botox, 49.3% demonstrated 50% or more reduction in the frequency of headache days after the first injection with an additional 11% and 10% increase in response observed during the second and third cycle of injections. In another study that focused on patients with migraine and medication overuse headaches [42], treatment with Botox decreased the frequency of headache and migraine days, headache intensity, number of severe headache days and percentage of patients with severe HIT-6 scores (poor quality of life). The authors concluded that Botox treatment is effective in patients with chronic migraine and medication overuse.

In recent years, a number of authors have investigated the utility of Botox therapy in migraine outside clinical trials and in real-life situations. These studies [43, 44], have confirmed the positive results of clinical trials of Botox therapy in chronic migraine. A large survey conducted in 28 Italian health centers also concurred with the conclusion of these real-life studies [45].

Sites of Botox Injection, Recommended Dose per Site and per Session

The most common injection technique currently used for treatment of chronic migraine is the one used in the PREEMPT studies. The PREEMPT protocol recommends injecting five pericranial (around the head) muscles, one muscle in the upper neck (splenius,) and one in shoulder muscle (trapezius). The pericranial muscles consist of three forehead muscles (corrugator, procerus, and frontalis), one muscle at each temple (temporalis) and one muscle at the back of the head (occipitalis) (Fig. 4.1). The function of these muscles and the number of injections per muscle

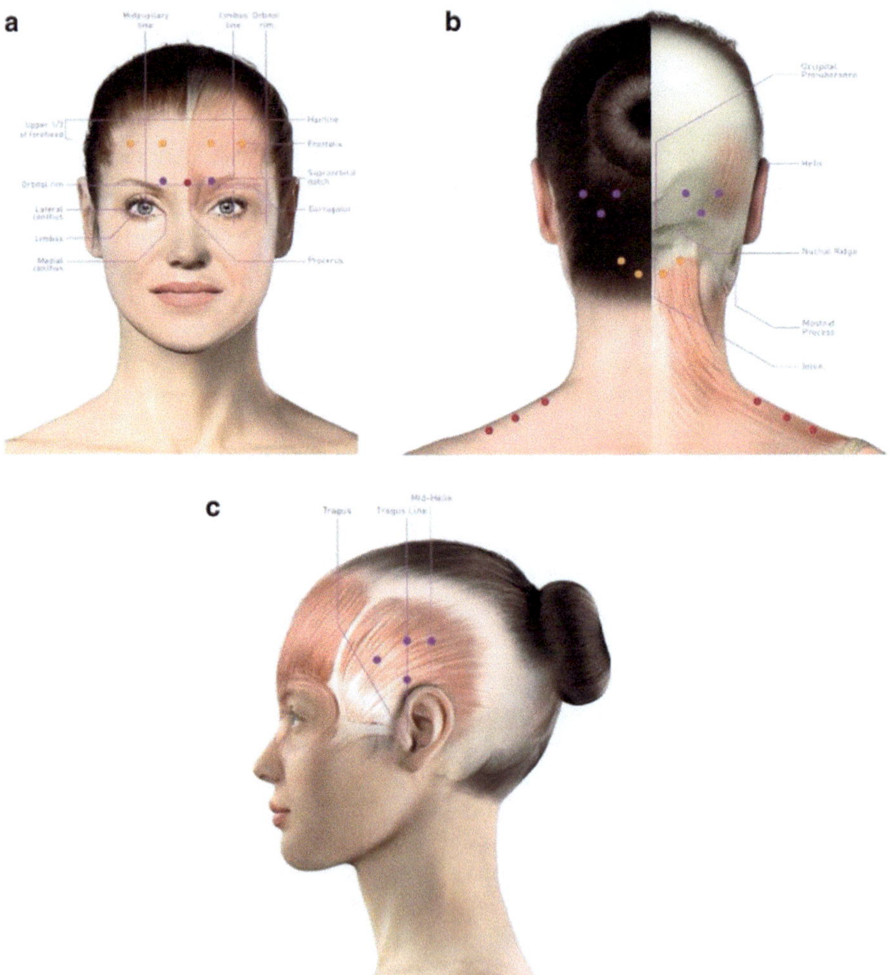

Fig. 4.1 Sites of Botox injections for treatment of chronic migraine as recommended by the PREEMPT Study group. From Blumenfeld et al. 2017 [46]. In Headaches. With permission from the Publisher, Wiley)

Table 4.2 Injection paradigm recommended by PREEMPT study. Injected muscles, muscle location, muscle function, number of injection sites and the dose injected per site

Muscle	Location	Function of muscle	Number of injection sites	Dose per injected site
Corrugator	Above the medial edge of eyebrow	Draws the eyes together and downward	One on each side	5 units
Procerus	Between two eyebrows	Pulls the eyebrows together	One injection at midline	5 units
Frontalis	Forehead	Moves eyebrows up	Four sites	5 units
Occipitalis	Back of the head	Moves the scalp back	Three on each side	5 units
Splenius	Upper neck	Turns and tilts the head to the same side	Two on each side	5 units
Trapezius	Shoulder	Moves the shoulder up	Thee on each side	5 units

and the dose per injection site are presented in Table 4.2. The total dose per session is 165 units of Botox with an option to increase it to 195 units, per discretion of the injecting physician.

In recent years, investigator from PREEMPT study group have shed more light on different aspects of chronic migraine's response to Botox injection. In regard to the onset of response, comparing 688 patient receiving Botox and 698 patients receiving placebo, one study found that even at week 1 after Botox injection the difference between the two groups was statistically and significantly in favor of Botox [47]. Furthermore, another study performed on close to 1400 patients who participated in the PREEMPT study demonstrated that response to Botox was well beyond improvement of headache and encompassed improvement of many aspects of quality of life [48].

In practice, from the patients' point of view, one of the major issues with Botox treatment of chronic migraine is the number of injections—31 injections was advocated in the PREEMPT protocol. Although the patients are generally pleased with the outcome and return every 3–4 months for reinjection, they do complain of the number of injections. I have designed an injection paradigm that encompasses 21 injected sites. This protocol which was conducted initially at Walter Reed Army Medical Center in Washington DC and then at Yale University in New Haven, CT over nearly 20 years produced very comparable results with that of PREEMPT protocol. In this protocol, temple injections are reduced from 4 to 2 on each side (using a larger dose of 15 units per site) and the occipital injections are reduced from 3 to 1 on each side using a larger dose of 10 units per site. The six injections into trapezius muscle are eliminated. For neck muscles, 3 injections, of 10 units each are given into the posterior neck muscle (splenius), on each side (Fig. 4.2) [49]. Although some authors have expressed concern that injection of higher doses into the temporal and neck muscles may cause undesirable muscle weakness, we have not noticed appreciable weakness of neck or temporalis muscle after thousands of Botox injection sessions performed for treatment of chronic migraine. The total

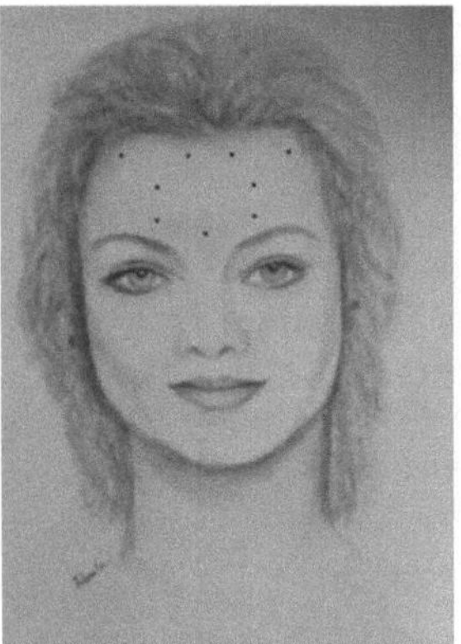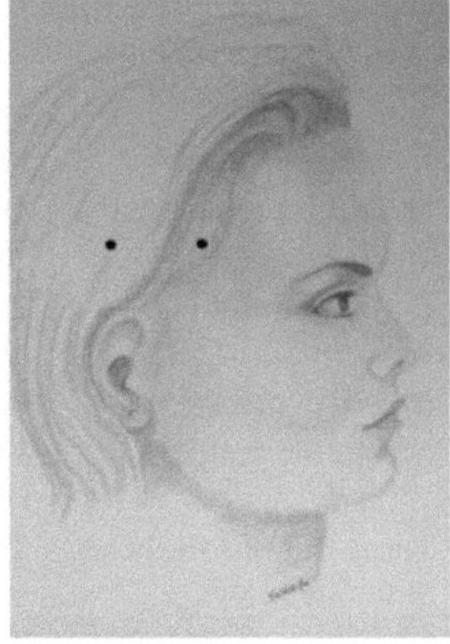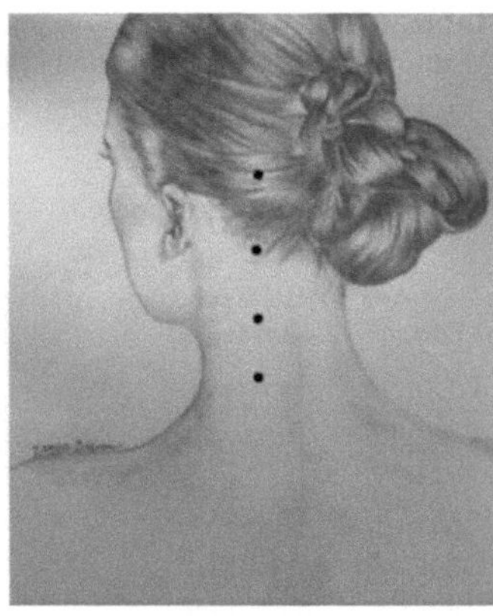

Fig. 4.2 The site of injections in the method used by Yale group for treatment of chronic migraine [49]. (Drawings courtesy of Tahereh Mousavi M.D. and Damoun Safarpour M.D.)

dose per session 185 units of Botox is slightly higher of PREEMPT. In patients with a very small neck, the neck dose was is reduced to 5 units per site making a total dose per session of 165 units.

Injection Method

Botox comes in small vials with the active powdered ingredient sitting at the bottom of the vial; it has to be mixed with normal saline (salt water) before injection. Some injectors like to add 1 cc and some add 2 cc of normal saline into the Botox vial containing 100 units of the toxin. This author for most indications prefers 1 cc dilution which allows injecting smaller volumes per site. After adding saline into the Botox vial, the solution is shaken gently and then is drawn into a small, thin 1 cc syringe with 10 divisions each representing 0.1 cc. When using 1 cc dilution, each of the 10 divisions of the syringe will contain 10 units of Botox (if using vials containing 100 units). Botox injections into the skin and muscles for migraine are superficial and performed with a small and thin needle (¾ inch, 27 or 30 guage needle). In experienced hands, injections into pericranial sites, upper neck and shoulder muscles cause minor discomfort. Usually there is no bleeding, but when there is minor bleeding, it stops quickly when wiped by a dry gauze. The injections can be done with the patient lying down or sitting up. This author prefers injecting migraine patients in the sitting up position. The whole procedure takes approximately 15 min.

Accuracy of dilution is very important in botulinum toxin therapy. This is particularly true when treating migraine patients since several muscles are small, hence, inaccurate dilution leads to overdosing and unpleasant side effects. For instance, small corrugator and procerus muscles are too close to the eye (see Figs. 4.1 and

4.2), and wrong dilution can lead to weakening of small muscles around the eye causing drooping of the eyelid or double vision that could last for 2-3 months. If the Botox solution is prepared and dilution is done by someone other than the injecting physician, it is the responsibility of the injecting physician to double check the accuracy of the dilution before injecting the patient.

Side Effects of Botox Therapy in Chronic Migraine

Side effects that develop following Botox treatment of migraine are minor and transient. In the large PREEMPT study consisting of 1384 patients, temporary pain at the site of injection, minor local bleedings (when the tip of the needle nicks a small blood vessel), mild muscle weakness and eyelid drooping occurred in 2–6% of the patients [39]. Drooping of the upper eyelid can last for several weeks, but in my experience, can be easily avoided by careful placement of the thin needle into the lower forehead muscles (procerus and corrugator—see Figs. 4.1 and 4.2), away from the upper eye lid. PREEMPT authors reported no serious side effects, safety and tolerability issues that concurred with the experience of clinicians in real-life situations (not a clinical trial).

Several studies have compared the preventive effect of Botox therapy in chronic migraine with the effect of two major headache preventive drugs, topiramate and divalproex. Side effects were more common in topiramate and divalproex groups. More patients in the topiramate and divalproex groups discontinued treatment due to undesirable side effects than the group that received Botox (24% versus 7% and 27% versus 3% for topiramate versus Botox and divalproex versus Botox, respectively) [50, 51].

Comparative data are now needed between CGRP inhibitors and Botox regarding degree of efficacy, side effects and endurance of therapeutic effects. In one retrospective observation over 6–8 months and after 2 cycles of Botox treatment (3–4 months apart) more patients with erunumab (the most widely used CGRP inhibitor) dropped out of the study compared to Botox (27% versus 3%) [52]. In some patients of this study, and in a recent study adding erunumab to Botox (combined therapy) improved efficacy of response and the patient's quality of life and [53]. According to a recent review, currently, the longterm safety data are only available for Botox and not for erumumab [54].

Episodic Migraine

The term episodic migraine defines headaches with a frequency of less than 15 times per month. Seven high quality, blinded Class I and II studies (see Chap. 3 for definition of study class) assessed the efficacy of botulinum toxin therapy in episodic migraine. Three of the seven studies have used similar or higher doses than

PREEMPT studies. All studies failed to show efficacy of botulinum toxin treatment in episodic migraine. Based on these data, in 2016, the Development Guideline Subcommittee of the American Academy of Neurology (AAN), defined botulinum toxin treatment as ineffective in management of episodic migraine [55]. However, a recent phase three quality study (see Chap. 3 for definition of research phases) has shown that Botox is effective in reducing pain days and improving quality of life in the high frequency tension headaches (11–13 pain days per month) [56].

Tension-Type Headaches

Tension Type Headaches (TTH) are the most common type of headaches with a prevalence of 38% in the US population [57]. Compared to migraine, tension headaches are more often bilateral and associated with scalp tenderness and less often associated with nausea and vomiting. Also, most tension headaches are less severe than migraine. The prevalence of chronic TTH (15 or more headaches per month) is similar to that of chronic migraine at 2% in the general population [58].

Treatment of TTH should start with behavior modification, psychotherapy and biofeedback aiming at reducing stress. For chronic TTHs, amitriptyline is often prescribed [58]. European guidelines also advocates the use of medications such as venlafaxine and mirtazapine that reduce the function of serotonin and norepinephrine [59].

The literature on quality studies (controlled and blinded) in regard to botulinum toxin therapy for TTHs contains contradictory data and is not convincing. In 2016, based on these contradictory results, the Guideline and Assessment Committee of the American Academy of Neurology stated the use of botulinum toxins in TTH "probably ineffective" [55]. However a recent review of this subject [60] expresses a different view. In this study [60], the authors performed meta-analysis on the data derived from 11 reported quality studies [61–71]. Meta-analysis is considered the most accurate form of statistical analysis; it merges and synthetizes the independent data from different studies. The authors' meta-analysis of literature in chronic TTH concluded that botulinum toxin therapy significantly ($P < 0.05$) reduced intensity, frequency, duration of headaches per day as well as the amount of the headache medications needed to control severe TTH. The results of this single study, though comprehensive, needs verification by future similar studies. The problem with the literature in this area is that none of the reported quality studies used the dose and treatment scheme of PREEMPT study which had proven effective in chronic migraine and led to FDA approval of Botox for this indication. There is an urgent need for such a study in chronic tension headaches using PREEMPT study design which had proven successful for chronic migraine. At the present time, botulinum toxin therapy is not FDA approved for treatment of tension-type headaches.

Secondary Headaches

The international society of headaches classifies headaches into primary and secondary types. Primary headaches include migraine, episodic headaches and tension type headaches. Secondary headaches are secondary to a defined cause such as head injury or stroke. There is no population-based data on acute secondary headaches [72]. In a selected population of 30,000 individuals 30 to 44 years of age, 2.14% reported having persistent secondary headaches [73]. Approximately 14% of patients with stroke complain of headache at the onset of stroke, while up to 50% complain of headaches after bleeding inside the brain [74]. Brain tumor related headaches occur in 5% of the patients and have no particular characteristics [75]. In one study, 38% of soldiers returning from combat complained of headaches related to head injury (post-traumatic headaches—PTH) [76]. Among patients with PTH, 18–22% continue to have headaches beyond 1 year after the head trauma [77].

A small group of published literature suggests that injection of botulinum toxin into scalp, using the PREEMPT method as used for treatment of chronic migraine, can alleviate persistent headaches after head injury. Zirovich and co-workers [78] conducted a placebo-controlled and blinded study using Dysport injections in 40 patients with PTHs. Dysport is a type A botulinum toxin similar to Botox. The study showed that the group receiving Dysport injection demonstrated a significant decrease in headache days per week as well as a decrease in headache intensity compared to the placebo group. The total dose of Dysport used was 387 units, approximately equivalent to 150 units of Botox. Furthermore, in an open label study (not placebo controlled) of 64 patients, the authors found that following Botox injections into the scalp (using the PREEMPT method), 64.1% of 64 patients reported significant improvement of post-traumtic headaches [79]. These encouraging data warrant conduction of more in depth studies to define the role of botulinum toxin treatment in patients suffering from persistent headaches after head injury.

Economic Issues

Several recent studies have shown that Botox treatment of chronic migraine (despite high cost of Botox) is economically sound and advantageous for the patients. In a study of 230 patients with chronic migraine [80], treatment with Botox over a 6-month period resulted in 55% and 57% reduction in emergency department visits and hospitalizations, respectively. The investigators reported a cost reduction (saving) of $1219 per patient over the six-month period of Botox treatment. Furthermore, Hepp and co-workers [81] have assessed headache-related health care utilization at 6, 9 and 12 months in a group of chronic migraine patients treated with Botox and compared the results with a group of patients treated with oral migraine prophylactic medications (OMPM). Using a regression analysis method (a form of statistical method), they found that the group on Botox had 20%, 21%, and 19% less emergency department visits over 6, 9 and 12 months and also 47%, 48%, 56% less hospitalizations compared to the OMPM group, respectively.

As described above, the newly introduced calcitonin gene related peptide (CGRP) inhibitors are now widely used for treatment of episodic and chronic migraine. Treatment of chronic migraine with these drugs, however, is more expensive than treatment with Botox. A comparative report published in 2018 shows the monthly cost of Botox treatment for chronic migrain as $ 310.52 versus $ 575 for erunumab (the most commonly used CGRP inhibitor drug) [82].

Discussion

Since 2010 (the date of FDA approval), Botox has been the first line drug for treatment of chronic migraine (CM) (15 or more headache days/month). It has proven to be safe and it provides sustained efficacy over years of treatment [54]. With introduction of CGRP inhibitors to the market (2018) (Table 4.1), the role of Botox as the first line of treatment for CM has been challenged. These drugs, like Botox are efficacious in CM, provide a sustained effect while possessing a low side effect profile [83]. CGRP inhibitor therapy, however, is more expensive than treatment with Botox in CM (see above). High quality studies are needed to compare the efficacy of these two different modes of therapy in CM preferably providing longterm data. Additional studies are also needed to assess the efficacy of other types of botulinum toxin A (for example Xeomin or Dysport) or botulinum toxin type B (Myobloc) in management of chronic migraine. Finally, some studies have shown that in recalcitrant cases of chronic migraine, combination of Botox and erunumab (the most commonly used CGRP inhibitor) provides better results than each mode of treatment alone [84]. There is a need for further exploration of this combination therapy that may help patients with severe CM.

References

1. Müller B, Gaul C, Reis O, Jürgens TP, Kropp P, Ruscheweyh R, Straube A, Brähler E, Förderreuther S, Schroth J, Dresler T. Headache impact and socioeconomic status: findings from a study of the German Migraine and Headache Society (DMKG). J Headache Pain. 2023 Apr 4;24(1):37. https://doi.org/10.1186/s10194-023-01564-7. PMID: 37016306; PMCID: PMC10071716.
2. The International Classification of Headache Disorders 3rd ed. (ICHD-3); 2017
3. Lipton RB, Bigal ME, Diamond M, et al. Migraine prevalence, disease burden, and the need for preventive therapy. Neurology. 2007;68:343–9.
4. GBD 2015 Disease and Injury Incidence and Prevalence Collaborators. Global, regional, and national incidence, prevalence, and years lived with disability for 310 diseases and injuries, 1990–2015: a systematic analysis for the Global Burden of Disease Study 2015. Lancet. 2016;388:1545–602.

5. Steiner TJ, Stovner LJ, Jensen R, Uluduz D, Katsarava Z. Lifting the burden: the global campaign against headache. Migraine remains second among the world's causes of disability, and first among young women: findings from GBD2019. J Headache Pain. 2020 Dec 2;21(1):137. https://doi.org/10.1186/s10194-020-01208-0. PMID: 33267788; PMCID: PMC7708887.
6. Charles A. Migraine. NEGM. 2017;377:553–61.
7. Ogunlaja OI, Goadsby PJ. Headache: treatment update. eNeurologicalSci. 2022 Aug 17;29:100420. https://doi.org/10.1016/j.ensci.2022.100420. PMID: 36636337; PMCID: PMC9830470.
8. Kuca B, Silberstein SD, Wietecha L, Berg PH, Dozier G, Lipton RB, COL MIG-301 Study Group. Lasmiditan is an effective acute treatment for migraine: a phase 3 randomized study. Neurology. 2018 Dec 11;91(24):e2222–32. https://doi.org/10.1212/WNL.0000000000006641. Epub 2018 Nov 16. PMID: 30446595; PMCID: PMC6329326.
9. Dodick DW, Lipton RB, Ailani J, Lu K, Finnegan M, Trugman JM, Szegedi A. Ubrogepant for the treatment of migraine. N Engl J Med. 2019 Dec 5;381(23):2230–41. https://doi.org/10.1056/NEJMoa1813049.
10. Ailani J, Lipton RB, Hutchinson S, Knievel K, Lu K, Butler M, Yu SY, Finnegan M, Severt L, Trugman JM. Long-term safety evaluation of ubrogepant for the acute treatment of migraine: phase 3, randomized, 52-week extension trial. Headache. 2020 Jan;60(1):141–52. https://doi.org/10.1111/head.13682. Erratum in: Headache. 2021 June;61(6):978-981. PMID: 31913519; PMCID: PMC7004213.
11. Tso AR, Gadsby PG. Anti-CGRP antibodies: the next era of migraine prevention? Curr Treat Options Neurol. 2017 Aug;19(8):27. https://doi.org/10.1007/s11940-0463-4.
12. Jabbbari B. Botulinum toxin treatment of pain disorders. 2nd ed. Cham: Springer Nature; 2022.
13. Sacco S, Bendtsen L, Ashina M, Reuter U, Terwindt G, Mitsikostas DD, Martelletti P. European headache federation guideline on the use of monoclonal antibodies acting on the calcitonin gene related peptide or its receptor for migraine prevention. J Headache Pain. 2019 Jan 16;20(1):6. https://doi.org/10.1186/s10194-018-0955-y. Erratum in: J Headache Pain. 2019 May 23;20(1):58. PMID: 30651064; PMCID: PMC6734227.
14. Huang IH, Wu PC, Lin EY, Chen CY, Kang YN. Effects of anti-calcitonin gene-related peptide for migraines: a systematic review with meta-analysis of randomized clinical trials. Int J Mol Sci. 2019 July 18;20(14):3527. https://doi.org/10.3390/ijms20143527. PMID: 31323828; PMCID: PMC6678090.
15. Silberstein S, Mathew N, Saper J, Jemkins S. Botulinum toxin type A as migraine preventive treatment. For the Botox migraine clinical research group. Headache. 2000;4:445–50.
16. Foster L, Clapp L, Erickson M, Jabbari B. Botulinum toxin A and chronic low back pain: a randomized, double-blind study. Neurology. 2001 May 22;56(10):1290–3. https://doi.org/10.1212/wnl.56.10.1290.
17. Borodic GE, Acquadro MA. The use of botulinum toxin for the treatment of chronic facial pain. J Pain. 2002 Feb;3(1):21–7. https://doi.org/10.1054/jpai.2002.27142.
18. Keizer SB, Rutten HP, Pilot P, Morré HH, v Os JJ, Verburg AD. Botulinum toxin injection versus surgical treatment for tennis elbow: a randomized pilot study. Clin Orthop Relat Res. 2002 Aug;401:125–31. https://doi.org/10.1097/00003086-200208000-00015.
19. Restivo DA, Tinazzi M, Patti F, Palmeri A, Maimone D. Botulinum toxin treatment of painful tonic spasms in multiple sclerosis. Neurology. 2003 Sept 9;61(5):719–20. https://doi.org/10.1212/01.wnl.0000080081.74117.e4.
20. Yuan RY, Sheu JJ, Yu JM, Chen WT, Tseng IJ, Chang HH, Hu CJ. Botulinum toxin for diabetic neuropathic pain: a randomized double-blind crossover trial. Neurology. 2009 Apr 28;72(17):1473–8. https://doi.org/10.1212/01.wnl.0000345968.05959.cf. Epub 2009 Feb 25.
21. Smith CP, Radziszewski P, Borkowski A, Somogyi GT, Boone TB, Chancellor MB. Botulinum toxin a has antinociceptive effects in treating interstitial cystitis. Urology. 2004 Nov;64(5):871–5; discussion 875. https://doi.org/10.1016/j.urology.2004.06.073.
22. Layeeque R, Hochberg J, Siegel E, Kunkel K, Kepple J, Henry-Tillman RS, Dunlap M, Seibert J, Klimberg VS. Botulinum toxin infiltration for pain control after mastectomy and

expander reconstruction. Ann Surg. 2004 Oct;240(4):608–13; discussion 613-4. https://doi. org/10.1097/01.sla.0000141156.56314.1f. PMID: 15383788; PMCID: PMC1356462.

23. Jarvis SK, Abbott JA, Lenart MB, Steensma A, Vancaillie TG. Pilot study of botulinum toxin type A in the treatment of chronic pelvic pain associated with spasm of the levator ani muscles. Aust N Z J Obstet Gynaecol. 2004 Feb;44(1):46–50. https://doi.org/10.1111/j.1479-828 X.2004.00163.x.

24. Braker C, Yariv S, Adler R, Badarny S, Eisenberg E. The analgesic effect of botulinum-toxin A on postwhiplash neck pain. Clin J Pain. 2008 Jan;24(1):5–10. https://doi.org/10.1097/ AJP.0b013e318156d90c.

25. Babcock MS, Foster L, Pasquina P, Jabbari B. Treatment of pain attributed to plantar fasciitis with botulinum toxin A: a short-term, randomized, placebo-controlled, double-blind study. Am J Phys Med Rehabil. 2005 Sept;84(9):649–54. https://doi.org/10.1097/01. phm.0000176339.73591.d7.

26. Kesary Y, Singh V, Frenkel-Rutenberg T, Greenberg A, Dekel S, Schwarzkopf R, Snir N. Botulinum toxin injections as salvage therapy is beneficial for management of patello-femoral pain syndrome. Knee Surg Relat Res. 2021 Oct 29;33(1):39. https://doi.org/10.1186/ s43019-021-00121-3. Erratum in: Knee Surg Relat Res. 2022 Feb 1;34(1):2. PMID: 34715941; PMCID: PMC8555335.

27. Allam N, Brasil-Neto JP, Brown G, Tomaz C. Injections of botulinum toxin type a produce pain alleviation in intractable trigeminal neuralgia. Clin J Pain. 2005 Mar-Apr;21(2):182–4. https://doi.org/10.1097/00002508-200503000-00010.

28. Wittekindt C, Liu WC, Preuss SF, Guntinas-Lichius O. Botulinum toxin A for neuropathic pain after neck dissection: a dose-finding study. Laryngoscope. 2006 July;116(7):1168–71. https:// doi.org/10.1097/01.mlg.0000217797.05523.75.

29. Mahowald ML, Singh JA, Dykstra D. Long term effects of intra-articular botulinum toxin A for refractory joint pain. Neurotox Res. 2006 Apr;9(2–3):179–88. https://doi.org/10.1007/ BF03033937.

30. Cui M, Khanijou S, Rubino J, Aoki KR. Subcutaneous administration of botulinum toxin A reduces formalin-induced pain. Pain. 2004 Jan;107(1-2):125–33. https://doi.org/10.1016/j. pain.2003.10.008.

31. Meng J, Ovsepian SV, Wang J, Pickering M, Sasse A, Aoki KR, Lawrence GW, Dolly JO. Activation of TRPV1 mediates calcitonin gene-related peptide release, which excites trigeminal sensory neurons and is attenuated by a retargeted botulinum toxin with anti-nociceptive potential. J Neurosci. 2009 Apr 15;29(15):4981–92. https://doi.org/10.1523/ JNEUROSCI.5490-08.2009. PMID: 19369567; PMCID: PMC6665337.

32. Gazerani P, Au S, Dong X, Kumar U, Arendt-Nielsen L, Cairns BE. Botulinum neurotoxin type A (BoNTA) decreases the mechanical sensitivity of nociceptors and inhibits neurogenic vasodilation in a craniofacial muscle targeted for migraine prophylaxis. Pain. 2010 Dec;151(3):606–16. https://doi.org/10.1016/j.pain.2010.07.029. Epub 2010 Aug 21.

33. Aoki KR. Evidence for antinociceptive activity of botulinum toxin type A in pain management. Headache. 2003 July–Aug;43(Suppl 1):S9–15. https://doi.org/10.1046/j.1526-4610.43.7s.3.x.

34. Bach-Rojecky L, Relja M, Lacković Z. Botulinum toxin type A in experimental neuropathic pain. J Neural Transm (Vienna). 2005 Feb;112(2):215–9. https://doi.org/10.1007/ s00702-004-0265-1.

35. Shuhendler AJ, Lee S, Siu M, Ondovcik S, Lam K, Alabdullatif A, Zhang X, Machado M, Einarson TR. Efficacy of botulinum toxin type A for the prophylaxis of episodic migraine headaches: a meta-analysis of randomized, double-blind, placebo-controlled trials. Pharmacotherapy. 2009 July;29(7):784–91. https://doi.org/10.1592/phco.29.7.784.

36. Aurora SK, Dodick DW, Turkel CC, DeGryse RE, Silberstein SD, Lipton RB, Diener HC, Brin MF, PREEMPT 1 Chronic Migraine Study Group. OnabotulinumtoxinA for treatment of chronic migraine: results from the double-blind, randomized, placebo-controlled phase of the PREEMPT 1 trial. Cephalalgia. 2010 July;30(7):793–803. https://doi. org/10.1177/0333102410364676. Epub 2010 Mar 17.

37. Diener HC, Dodick DW, Aurora SK, Turkel CC, DeGryse RE, Lipton RB, Silberstein SD, Brin MF, PREEMPT 2 Chronic Migraine Study Group. OnabotulinumtoxinA for treatment of chronic migraine: results from the double-blind, randomized, placebo-controlled phase of the PREEMPT 2 trial. Cephalalgia. 2010 July;30(7):804–14. https://doi.org/10.1177/0333102410364677. Epub 2010 Mar 17.

38. Dodick DW, Turkel CC, DeGryse RE, Aurora SK, Silberstein SD, Lipton RB, Diener HC, Brin MF, PREEMPT Chronic Migraine Study Group. OnabotulinumtoxinA for treatment of chronic migraine: pooled results from the double-blind, randomized, placebo-controlled phases of the PREEMPT clinical program. Headache. 2010 June;50(6):921–36. https://doi.org/10.1111/j.1526-4610.2010.01678.x. Epub 2010 May 7.

39. Aurora SK, Dodick DW, Diener HC, et al. OnabotulinumtoxinA for chronic migraine: efficacy, safety and tolerability in patients who received all five treatment cycles in the PREEMPT clinical program. Acta Neurol Scand. 2014;129:61–70.

40. Lipton RB, Rosen NL, Ailani J, et al. OnabotulinumtoxinA improves quality of life and reduces impact of chronic migraine over one year of treatment: pooled results of the PREEMPT randomized clinical trial program. Cephalalgia. 2016;36:899–908.

41. Silberstein SD, Dodick DW, Aurora SK, et al. Per cent of patients with chronic migraine who responded per onabotulinumtoxinA treatment cycle: PREEMPT. J Neurol Neurosurg Psychiatry. 2015;86:996–1001.

42. Silberstein SD, Blumenfeld AM, Cady RK, et al. OnabotulinumtoxinA for treatment of chronic migraine: PREEMPT 24-weel pooled subgroup analysis of patients who had acute headache medication overuse at baseline. J Neurol Sci. 2013;331:48–56.

43. Khalil M, Zafar HW, Quarshie V, Ahmed F. Prospective analysis of the use of onabotulinumtoxinA (BOTOX) in the treatment of chronic migraine; real-life data in 254 patients from Hull, U.K. J Headache Pain. 2014;15:54.

44. Kollewe K, Escher CM, Wulff DU, et al. Long-term treatment of chronic migraine with OnabotulinumtoxinA: efficacy, quality of life and tolerability in a real-life setting. J Neural Transm (Vienna). 2016;123:533–40.

45. Tassorelli C, Aguggia M, De Tommaso M, et al. OnabotulinumtoxinA for the management of chronic migraine in current clinical practice: results of a survey of sixty-three Italian headache centers. J Headache Pain. 2017;18:66.

46. Blumenfeld AM, Silberstein SD, Dodick DM, et al. Insights into the functional anatomy behind the PREEMPT injection program: guidance on achieving optimum outcomes. Headache. 2017;57:766–77.

47. Dodick DW, Silberstein SD, Lipton RB, DeGryse RE, Adams AM, Diener HC. Early onset of effect of onabotulinumtoxinA for chronic migraine treatment: analysis of PREEMPT data. Cephalalgia. 2019 July;39(8):945–56. https://doi.org/10.1177/0333102418825382. Epub 2019 May 21.

48. Diener HC, Dodick DW, Lipton RB, Manack Adams A, DeGryse RE, Silberstein SD. Benefits beyond headache days with onabotulinumtoxinA treatment: a pooled PREEMPT analysis. Pain Ther. 2020 Dec;9(2):683–94. https://doi.org/10.1007/s40122-020-00198-w. Epub 2020 Oct 7. PMID: 33026631; PMCID: PMC7648806.

49. Schaefer SM, Gottschalk CH, Jabbari B. Treatment of chronic migraine with focus on botulinum neurotoxins. Toxins (Basel). 2015;7:2615–28.

50. Cady RK, Schreiber CP, Porter JA, et al. A multi-center doube-blind pilot comparison of onabotulinumtoxina and topiramate for the prophylactic treatment of chronic migraine. Headache. 2011;51:21–32.

51. Blumenfeld AM, Schim JD, Chippendale TJ. Botulinum toxin type a and divalproex sodium for prophylactic treatment of episodic or chronic migraine. Headache. 2008;48:210–20.

52. Blumenfeld AM, Frishberg BM, Schim JD, Iannone A, Schneider G, Yedigarova L, Manack Adams A. Real-world evidence for control of chronic migraine patients receiving CGRP monoclonal antibody therapy added to onabotulinumtoxinA: a retrospective chart review. Pain

Ther. 2021 Dec;10(2):809–26. https://doi.org/10.1007/s40122-021-00264-x. Epub 2021 Apr 21. PMID: 33880725; PMCID: PMC8586140.

53. Armanious M, Khalil N, Lu Y, Jimenez-Sanders R. Erenumab and onabotulinumtoxinA combination therapy for the prevention of intractable chronic migraine without aura: a retrospective analysis. J Pain Palliat Care Pharmacother. 2021 Mar;35(1):1–6. https://doi.org/10.1080/15360288.2020.1829249. Epub 2020 Oct 30.

54. Blumenfeld AM, Kaur G, Mahajan A, Shukla H, Sommer K, Tung A, Knievel KL. Effectiveness and safety of chronic migraine preventive treatments: a systematic literature review. Pain Ther. 2023 Feb;12(1):251–74. https://doi.org/10.1007/s40122-022-00452-3. Epub 2022 Nov 22. PMID: 36417165; PMCID: PMC9845441.

55. Simpson DM, Hallett M, Ashman EJ, Comella CL, et al. Practice guideline update summary: botulinum neurotoxin for the treatment of blepharospasm, cervical dystonia, adult spasticity, and headache: report of the guideline development Subcommittee of the American Academy of neurology. Neurology. 2016;86:1818–26.

56. Martinelli D, Arceri S, De Icco R, Allena M, Guaschino E, Ghiotto N, Bitetto V, Castellazzi G, Cosentino G, Sances G, Tassorelli C. BoNT-A efficacy in high frequency migraine: an open label, single arm, exploratory study applying the PREEMPT paradigm. Cephalalgia 2022 Feb;42(2):170–75. https://doi.org/10.1177/03331024211034508. Epub 2021 Aug 18.

57. Schwartz BS, Stewart WF, Simon D, Lipton RB. Epidemiology of tension-type headache. JAMA. 1998;270:3881–383.

58. Freitag F. Managing and treating tension -type headache. Med Clin North Am. 2013;97:281–92.

59. Bendtsen L, Evers S, Linde M, Mitsikostas DD, Sandrini G, Schoenen J, EFNS. EFNS guideline on the treatment of tension-type headache – report of an EFNS task force. Eur J Neurol. 2010 Nov;17(11):1318–25. https://doi.org/10.1111/j.1468-1331.2010.03070.x.

60. Dhanasekara CS, Payberah D, Chyu JY, Shen CL, Kahathuduwa CN. The effectiveness of botulinum toxin for chronic tension-type headache prophylaxis: a systematic review and meta-analysis. Cephalalgia. 2023 Mar;43(3):3331024221150231. https://doi.org/10.1177/03331024221150231.

61. Hamdy SM, Samir H, El-Sayed M, Adel N, Hasan R. Botulinum toxin: could it be an effective treatment for chronic tension-type headache? J Headache Pain. 2009 Feb;10(1):27–34. https://doi.org/10.1007/s10194-008-0082-2. Epub 2008 Nov 22. PMID: 19030947; PMCID: PMC3451761.

62. Harden RN, Cottrill J, Gagnon CM, Smitherman TA, Weinland SR, Tann B, Joseph P, Lee TS, Houle TT. Botulinum toxin a in the treatment of chronic tension-type headache with cervical myofascial trigger points: a randomized, double-blind, placebo-controlled pilot study. Headache. 2009 May;49(5):732–43. https://doi.org/10.1111/j.1526-4610.2008.01286.x. Epub 2008 Oct 24.

63. Kokoska MS, Glaser DA, Burch CM, et al. Botulinum toxin injections for the treatment of frontal tension headache. J Headache Pain. 2004;5:103–9.

64. Padberg M, de Bruijn SF, de Haan RJ, et al. Treatment of chronic tension-type headache with botulinum toxin: a double-blind, placebo-controlled clinical trial. Cephalalgia. 2004;24:675–80.

65. Porta M. Comparative trial of botulinum toxin type a and methylprednisolone for the treatment of tension-type headache. Curr Rev Pain. 2000;4:31–5.

66. Rollnik JD, Tanneberger O, Schubert M, et al. Treatment of tension-type headache with botulinum toxin type A: a double-blind, placebo-controlled study. Headache. 2000;40:300–5.

67. Schmitt WJ, Slowey E, Fravi N, et al. Effect of botulinum toxin A injections in the treatment of chronic tension-type headache: a double-blind, placebo-controlled trial. Headache. 2001;41:658–64.

68. Schulte-Mattler WJ, Krack P, Group BS. Treatment of chronic tension-type headache with botulinum toxin A: a randomized, double-blind, placebo-controlled multicenter study. Pain. 2004;109:110–4.

69. Silberstein SD, Göbel H, Jensen R, et al. Botulinum toxin type A in the prophylactic treatment of chronic tension-type headache: a multicentre, double-blind, randomized, placebo-controlled, parallel-group study. Cephalalgia. 2006;26:790–800.
70. Smuts JA, Baker MK, Smuts HM, et al. Prophylactic treatment of chronic tension-type headache using botulinum toxin type A. Eur J Neurol. 1999;6:s99–s102.
71. Straube A, Empl M, Ceballos-Baumann A, et al. Pericranial injection of botulinum toxin type A (Dysport) for tension-type headache – a multicentre, double-blind, randomized, placebo-controlled study. Eur J Neurol. 2008;15:205–13.
72. Bahra A, Evans RW. The secondary headaches. Cephalalgia. 2021 Apr;41(4):427–30. https://doi.org/10.1177/0333102421999996. Epub 2021 Mar 16.
73. Aaseth K, Grande RB, Kvaerner KJ, et al. Prevalence of secondary chronic headaches in a population-based sample of 30–44-year-old persons. The Akershus study of chronic headache. Cephalalgia. 2008;28:705–13.
74. Rothrock JF, Diener H-C. Headache secondary to cerebrovascular disease. Cephalalgia. 2020; https://doi.org/10.1177/0333102421999045.
75. Palmieri A, Valentinis L, Zanchin G. Update on headache and brain tumors. Cephalalgia. 28 November 2020;41(4):431–437.
76. Theeler BJ, Flynn FG, Erickson JC. Headaches after concussion in US soldiers returning from Iraq or Afghanistan. Headache. 2010 Sept;50(8):1262–72. https://doi.org/10.1111/j.1526-4610.2010.01700.x. 2010 June 10.
77. Dwyer B. Posttraumatic headache. Semin Neurol. 2018 Dec;38(6):619–26. https://doi.org/10.1055/s-0038-1673692. Epub 2018 Dec 6.
78. Zirovich MD, Pangarkar SS, Manh C, Chen L, Vangala S, Elashoff DA, Izuchukwu IS. Botulinum toxin type A for the treatment of post-traumatic headache: a randomized, placebo-controlled, cross-over study. Mil Med. 2021 May 3;186(5–6):493–9. https://doi.org/10.1093/milmed/usaa391.
79. Yerry JA, Kuehn D, Finkel AG. Onabotulinum toxin a for the treatment of headache in service members with a history of mild traumatic brain injury: a cohort study. Headache. 2015 Mar;55(3):395–406. https://doi.org/10.1111/head.12495. Epub 2015 Feb 3.
80. Rothrock JF, Bloudek LM, Houle TT, et al. Real-world economic impact of onabotulinumtoxinA in patients wth chronic migraine. Headache. 2014;54(10):1565–73.
81. Hepp Z, Rosen NL, Gillard PG, et al. Comparative effectiveness of onabotulinumtoxinA versus oral migraine prophylactic medications on headache-related resource utilization in the management of chronic migraine: retrospective analysis of a US-based insurance data base. Cephalalgia. 2016;36(9):862–74.
82. Sussman M, Benner J, Neumann P, Menzin J. Cost-effectiveness analysis of erenumab for the preventive treatment of episodic and chronic migraine: results from the US societal and payer perspectives. Cephalalgia. 2018 Sept;38(10):1644–57. https://doi.org/10.1177/0333102418796842. Epub 2018 Aug 24.
83. Ashina M, Goadsby PJ, Reuter U, Silberstein S, Dodick DW, Xue F, Zhang F, Paiva da Silva Lima G, Cheng S, Mikol DD. Long-term efficacy and safety of erenumab in migraine prevention: results from a 5-year, open-label treatment phase of a randomized clinical trial. Eur J Neurol. 2021 May;28(5):1716–1725. https://doi.org/10.1111/ene.14715. Epub 2021 Jan 20. PMID: 33400330; PMCID: PMC8248354.
84. Scuteri D, Tonin P, Nicotera P, Vulnera M, Altieri GC, Tarsitano A, Bagetta G, Corasaniti MT. Pooled analysis of real-world evidence supports anti-CGRP mAbs and onabotulinumtoxinA combined trial in chronic migraine. Toxins (Basel). 2022 Aug 1;14(8):529. https://doi.org/10.3390/toxins14080529. PMID: 36006191; PMCID: PMC9413678. Combination therapy more effective.

Chapter 5
Pain Disorders other than Migraine

Abstract Following injection into the muscle or skin, botulinum toxin blocks the release of pain transmitters and modulators and lead to reduction of pain perception. Botulinum toxin treatment (with Botox) is now approved by FDA for treatment of chronic migraine (Chap. 4). High quality studies have shown efficacy of botulinum toxins in several pain syndromes including local pain in diabetic neuropathy, pain after shingles (post-herpetic neuralgia), pain after trauma to the limb, face pain in trigeminal neuralgia, heal pain in plantar fasciitis, non-surgical low back pain, pain associated with Raynaud syndrome and deep buttock pain in piriformis syndrome. Preliminary studies in several other pain syndrome have also demonstrated encouraging results. At the present time, none of these potential pain indications are FDA approved.

Keywords Botulinum toxin · Botulinum neurotoxin · Pain · Diabetic neuropathy · Neuralgia · Low back pain · Plantar faciitis · Raynaud syndrome

Introduction

Pain is the most common human medical complaint. International Association for the Study of Pain (IASP) defines chronic pain as a pain that persists 3 months or longer [1]. The prevalence of chronic pain in US is reported as 20% [2] comparable with that of Europe (19%) [3], where the highest prevalence for pain (30%) is reported for Poland [3]. Patient with chronic pain suffer from impaired quality of life [4]. In US, a report published in 2011, estimated the cost of chronic pain management (including direct health care cost and lost productivity) ranging from 560 to 635 billion dollars annually [5].

In most patients, pain is generated from a noxious stimulus which irritates the skin and peripheral nerves (peripheral pain). Central pain is uncommon. Less than 10% of pain experienced by the general population, is generated from a disease or disorder of the central nervous system (spinal cord or brain). This central pain can be seen is conditions such as stroke, multiple sclerosis or trauma to the brain or spinal cord.

B. Jabbari, *Botulinum Toxin Treatment*,
https://doi.org/10.1007/978-3-031-54471-2_5

In this chapter, we will briefly discuss the anatomy of pain pathways and the biologic and chemical substances which are essential in initiation and maintenance of pain. This will be followed by a brief description of animal studies that have shown how botulinum toxins can reduce pain by inhibiting pain transmitters and modulators. Finally, this chapter is predominantly devoted to discussion of the role and potential of botulinum toxin therapy in different human pain conditions.

Anatomy of Pain Pathways

The nerves in the body are of two major types, motor or sensory. A third type, autonomic nerves which consists of very thin fibers, deal with the function of the viscera and glands. Sensory nerves convey sensations, including pain to the brain. Perception of pain requires a cascade of events which includes four phases: transduction, transmission, modulation and perception:

Transduction

In this first phase of pain pathway, a noxious peripheral stimulus (thermal, mechanical, chemical) stimulates the peripheral sensory nerve endings which are scattered in the skin, muscle and joints. Located on these sensory nerve endings, are small receptors capable of sensing various types of the peripheral stimulation (heat, pressure, chemical). These receptors which are called nociceptive (related to pain) receptors are also present on the body of the central sensory nerve cells (neurons) in the spinal cord. The pain which arises from damage to the tissue (skin, muscle, joint) is called nociceptive pain, whereas the term neuropathic pain is applied to pain arising from damage to a peripheral nerve or the sensory pathways in the central nervous system.

Noxious stimulation of sensory nerve endings causes local secretion of several chemicals from the nerve endings which elicit stimulation of specific pain receptors. Furthermore, local tissue inflammation caused by accumulation of these chemicals leads to more stimulation of the nerve endings resulting in peripheral sensitization. Some of these chemicals such as histamine, bradykinin, Substance P and calcitonin gene-related peptide (CGRP) are well known; several others are currently under investigation.

Transmission

During this phase, electrical activity that is generated from stimulation of the above-mentioned receptors travels along the sensory nerve. Sensory nerve fibers have different sizes. The fibers that convey the pain modality are thin (A-delta fiber) or very thin (C fibers). A-delta fibers conduct faster and are responsible for the short lasting and very sharp initial pain felt after exposure to a noxious stimulus. Slow conducting, C fibers produce the less intense, but longer lasting pain that follows the initial sharp pain (Fig. 5.1, lower right).

On the path of the sensory pain fibers from periphery to the cortex (where the pain is perceived by cortical brain cells), there are three distinct sensory stations (Fig. 5.1). Each sensory station contains nerve cells that receive sensory fibers from the periphery and project their own sensory fibers more centrally to the next station and toward the cortex. The first sensory station is located in the dorsal nerve root close to the spine and is called dorsal root ganglion or DRG (Fig. 5.1, lower right).

The cells of DRG have a T shaped structure with a peripheral and central sensory fiber (axon). The peripheral axon of DRG receives sensory information (including pain) from the nerve ending via the previously described phenomenon of transduction. The central axon of nerve cell in DRG, enters the spinal cord, and connects (synapse) with the second sensory neuron in the dorsal part of the spinal cord (Fig. 5.1). The axon of this spinal sensory neuron crosses the cord and travels in the opposite side up to the lower part of the brain (medulla and mid-brain) (Fig. 5.1) where it gives collateral branches to a network of cells (reticular formation), involved in pain modulation (colored blue in Fig. 5.1). Higher, deep in the brain the sensory information from spinal nerve cells arrives in the third sensory station, named thalamus (Fig. 5.1, upper section). The sensory cells of the thalamus are in direct contact with the sensory cells of the cortex. There are several chemical agents which are involved in pain transmission through to the central nervous system at spinal cord, thalamus and cortex levels. The tree best known of these agents are glutamate, Substance P and calcitonin gene-related peptide (CGRP).

Pain Modulation

Human cortex exerts some control over the incoming pain volleys to the cortex. This is done through a descending sensory system which originates from the cortex and makes multiple synapses (contacts) with the nerve cells scattered in the medulla and midbrain within a netlike structure called reticular formation (Fig. 5.1). These cells receive collateral connections from the ascending sensory fibers as they travel within medulla and mid-brain toward the cortex. This modulatory effect is probably a safety mechanism which protects the cortex from excessive stimulation. The chemicals believed to be involved in pain modulation are noradrenaline (a hormone) and serotonin.

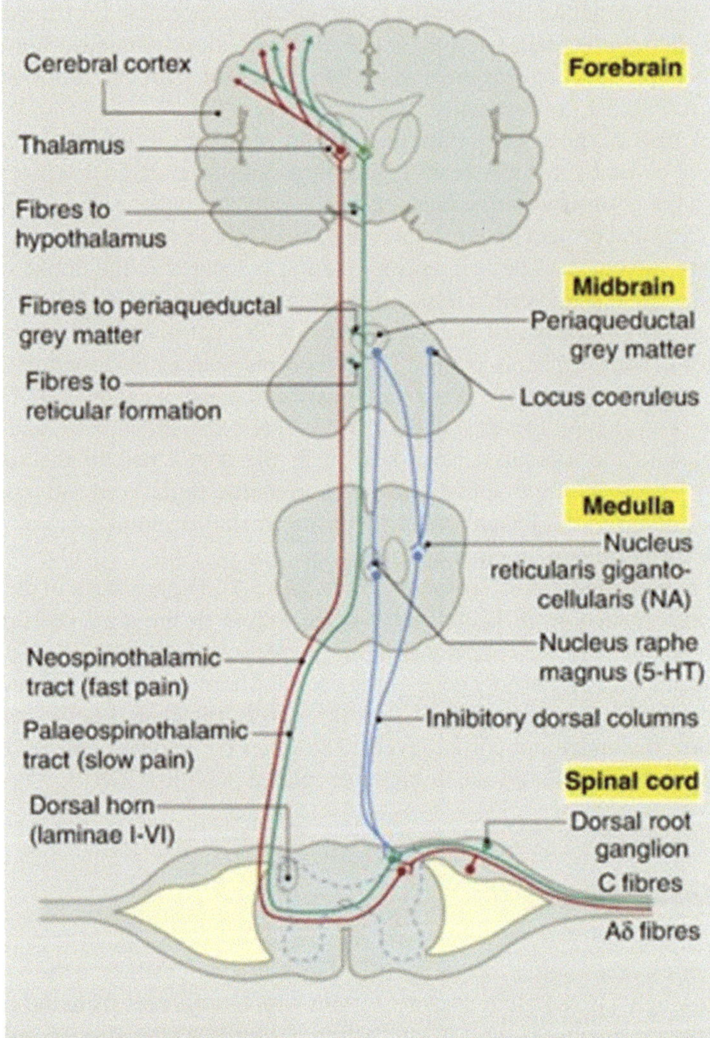

Fig. 5.1 Pain pathways. (From Steeds Anatomy and Physiology of Pain, Surgery (Oxford) 2016—Reprinted with permission from Elsevier)

Pain Perception

The pain signals which reach the thalamus from the periphery reach three areas of the cerebral cortex (a layer of cells that cover the brain) (Fig. 5.2): the somatosensory cortex which is located in the parietal lobe and localizes the physical sensations including pain, the limbic system consisting of a group of cells located in the medial aspect of the temporal and the frontal lobes dealing with the emotional aspect of

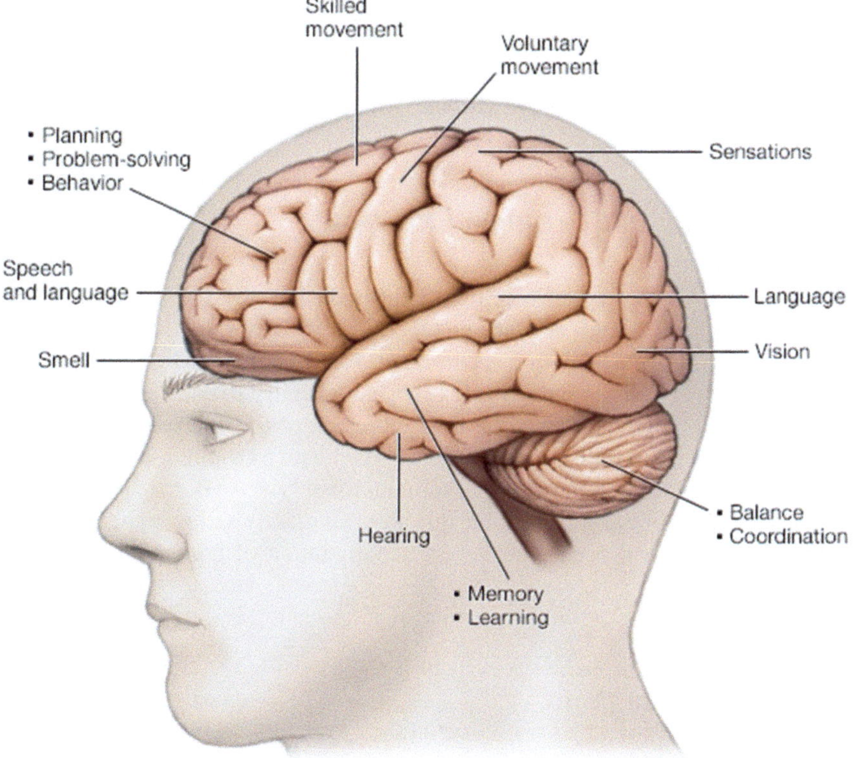

Fig. 5.2 Four lobes of the brain representing different functions. The lobe located in front of the head is the frontal lobe. Posterior to that is parietal lobe that deals with sensations including pain. The temporal lobe in in the temple region deals with memory and hearing among other functions

painful stimuli and the frontal cortex that processes meaning and cognition of nociception (pain). The perception of pain therefore, involves multiple cortical structures which combine sensation, emotion and conscious thought.

A Brief Review of Animal Studies of Botulinum Toxins in the Field of Pain

Over the past 30 years, a large number of animal studies have shown that injection of botulinum toxins to animals can inhibit secretion of pain transmitters and prevent or reduce the pain behavior. Although most of these studies have been performed with onabotulinumtoxinA (Botox), studies with other type A toxins and with the type B toxin are also forthcoming (see Chaps. 2 and 3 for definition of different botulinum toxins). These studies have demonstrated that botulinum toxins can affect pain transmission via their influence upon nerve endings, dorsal root ganglia (DRG) and spinal cord sensory neurons.

Nerve Endings and Peripheral Receptors

In formalin model of pain, injection of formalin into the rat's paw causes severe sharp pain which lasts for seconds and then a less severe pain that last longer, minutes to hours. The first peak of this pain is due to the acute irritation of nerve endings by formalin, whereas the second pain represents the irritating effect of local inflammation caused by formalin injection. Examination of the injected tissue (rat's paw) shows local accumulation of glutamate, a known pain transmitter and local presence of inflammatory cells. Injection of botulinum toxin type A (Botox) and type B toxin (Myobloc), 5 days before formalin injection, markedly reduces the inflammatory peak of pain (second peak) and lowers accumulation of glutamate at the injected tissue [6, 7].

Dorsal Root Ganglion

When cultured, nerves cells of dorsal root ganglia (DRG), the first sensory nerve cell (neurons) (Fig. 5.1, lower right) which receive pain signals from the periphery, secrets substance P, a pain transmitter. Adding Botox to this culture inhibits the release of substance P from DRG nerve cultures [8].

Spinal Cord Sensory Neurons

It has been shown, in animals, that after intramuscular injection, the receptor protein that receives Botox at nerve-muscle junction (SNAP 25, see Chap. 1 for more detailed description) travels to the spinal cord and influences the spinal sensory nerve cells (second sensory neurons which receive pain signals) [9]. Furthermore, injection of botulinum toxin B into the paw of the rat reduces release of substance P (a chemical pain transmitter) from the spinal neurons after formalin activation [7].

Several other studies, both in animals and in human, have shown that injection of botulinum toxin into muscle or skin can diminish induced pain sensation by influencing the pain transmitters at or above the spinal cord level [7, 10–15].

Human Pain Syndromes

Botulinum toxins have shown efficacy after intramuscular or subcutaneous (under the skin) injection in a variety of human pain syndromes. In this section, we will describe those pain syndromes in which research from high quality studies has provided compelling evidence for their efficacy.

Chronic Low Back Pain

Low back pain is defined as a pain that occurs between 12th rib (last and the lowest rib) and the end of the lumbar spine at the region of iliac crest. Epidemiological studies have demonstrated that 75–80% of all people suffer from low back pain sometime during their lifetime [16]. Chronic low back pain is defined as a low back pain that lasts more than 6 months. Between 2% and 7% of patients with acute low back pain develop chronic low back pain. Low back pain is a major burden to the US and European economy with a disability rate of 11–12% [17].

Low back pain has different causes and can arise from ailment of different structures in the low back area. Lumbar spine consists of five bones (vertebrae) each separated by a soft disc and wrapped by several layers of muscles and tendons which maintain its stability. The spinal cord which is located inside the spinal column ends just above the lumbar spine but nerve fibers that supply motor and sensory function of the legs emerge from the end of the spinal cord and travel to the legs after passing between the five lumbar vertebrae. These nerve roots after leaving lumbar column (vertebrae) join together and constitute the major nerve supply of the leg. For instance, sciatic nerve is made from nerve roots that come from fourth and fifth lumbar roots joining with the first three sacral roots (sacrum is part of the pelvis).

Structural damage to the lumbar bones (trauma, tumor, infection) or herniated discs can apply pressure to the nerve roots and cause low back pain. Congenital spinal stenosis (narrowing) can also cause low back pain at some point in life. Low back pain can also arise from tightness of the muscles that surround the lumbar column. Sometimes these muscles on examination, demonstrate areas sensitive to pressure which are termed trigger points (pressure upon them triggers pain). Unfortunately, in most patients with chronic low back pain radiological procedures such as CT scan or MRI do not disclose significant lesions (herniated disc or other abnormalities) amenable to surgical remedy. Non-specific findings such as bone degeneration are often found in the elderly's individual examinations.

Management of chronic low back pain is a major medical challenge. A recent review of this subject details pharmacological and non-pharmacological approaches for treatment of low back pain [18]. Non-pharmacological approaches include behavioural management, special exercises, massage, superficial heat, acupuncture, yoga, Tai chi, operant (psychological) therapy and chiropractic manipulation.

Pharmacological therapy starts with non-steroidal, anti-inflammatory drugs (aspirin, tylenol, others). The American College of Physicians' guidelines recommend duloxetine and tramadol as secondary line of treatment for chronic low back pain. When the pain is neuropathic (secondary to peripheral nerve or spinal cord damage, often with a burning quality) gabapentin is recommended. Opioids are effective, but due to their potential for addiction, should be kept as the last resort and used sparingly. Lumbar epidural steroid injection may provide temporary pain relief, but reinjections are often required. Radiofrequency sacroiliac joint stimulation and spinal cord stimulation may provide temporary relief as well. Surgery is indicated in a limited number of patients more often in patients with acute low back pain related to herniated disc. Failure after surgery is not uncommon. The term failed back syndrome is used for low back pain continuing after surgery.

Botulinum Toxin Treatment of Chronic Low Back Pain

Botulinum toxin treatment of chronic low back pain is based on the premise that intramuscular injection of botulinum toxin can relax the tense muscles by blocking the release of acetylcholine from nerve terminals at nerve-muscle junction. As described before, acetylcholine that is released from the end of peripheral nerves activates the muscle leading to muscle movement and muscle contraction. Furthermore, as described above, injection of botulinum toxin into the muscle or skin can diminish or abolish pain by reducing the function of pain transmitters and pain modulators. For these reasons, over the past 25 years, several investigators have explored the efficacy of botulinum toxin therapy in chronic low back pain. These studies were done with different toxins and under different protocols. Among different studies, two high quality studies (albeit including small number of patients), statistically produced significant improvement of chronic low back pain not amenable to surgery. This research was conducted first at the Walter Reed Army Medical Center at Washington DC and then was repeated, with the same design, at the Yale University in New haven, CT.

Walter Reed-Yale Protocol

This protocol is based on the premise that in chronic low back pain not amenable to surgery tightness of extensor back muscles (also called erector spinae-ES, Fig. 5.3) plays a pivotal role in chronicity of pain. Increased tone of these muscles can be seen in recording of these muscles electrical activity at rest by electromyography and even sometimes, by palpation during clinical examination. Extension of the spine results from the function a powerful muscle in the lumbar region called erector spinae (ES). Erector spinae is made from three long muscles that originate from the base of the neck and after traveling through the upper back join together at level of the upper lumbar region. The lower end of ES attaches to the pelvic bone (Fig. 5.3). This single bulk of the three joined muscles (ES), extends and straightens the spine. The Walter Reed-Yale protocol calls for five injections into the ES, one at

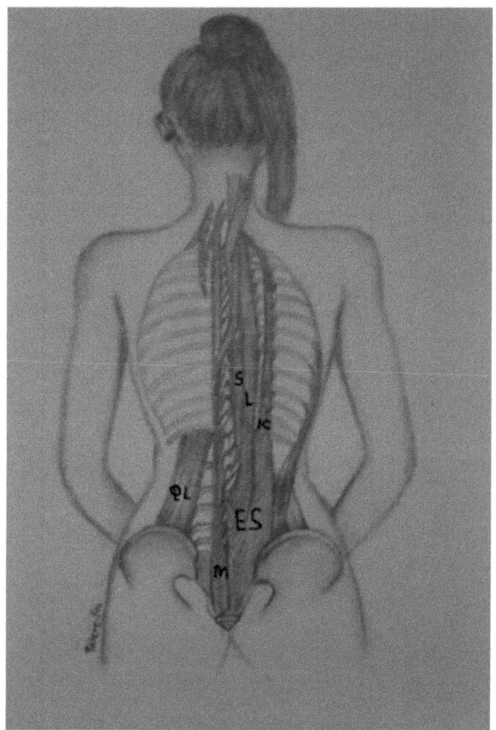

Fig. 5.3 Major muscles of low back: superficial layer (ES-shown on the right); deep layer; quadratus lumborum (QL) and multifidus (M) shown on the left. The spinalis (marked S), longisimus (marked L) and iliocostalis (IC) join at T12-L1 level to form a single mass, the erector spinae (ES) at the lumbar region. (Drawing, courtesy of Tahere Mousavi. M.D.)

each lumbar level (L1 to L5). The injections are carried under the guidance of electromyography (EMG), a technique that monitors the electrical activity of the muscle. The injections are performed with a special thin and hollow needle connected to EMG unit and the syringe that contains the botulinum toxin. Patients are instructed to extend their backs. If needle is inserted properly in the extensor muscle, the noise of the muscle activity on EMG ascertains its proper placement into the extensor muscle and the botulinum toxin is then injected through the same needle into the muscle.

Using this technique, Jabbari and co-workers have investigated the effect of botulinum toxin injection into ES muscles via two double-blind, placebo-controlled studies in patients with chronic low back pain [19, 20]. All patients had failed treatment with three or more medications for low back pain previously and had low back pain for more than 6 months. None had surgery and their CT or MRI showed no significant lesion(s) requiring surgery. The first study was conducted with Botox on 27 patients at Walter Reed Army Medical Center in Washington DC [19]. The second study was performed 10 years later at Yale University, using an identical protocol and technique on 33 patients [20]. The toxin used for the second study was Dysport, another type A toxin similar to Botox (for definition of toxin types see Chap. 3). Each unit of Botox equals approximately 2.5–3 units of Dysport. The first study was on patients with unilateral, or predominantly unilateral, low back pain. Patients received 40 units of Botox into the ES muscle at each of the 5 lumbar levels (total of 200 units). In the second study (Yale study), some patients had unilateral, whereas others had bilateral low back pain. They received 100 units of Dysport (approximately 40 units of Botox) into ES at each lumbar level. In unilateral low back pain, the total dose of Dysport was 500 and in bilateral low back pain it was 1000 units.

The results of the two studies were almost identical. Significant pain relief was reported by 52% and 54% of the patients who received botulinum toxin, respectively. Majority of the patients in the toxin groups (but not in the placebo group) also reported improvement of their quality of life. Patients who were injected with botulinum toxin did not experience any significant side effects (weakness of the back or legs) in either of the two studies. A few patients (5%) developed a transient, mild flu like syndrome lasting a few days which is expected to happen in small percentage of patients after botulinum toxin therapy. In an open label study (not blinded), Jabbari and his colleagues treated 75 patients suffering from chronic low back pain with the same protocol over 14 months. Patients received botulinum toxin injections for low back pain every 3–4 months. Again, over 50% of patients reported significant pain relief. The positive effect of treatment was sustained over 14 months [21]. In a smaller study using Dysport and Walter Reed-Yale technique, authors reported that 76% of patients who received Dysport reported significant pain relief after 3 weeks versus 20% of those who received placebo [22]. Another study with follow up of 6 months also found injection of botulinum toxin in low back muscles was beneficial to the patients for management of low back pain with a low incidence of side effects (two patients reported mild pain at the site of injection) [23].

Other investigators who have not used Walter Reed-Yale Technique and used lower doses of Botox did not report significant improvement of low back pain [24]. Likewise injection of deeper muscles of the back (quadratus lumborum and iliopsoas—see Fig. 5.3) with Botox failed to improve low back pain [25].

Patient Observation

A 65 year-old man who had experienced low back pain for several years was referred to Yale Botulinum Toxin Clinic for evaluation. There was no history of back injury or surgical intervention. The pain affected the low back in the mid-lumbar region with no radiation to the lower limbs. A magnetic resonance imaging of the back showed diffuse degenerative spine disease but no acute pathology. Treatment with a large number of painkillers had not been helpful. The patient's examination was normal except for slightly increased muscle tone in the low back area. Since the pain was predominantly on the right side, the patient was injected on the right side only (Fig. 5.4). The injection was into the extensors of the spine (erector spinae muscle) and performed at five lumbar levels. The dose of Botox was 40 units per injection site for a total of 200 units. After a week, patient reported significant improvement of his low back pain. Over a 3 year period of follow up, he received Botox injections every 3–4 months and each time reported satisfaction with the therapy. He experienced no side effects.

Fig. 5.4 The site of lumbar injections into ES (erector Spinae-extensor of spine). (Drawing courtesy of Dr. Damoun Safarpour)

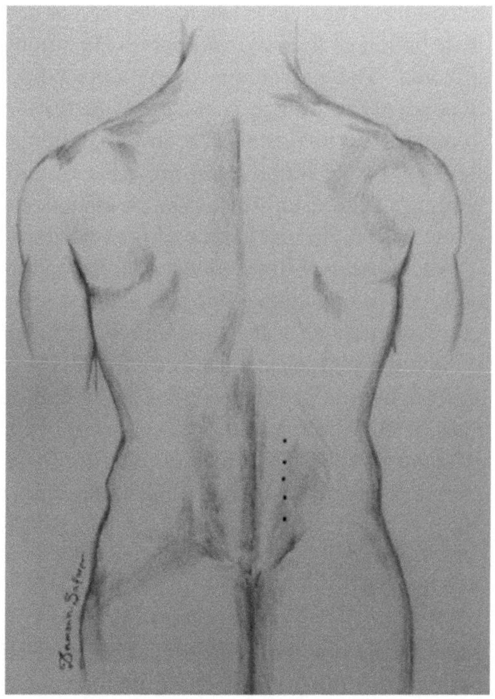

At present, using the criteria of the Guidance Development Subcommittee of the American Academy of Neurology [26, 27] the efficacy for botulinum toxin therapy is at level B (probably effective) based on two class II studies (high quality studies with small size of cohorts). Based on these data, botulinum toxin therapy should be considered for patients with chronic low back pain who are not candidates for surgery and have repeatedly failed medications. It has to be done however by injectors with considerable knowledge of back anatomy and botulinum toxin injection technique. It is currently not a FDA approved indication.

Pain After Shingles (Post-Herpetic Neuralgia (PHN))

Shingles (Herpes Zoster) results from reactivation of childhood chicken pox virus in the later years of life. The disease starts with eruption of small vesicles over the skin with a typical distribution pattern along the course of the nerve routes or peripheral nerves. Back, chest and limbs are commonly involved but, in some cases, eruptions occur on the face. In the early stage, when vesicles have erupted on the skin, itch is the most disturbing complaint. After a few weeks, the vesicles dry up and leave scars and cause skin discoloration. Some patients with shingles may develop pain either during the acute phase or more often after skin lesions heal (post-herpetic neuralgia). The pain is often described as severe, sharp and jabbing and is felt in the distribution of the involved nerves. In some patients, large parts of the body can be affected. The percentage of patients who develop pain after shingles is highly dependent on the age at the onset of their symptoms; it is 5% among individuals younger than 60% and 20% among patients who are 80 years of age or older [28]. Severity of the initial pain, presence of another type of neuropathy at the time of shingle's skin lesions and slow clearance of shingle's virus from the saliva also correlate with higher incidence of post-herpetic neuralgia (PHN) [29–31].

Vaccination with the newer vaccine against shingles (Shingrix) is more than 90% effective in preventing shingles and reducing the incidence of post-herpetic neuralgia. Treatment with steroids can reduce the pain during the acute phase, but does not reduce the incidence of developing PHN [32]. Early antiviral therapy (treatment against shingle's virus) reduces the risk of developing neuralgia after shingles [33]. Pain of shingles may last for months or even years and can severely incapacitate the affected patient. Therefore employing a treatment approach with low side effect profile is desirable in order to properly manage the post-herpetic neuralgia.

Treatment

Medical treatment of pain after shingles (PHN) consists mainly of administration of painkillers (analgesics). These include the commonly used over the counter drugs such as aspirin or acetaminophen or the types of painkillers that specifically promote pain inhibition in the central nervous system by enhancing the effects of the powerful inhibitory neurotransmitter GABA (Gaba aminobutyric acid), abundantly present at the junction of nerve cells (synapse). The major drugs in this category are carbamazepine (Tegretol), pregabalin (Lyrica) and baclofen (Liorisal). In more severe cases, a course of steroid therapy with prednisone may reduce the pain intensity. Inducing nerve block by injection of anaesthetic medications such as lidocaine into the sensitive skin regions, electrical stimulation of skin nerves or even spinal cord electrical stimulation has been employed for management of recalcitrant pain after shingles. Unfortunately, despite these medical measures, a sizeable proportion of patients with shingles, continue to experience disabling pain and live with impaired (often severely) quality of life. In some cases of shingles, poor response to pain treatment may be a reflection of extension of shingle lesions beyond the nerve roots and peripheral nerves. It has been shown that, not infrequently, the shingle's virus can travel from the peripheral nerves centrally and through the nerve roots into the spinal cord. In many such cases, examination of the cerebrospinal fluid demonstrates presence of the inflammatory cells indicating spread of the inflammation to the central nervous system.

Botulinum Toxin Therapy in PHN

Animal studies and studies of human volunteers have shown that injection of botulinum toxins into or under the skin alleviates experimentally induced pain [34, 35]. This pain relieving effect of the BoNTs is attributed to the inhibitory effect of the toxin upon pain transmitters such as glutamate, substance p and Calcitonin Gene-related peptide (CGRP) [36, 37].

Several studies have reported the efficacy of botulinum toxin treatment in PHN. Among them are two high quality, double-blind, placebo-controlled, class I investigations (see definition of study classes in Chap. 3) that have demonstrated substantial improvement of pain in a high percentage of patients after injection of botulinum toxin injection under skin at painful areas [38, 39]. One study used Botox and the other a Chinese Botulinum toxin A (Prosigne) similar to Botox. In each patient, 12–20 sites were injected. Botulinum toxin therapy also improved patients' sleep in patients with PDN. The patients in the toxin group also used less opioids for pain control. This experience is shared by several other investigators who found similar results in the open label (not blinded) observations [40, 41]. In a recent study, investigators found that injection of botulinum toxin into the skin relieved pain both during the active phase of the infection and after infection (PHN), but it was more effective in the latter (PHN) [42]. Another study, through meta-analysis (a sophisticated statistical method), compared the effectiveness of botulinum toxin therapy injection with lidocaine injection in a group of patients with PHN. Investigators of this study, reviewed data from 7 high quality reported studies on this subject comprising 742 patients. They found that the efficacy rate (analgesic effect) was significantly higher in the group that had received botulinum toxin injections. There was no difference between the two groups regarding adverse effects [43].

The injections are given through a short (¾ in.), thin (gauge 30) needle. Since injections are uncomfortable due to skin sensitivity, an anaesthetic cream (Emla) may be applied an hour before the injections. The skin may be further numbed by an anaesthetic spray during the injections. The Botox dose per injection site is small, 2.5–5 units, for a total dose of 20–200 units depending on the extent of skin involvement. The pain relieving effect of Botox appears in 3–5 days and can last for 3 or more months. If shingles involves the face, the dose and number of injections need to be limited to a minimum in order to avoid facial weakness. This is, however, an uncommon side effect since the dose per site is small usually 2–2.5 units and injections are superficial. The facial weakness, if it develops, is mild and usually disappears within 2–3 months.

Sample Case

A 62-year-old female presented with severe pain behind the left ear of nearly 2 years duration. Two years ago, she had developed shingles which was characterized by skin lesions in the back of the head and behind the left ear. The affected area was painful and the pain was intensified by the passage of time. She described the pain as jabbing and stabbing, resulting in loss of sleep, causing marked apprehension in anticipation of the next bout. Some episodes were described as "torture and unbearable." Treatment with a medication against herpes virus (acyclovir) improved the skin lesions but did not alter the pain. More severe bouts of pain were followed by disabling headaches. Painkillers such as gabapentin, pregabalin and oxycodone (narcotic) offered little help.

The patient was referred to Yale University Botulinum Toxin Clinic where her examination showed residual scars of zoster infection behind her left ear. The skin in this area was sensitive to touch. A total of 48 units of Botox was injected in a grid-like pattern under the skin, behind the left ear, at 16 points (3 units/point), using a thin 30-gauge needle (Fig. 5.5). The Botox dilution was 100 units per 2 cc of saline. Patient reported a sharp drop in pain frequency and intensity 5 days after the injections. The pain then completely disappeared at week 2 post-injection, but gradually returned at 2.5 months post-injection. Over the next 2 years following the first treatment, patient received Botox injections every 3–4 months. During the third year, pain relief after Botox injections lasted 6 months. In her last follow up (4 years after the first treatment), she had no pain for 9 months and the returned pain was described as subtle and insignificant. She was very pleased with the outcome.

Trigeminal Neuralgia (TN)

This term applies to facial pain that is felt in the distribution of trigeminal nerve. The trigeminal nerve, the fifth cranial nerve (one of 12 cranial nerves that supply the eyes, tongue, throat, head and face), is a pure sensory nerve. It supplies sensation of

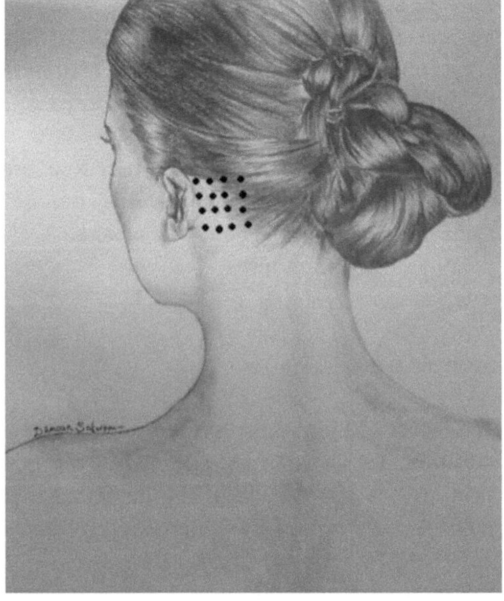

Fig. 5.5 Site of Botox injections for the above described patient with post-herpetic neuralgia. (Drawing, courtesy of Damoun Safarpour M.D.)

the upper, middle and lower face regions. Face pain in TN is sharp, jabbing and short lasting often occurring several times during the day and unnerves the patient. It is usually felt on one side of the face sparing the forehead. In some cases, pain radiates to the gums and inside the mouth.

Trigeminal neuralgia is usually a problem of middle or old age and rarely affects young people. The age of onset in most patients is between 50 and 60 years. It has a prevalence of 4/100,000 in the US [44]. If a young person develops TN, multiple sclerosis or a tumor at the base of the brain (brain stem) should to be suspected. Among older individuals, the cause of TN in some patients is compression of a small blood vessel against the trigeminal nerve deep in the brain, Treatment is medical or, in some cases surgical. Medical treatment includes medications which are commonly used for treatment of epilepsy that slow down sensory nerve conduction and have analgesic effect. The commonly used such drugs are phenytoin, carbamazepine (tegretol), gabapentin (neurontin), pregabaline, levitracetam and lamotrigine. Although partially effective, side effects are not uncommon (dizziness, nausea, confusion) leading to unsuccessful longterm use.

The most popular surgery for TN is called microvascular surgery. In this procedure the surgeon opens the back of the skull and separates nerve from the culprit blood vessel that pressing against it. It is effective, but the pain can recur after several years. Furthermore, the surgical procedure is a major task with potential serious side effects such as loss of hearing and balance. Radiofrequency stimulation and Gamma knife surgery are also performed with some degree of success in patients with TN. Peripheral nerve electrical stimulation, deep brain stimulation and transcranial magnetic stimulation are under investigation. In a few patients, focused ultrasound relieved the pain by causing microlesions deep in the specific sensory part of the brain [45].

Botulinum Toxin Treatment

Two high quality class I (see definition in Chap. 3), double-blind, placebo-controlled studies have demonstrated the efficacy of botulinum toxin therapy in management of trigeminal neuralgia [46, 47]. Both investigations used a Chinese botulinum toxin type A similar to Botox (Prosigne). Prosigne's units are believed to approximate Botox's units. The investigators in both studies injected the involved skin of the face in a grid-like pattern at 12–16 sites. Injections not only improved pain but also significantly improved the patients' quality of life. One of these two studies [47] compared the results of low dose (25 units) with high dose (75 units) of Prosigne for pain relief in TN. The authors concluded that 25 units is as effective as 75 units for pain relief and suggested using the low dose of 25 units in order to avoid facial weakness. The author of this chapter has injected 8 patients suffering from TN with Botox using a method similar to that described above. Five of the eight patients experienced a satisfactory response.

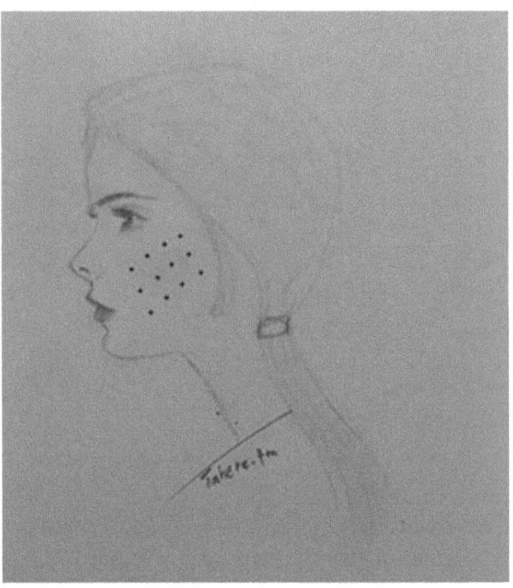

Fig. 5.6 The sites of Botox injections in author's patient with trigeminal neuralgia. (Drawing, courtesy of Tahereh Mousavi, M.D.)

Sample Case

A 41-year old female complained of severe, intermittent jabbing pain in the left face for 9 months. The pain involved mainly the middle of the face, but often radiated to the left ear. It lasted 5–30 s, but recurred frequently, sometimes 5–10 times/day. Treatment with different painkillers offered no relief. Patient stated the sharp pain often depresses her as there seems to be no remedy for it. Injection of Botox into the left side of her face at 12 points (2 units per point- Fig. 5.6) resulted in marked reduction of pain frequency (from 3 to 4/day to 1 to 2/month). The recurring pain was considerably lighter in intensity compared to its predecessors. Repeated injections every 4 months had the same effect.

Diabetic Neuropathy(DN)

Neuropathy means a diseased peripheral nerve. Diabetes can damage peripheral nerves and cause diabetic neuropathy. Diabetic neuropathy affects 25–26% of individuals with type 2 (late onset) and 16% of individuals with type 1 (early onset) diabetes [48]. Patients with DN complain of pain, numbness and, in advanced cases, weakness in the feet or hands. These symptoms are more prominent in the lower limbs. The skin in the affected areas is sensitive to touch (hyperesthesia) and sometimes touch evokes pain (allodynia). Pain may develop spontaneously and interfere with patients' rest and sleep. The pain of diabetic neuropathy has the characteristic of a neuropathic pain. Neuropathic pain is sharp and burning and is often associated with allodynia (skin sensitivity to touch). Areas most commonly affected in diabetic neuropathy are top of the foot and toes. Painful diabetic neuropathy (PDN) affects 20–24% of the patients with diabetes [49].

On examination, the patients often demonstrate decreased sensations to heat, cold, touch and position in the affected limbs. Diabetic neuropathy is usually bilateral and involves both sides. The symptoms are more severe in the distal parts of the lower limbs, feet and toes. There may be discoloration of the skin overlying the affected areas.

Treatment of diabetic neuropathy consists of avoiding sugar, lowering blood sugar levels with medications and treating pain when present. Mild cases of painful neuropathy can be managed by over the counter pain killers, whereas more severe cases require prescribed medications with recognized efficacy in neuropathic pain syndromes. Gabapentinoids (gabapentin, pregabalin), tricyclic antidepressants (amitriptyline), as well as serotonin and norepinephrine reuptake inhibitors (SNRIs) (duloxetine, venlafaxine) are generally accepted as the first line of drugs for PDN [50]. Canadian guidelines (Diabetes Canada-DC) recommends pregabalin to be used before other agents [51]. Sodium channel blockers, such as carbamazepine, oxcarbazepine, lamotrigine, and lacosamide are also recommended by AAN as additional first line drugs [52]. Unfortunately, despite availability of the above-mentioned drugs for neuropathic pain, recalcitrant pain in DPN is not uncommon and when present, impairs the patients' quality of life significantly.

Botulinum Toxin Therapy for PDN

Efficacy of botulinum toxins against pain in PDN has been investigated in four double-blind, placebo-controlled studies [53–56]. Injections were performed with a thin and short needle (less than 1 in. in length, gauge 27.5 or 30) in a gride-like pattern covering the dorsum (top) of the foot (Fig. 5.7). The number of injected sites varied from 12 to 15 in different studies. Some studies used Botox, whereas others used Dysport. Dysport is another type A botulinum toxin similar to Botox. However, the unit strength of the two toxins is different. As described earlier, each unit of Botox approximates 2.5–3 units of Dysport. The dose per injection site was small, 2.5–5 units for Botox. In one study, toxin therapy not only improved pain but also improved the patients' sleep and quality of life [55]. In another recent study [57], injection of 30–100 units of Botulinum toxin A into calf muscles or flexors of the toes significantly improved muscle cramps in PDN, an effect that persisted for 20 weeks with repeated injections (every 3–4 months).

Plantar Fasciitis

Plantar fasciitis is related to damage to the plantar fascia (PF) from repeated trauma. Repeated trauma (running, certain sports and jobs) can cause micro-tears in the plantar fascia with concurrent inflammation. Plantar fascia is a superficially located

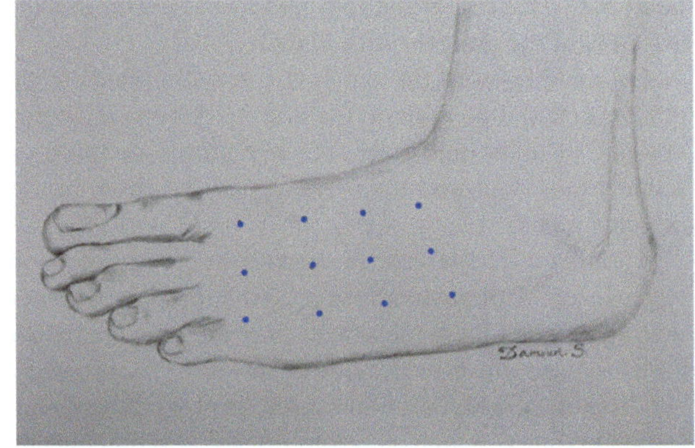

Fig. 5.7 Technique of skin injection for painful peripheral neuropathy in diabetic patients (Yuan and coworkers) [53]. Injections were performed on both feet. (Drawing, courtesy of Damoun Safarpour, M.D.)

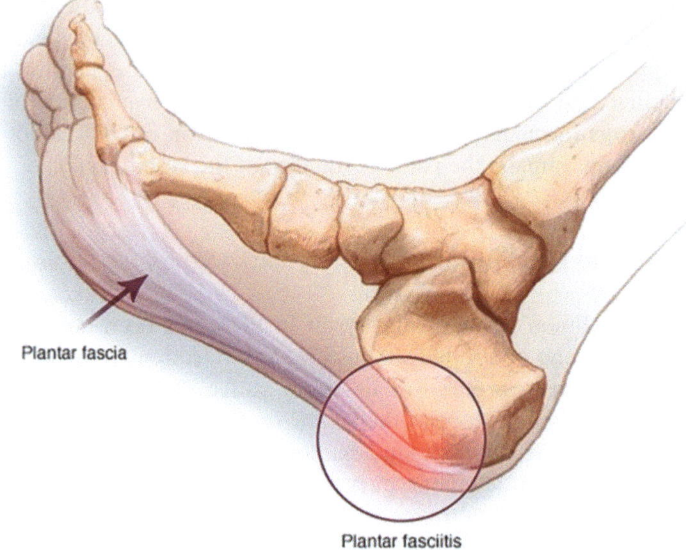

Fig. 5.8 Planter fascia and the area of pain (in red) in plantar fasciitis. (Courtesy of Mayo Foundation)

layer of fibrous tissue (just under the skin of the sole of the foot) that connects the medial part of the heel to the base of the toes (Fig. 5.8). It is thickest, close to its origin at the heel and it thins out as it approaches the toes. When it gets close to the toes, plantar fascia divides into five segments each connecting to the base of one toe. Under the PF, are located three muscles that flex the toes, one for three middle toes, one for the big toe and one for the small toe.

Damaged plantar fascia causes pain that is felt most often in the heel(s), but also sometimes at the bottom of the feet. Pain can be felt during exertion or after a period of rest. It can be severe, impair the quality of life and interfere with sleep. In many patients, stopping the culprit activity (running, long distance walking, heavy lifting) improves the condition and the pain gradually subsides. Other patients with plantar fasciitis, however, may continue experiencing pain despite stopping the responsible activity or a job that requires continuing heavy foot works such as football or running. Plantar fasciitis affects 10% of all runners and over two million people in the US [58].

Treatment of PF starts with simple measures such as stretching, taping, night splints, orthosis, non-steroidal, anti-inflammatory medications. In more persistent cases, steroid injections, ultrasound therapy, application of shock waves, acupuncture and cryosurgery (with freezing probes) are used. Unfortunately, the positive effect of these measures is often short lived. Furthermore, some of these therapeutic approaches are painful and hard to tolerate (i.e. shock wave therapy), while injection of steroids may cause rupture of the plantar fascia and make the situation more complicated. Clearly, an effective and safe treatment approach with less side effects is desirable for management of severe forms of PF.

Botox Treatment of Plantar Fasciitis (PF)

In 2005, author of this chapter and his colleagues conducted and published the results of the first prospective, placebo-controlled, double-blinded investigation on the efficacy of Botox in plantar fasciitis at the Walter Reed Army Medical Center (WRAMC) in Washington D.C. [59]. Twenty-seven patients with plantar fasciitis and chronic symptoms (lasting >6 months) completed the study. Study subjects received either Botox (70 units) or placebo (saline), 0.7 cc into two sites: (1) medial part of the heal(s), origin of plantar fascia 40 units of Botox or 0.4 cc of saline (2) into the bottom of the foot, at mid-point, between the heal and base of the toes (if Botox 30 units, if saline 0.3 cc) (Fig. 5.9).

Efficacy of the treatment was measured at 3 and 8 weeks following injections. The group that received Botox injections improved in several measures compared to the placebo: Maryland Foot Score ($P = 0.001$), Pain Relief measured by Visual Analog Scale, on the scale of 0–10 ($P < 0.0005$), and the Pressure Algometry Response ($P = 0.003$); in clinical research; P scores of less than 0.05 are considered statistically significant. No side effects were noted. Later, our group found through experience that adding an additional injection into the soleus muscle which is often tight in plantar fasciitis leads to more alleviation of pain (Fig. 5.10).

In 2010, Huang and co-workers [60], using a similar technique and a total dose of 50 units (Botox), reported very similar results in a blinded study of 50 patients with plantar fasciitis. Díaz-Llopis and coworkers [61] compared the efficacy of Botox injection in plantar fasciitis with a combined steroid (betamethasone) and lidocaine injection in plantar fasciitis. One month after injections, both groups described pain relief which was more notable among patients who had received Botox. At 6 months post-treatment, patients who had received Botox were still satisfied with the level of pain relief, whereas patients who had received steroids

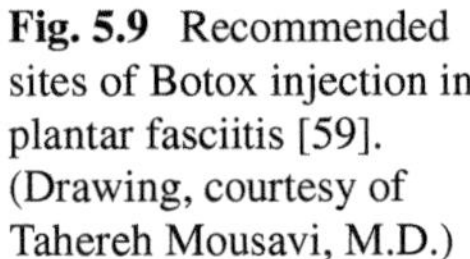

Fig. 5.9 Recommended
sites of Botox injection in
plantar fasciitis [59].
(Drawing, courtesy of
Tahereh Mousavi, M.D.)

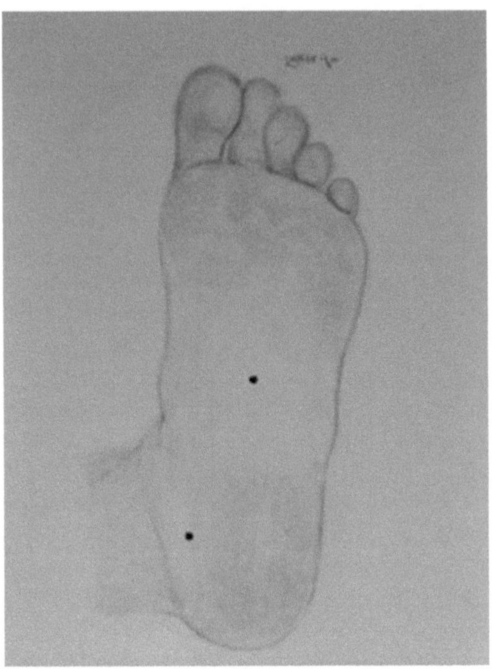

experienced recurrent pain. Similar result regarding superiority of Botox to steroid was noted in another comparative study where, in addition to heal injection authors also injected into the soleus muscle [62]. In 2017, improvement of pain and foot function was reported in patients with PF following Xeomin (another type of botulinum toxin A similar to Botox) injections into the painful sites of the foot [63]. The units of the Botox and Xeomin have approximately the same strength. In a more recent study [64], investigators compared the result of Botox injection with injection of an steroid (dexamethasone) or an anesthetic (lidocain) in patients with plantar fasciitis. Six months after injection, all three treatments improved pain in planter fasciitis and there was no significant difference between the three. This study did not include additional soleus injection. Considering the results of the studies cited above, botulinum toxin A (Botox or Xeomin) injections can relieve pain in plantar fasciitis and this treatment seems to be more effective than steroid injections if injection of the soleus muscle is included among the injection sites. Botox treatment seems to be safer and has less side effects than steroid therapy.

Sample Case

A 73 year-old man had noted discomfort at the bottom of his feet, 7–8 years prior to a visit to the Yale Botulinum Toxin Treatment clinic. He was an avid tennis player who felt the most foot discomfort on the days that he played longer games. The

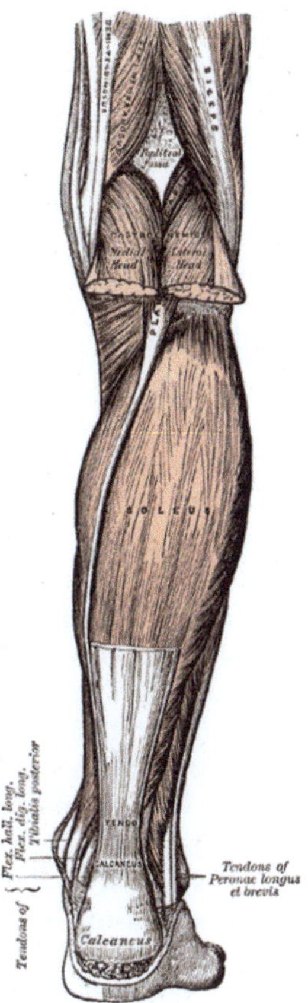

Fig. 5.10 Soleus muscle can be injected on the back of the calf. The injector should avoid injecting Achilles tendon (colored white below soleus) which easily ruptures. (Figure from Gray's anatomy provided by Wikimedia under Creative Commons Attribution-Share Alike 4.0 license)

discomfort gradually changed to pain which was felt at the heels and around the medial part of both feet. Over the years, he had tried a variety of treatments including stretching, orthosis, night splints, non-steroidal anti-inflammatory drugs, sessions of acupuncture and steroid injections. The latter two had helped some, but the results were short lived. He stated having more "bad" days recently during which the heel pain was severe and quite uncomfortable.

His neurological examination was normal. Botox was injected into both feet using the methodology described above. A total of 70 units was injected −40 units close to the heel and 30 units at the bottom of the foot (Fig. 5.9). Within days, the patient reported significant improvement of his heel pain; the pain relief lasted for 7 months. The second treatment also produced pain relief for 7–8 months. For the third and fourth treatments, an additional 30 units of Botox was injected into the soleus muscle which is located at the back of the lower leg and flexes the foot down via its attachment to Achilles tendon (10). It is often found to show increased tone in patients with PF. The third and fourth injections provided longer pain reliefs (9–10 months). Patient reported no side effects.

Pain After Trauma to the Peripheral Nerves (Post-traumatic Neuralgia)

Trauma to the peripheral nerves can cause sustained pain in the distribution of the injured nerves that sometimes, due to the intensity of pain, incapacitates the patient.

Case Report

A 56-year-old woman was referred to the Yale Botulinum Toxin Treatment Clinic for evaluation of severe post-traumatic neuralgia and to be considered for BoNT treatment. Twelve years earlier, her car was forcefully rear-ended when she braked hard in order to avoid hitting a car in front of her. The accident heavily bruised her right ankle and the lateral aspect of her right foot. The foot and ankle continued to ache and an area of intense allodynia (touch perceived as pain) developed over the lateral malleolus (bone at the ankle) extending up to the lower leg. A large number of medications failed to improve either the pain or the local allodynia. The most recent medications included gabapentin, pregabalin, tramadol, capsaicin ointment and coltran gel. In patient's own words: "The physical, emotional and psychological impact of my chronic pain defies description. Everynight, I have to take tylenol, advil, ambien, apply ankle soak, topical pain cream and heat wrap in order to be able to sleep. With all this, many nights I am unable to sleep due to persistent pain. Even the pressure of sheets, would cause the pain to flare up—sleeping on my side is impossible."

On examination, muscle strength was normal, but foot movements were slow and intensified the ankle pain. A large area of allodynia (tough causing pain) and hyperesthesia was present including the lateral aspect of the right foot extending 10 cm above the right ankle. The most intense allodynic region was over the lateral malleolus extending to 5 cm above the ankle (Fig. 5.11).

OnabotulinumtoxinA (ona-A) was injected subcutaneously into the dorsolateral aspect of the right foot (50 units; 20 sites—grid pattern) including the region of lateral malleolus. Patient reported 30% reduction of pain (VAS score went down to 7 from 10) a week after the first injection and 90% decrease after the second injection, 3 months later (VAS score went down to 1–2) 6 months later. Patient state that the effect after the second injection was astounding. "I stopped taking gabapentin and using pain wrap at night. I can now wear high heal shoes and clothes that rub against my ankle. I am looking forward to wearing boots for the first time in 12 years." An examination 3 months after the second injection showed marked reduction of allodynia which was now much less intense and limited to only a small area above the lateral malleolus.

Based on anecdotal observations such as the patient described above, and the animal studies that illustrated the analgesic effect of botulinum toxins in animal models [6–15], investigators began to assess the efficacy of botulinum toxin

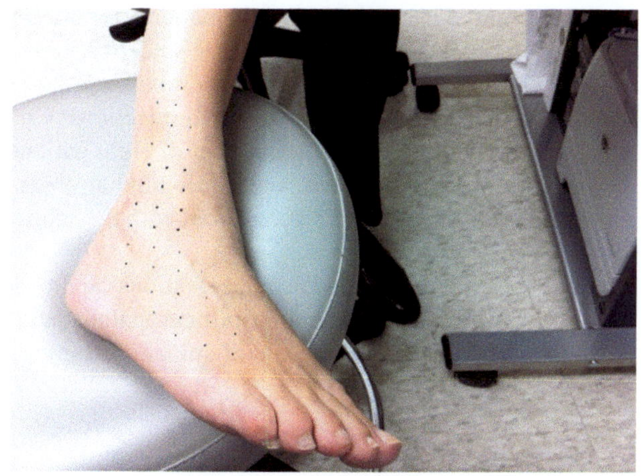

Fig. 5.11 Site of Botox injections for post-traumatic neuralgia. Darker dots illustrates areas of more intense pain. (From author's personal collection)

injections in human post-traumatic painful neuropathies through high quality studies. In 2008, Dr Ranoux and co-workers from France [65] studied 25 patients using a double-blind, placebo-controlled protocol. Patients had both surgical and non-surgical trauma to a single peripheral nerve. Botox injection were performed into the skin with a small needle over the area of pain at 20 points, 1 cm apart. The total dose per session ranged from 20 to 190 units based on the extent of the painful areas. The pain intensity started to decrease from 2 weeks post-injection in favor of Botox (versus saline/placebo) and the improvement lasted until week 14 (P = 0.03). No patient reported any side effects except seconds of pain at the time of injection. In 2017, the same group [66] looked at efficacy of repeated Botox injections in 64 patients (34 in BoNT group, 32 in saline group) with neuropathic pain at three research centers. Patients had two injections, 12 weeks apart. The method of injections was the same as that of the first study. The patient's response was evaluated at 4, 6, 12, 16 and 24 weeks after the first injection. Compared to placebo, self-reported pain intensity was significantly decreased after week 1 following after Botox injection and remained significantly decreased in each of the subsequent weeks through the duration of the study. The results of these two studies strongly support the usefulness of Botox injections into the skin in patients suffering from severe pain after trauma to the peripheral nerves.

Neuropathic Pain Secondary to Spinal Cord Injury

Han and coworkers [67] investigated the effect of BoNT injection in 40 patients who suffered from chronic neuropathic pain following spinal cord injury. The study was double-blind and placebo-controlled assessing the effect of 200 units of a South Korean type A botulinum toxin (Meditoxin, South Korea). The toxin was delivered in a checkerboard pattern under the skin at the region of pain. At 4 and 8 weeks post-injection, 55% and 45% of the patients reported pain relief of 20% or greater in the toxin injected group versus 15% and 10% in the placebo group. The quality of life was also improved more in the toxin injected group. No motor or sensory deficit was noted after botulinum toxin injections. Chun and colleagues [68] replicated these results in a smaller number of eight patients with local pain after spinal cord injury at lower thoracic and upper lumbar areas. In their study, Botox injections under the skin were also compared with the saline injections. The total injected dose of Botox was 200 units.

The above mentioned human observations on the analgesic effect of BoNT therapy for post-traumatic neuralgia in neuropathic pain after spinal cord injury are supported also in animal models of spinal cord injury with post-traumatic neuralgia [69].

Piriformis Syndrome (PS)

Piriformis syndrome is a clinical condition characterized by deep pain in the buttock related to tightness of piriformis muscle which is located deep in the buttock under gluteal muscles (large buttock muscles). Tightness of the triangular piriformis muscle can cause pain deep in the buttock due to its proximity to the roots of the sciatic nerve. The pain of piriformis muscle can be confused sometimes with low back pain due to a dislocated disc in the spinal column or with sciatica that results from irritation of the sciatic nerve itself in the thigh.

Diagnosis of piriformis syndrome is often difficult due to complexity of the involved anatomy. In mild cases, treatment with non-steroidal analgesics is helpful. For recalcitrant pain more aggressive treatment is required.

Botox injection into piriformis muscle has been shown to improve pain resulting from the piriformis syndrome. The largest placebo-controlled, blinded study was conducted by Fishman and co-workers who compared the results of Botox, lidocaine and placebo injections into the piriformis muscle of patients affected by PS. After injections, pain relief was noted in 67%, 32% and 6% of the three groups, respectively [70]. The technique of injection is laborious and needs to be performed under electromyographic guidance to ensure proper insertion of the injecting needle. Electromyography records the electrical activity of the muscle and, in case of piriformis syndrome, often demonstrates abnormal increased activity of this muscle at rest. For injection, a special hollow needle is used that both records the muscle activity and allows injection of botulinum toxin through its core. Unlike for most indications of botulinum toxin therapy that utilize a short needle (¾ to 1 in.), a long needle, 4.5–5 in., is needed for injections in PS in order to reach the deeply located piriformis muscle (Fig. 5.12). For Botox, usually a dose of 100 units is delivered in a single injection.

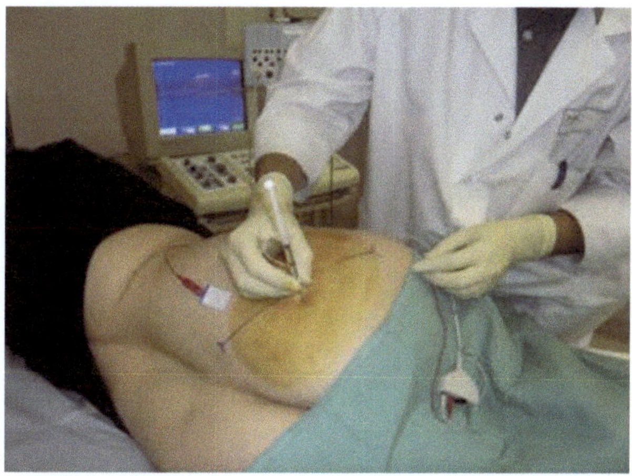

Fig. 5.12 Technique of botulinum toxin injection into the piriformis muscle. (Michel and co-workers 2013 [71]—Reproduced under https://creativecommons.org/licences/by/4.0. Courtesy of publisher Elsevier Masson SAS [71])

In a recent double -blind, placebo-controlled study of 84 patients, authors compared the results of botulinum toxin injection (under ultrasound guidance) with combined injection of ozone and steroids into the priformis muscle. Both effectively reduced the pain days after injection, but combination of ozone and steroid had more analgesic effect in short term. However, botulinum toxin analgesic effect surpassed the effect of combination therapy at 3 and 6 months [72].

There are several other pain syndromes in which there is scientific evidence for efficacy of botulinum toxin therapy. These include pain in arthritis, muscle pain associated with stroke, pain associated with involuntary neck movements (cervical dystonia), bladder and pelvic pain and pain associated with certain childhood surgeries. These are discussed in other chapters of this book.

Conclusion

Neuropathic pain (NP) comprise a large group of pain disorders that results from disturbance of peripheral nerves by trauma, pressure, infection and other factors. Less commonly, neuropathic pain is due to spinal cord injury (central pain). Although FDA has not yet approved botulinum toxin therapy for any of the categories of neuropathic pain discussed in this chapter, evidence from high quality studies strongly suggests efficacy of botulinum toxin therapy in several NP categories. In clinical medicine, insurance companies sometimes approve the use of a non-FDA approved drug based on strong evidence presented from published high quality (double-blind, placebo-controlled) studies.

References

1. Treede RD, Rief W, Barke A, Aziz Q, Bennett MI, Benoliel R, Cohen M, Evers S, Finnerup NB, First MB, Giamberardino MA, Kaasa S, Kosek E, Lavand'homme P, Nicholas M, Perrot S, Scholz J, Schug S, Smith BH, Svensson P, Vlaeyen JWS, Wang SJ. A classification of chronic pain for ICD-11. Pain. 2015;156(6):1003–7.
2. Yong RJ, Mullins PM, Bhattacharyya N. Prevalence of chronic pain among adults in the United States. Pain. 2022 Feb 1;163(2):e328–32. https://doi.org/10.1097/j.pain.0000000000002291.
3. Breivik H, Collett B, Ventafridda V, Cohen R, Gallacher D. Survey of chronic pain in Europe: prevalence, impact on daily life, and treatment. Eur J Pain. 2006;10(4):287–333. https://doi.org/10.1016/j.ejpain.2005.06.009.
4. Cohen SP, Vase L, Hooten WM. Chronic pain: an update on burden, best practices, and new advances. Lancet. 2021 May 29;397(10289):2082–97. https://doi.org/10.1016/S0140-6736(21)00393-7. PMID: 34062143.
5. Relieving pain in America a blueprint for transforming prevention, care, education, and research. Reli Pain Am A Bluepr Transform Prev Care Educ Res. 2011;26:1–364. Institute of Medicine (US) Committee on Advancing Pain Research, Care, and Education.
6. Cui M, Khanijou S, Rubino J, et al. Subcutaneous administration of botulinum toxin a reduces formalin-induced pain. Pain. 2004;107:125–33.
7. Marino MJ, Terashima T, Steinauer JJ, et al. Botulinum toxin B in the sensory afferent: transmitter release, spinal activation, and pain behavior. Pain. 2014;155:674–84.
8. Welch MJ, Purkiss JR, Foster KA. Sensitivity of embryonic rat dorsal root ganglia neurons to clostridium botulinum neurotoxins. Toxicon. 2000;38:245–58.
9. Matak I, Riederer P, Lacković Z. Botulinum toxin's axonal transport from periphery to the spinal cord. Neurochem Int. 2012 July;61(2):236–9. https://doi.org/10.1016/j.neuint.2012.05.001.
10. Hou YP, Zhang YP, Song YF, Zhu CM, Wang YC, Xie GL. Botulinum toxin type A inhibits rat pyloric myoelectrical activity and substance P release in vivo. Can J Physiol Pharmacol. 2007 Feb;85(2):209–14. https://doi.org/10.1139/y07-018.
11. Lucioni A, Bales GT, Lotan TL, McGehee DS, Cook SP, Rapp DE. Botulinum toxin type A inhibits sensory neuropeptide release in rat bladder models of acute injury and chronic inflammation. BJU Int. 2008;101:366–70.
12. Meng J, Wang J, Lawrence G, Dolly JO. Synaptobrevin I mediates exocytosis of CGRP from sensory neurons and inhibition by botulinum toxins reflects their anti-nociceptive potential. J Cell Sci. 2007;120:2864–74.
13. Meng J, Ovsepian SV, Wang J, Pickering M, Sasse A, Aoki KR, Lawrence GW, Dolly JO. Activation of TRPV1 mediates calcitonin gene-related peptide release, which excites trigeminal sensory neurons and is attenuated by a retargeted botulinum toxin with antinociceptive potential. J Neurosci. 2009;29:4981–92.
14. Matak I, Tékus V, Bölcskei K, Lacković Z, Helyes Z. Involvement of substance P in the antinociceptive effect of botulinum toxin type A: evidence from knockout mice. Neuroscience. 2017 Sept 1;358:137–45. https://doi.org/10.1016/j.neuroscience.2017.06.040. Epub 2017 July 1.
15. Tang M, Meng J, Wang J. New engineered-botulinum toxins inhibit the release of pain-related mediators. Int J Mol Sci. 2019 Dec 30;21(1):262. https://doi.org/10.3390/ijms21010262. PMID: 31906003; PMCID: PMC6981458.
16. Andersson GBJ. Epidemiological features of chronic low-back pain. Lancet. 1999;354:581–5.
17. Balagué F, Mannion AF, Pellisé F, Cedraschi C. Non-specific low back pain. Lancet. 2012 Feb 4;379(9814):482–91. https://doi.org/10.1016/S0140-6736(11)60610-7. Epub 2011 Oct 6.
18. Knezevic NN, Candido KD, Vlaeyen JWS, Van Zundert J, Cohen SP. Low back pain. Lancet. 2021 July 3;398(10294):78–92. https://doi.org/10.1016/S0140-6736(21)00733-9. Epub 2021 June 8.
19. Foster L, Clapp L, Erickson M, Jabbari B. Botulinum toxin A and chronic low back pain: a randomized, double-blind study. Neurology. 2001;56:1290–3.

20. Machado D, Kumar A, Jabbari B. Abobotulinum toxin A in the treatment of chronic low back pain. Toxins (Basel). 2016, Dec 15;8(12):pii: E374.
21. Jabbari B, Ney J, Sichani A, Monacci W, Foster L, Difazio M. Treatment of refractory, chronic low back pain with botulinum neurotoxin a: an open-label, pilot study. Pain Med. 2006 May–June;7(3):260–4. https://doi.org/10.1111/j.1526-4637.2006.00147.x.
22. Jazayeri SM, Ashraf A, Fini HM, Karimian H, Nasab MV. Efficacy of botulinum toxin type a for treating chronic low back pain. Anesth Pain Med. 2011 Fall;1(2):77–80. https://doi.org/10.5812/kowsar.22287523.1845. Epub 2011 Sept 26. PMID: 25729661; PMCID: PMC4335729.
23. Sahoo J, Jena D, Viswanath A, Barman A. Injection botulinum toxin A in treatment of resistant chronic low back pain: a prospective open-label study. Cureus. 2021 Sept 8;13(9):e17811. https://doi.org/10.7759/cureus.17811. PMID: 34660021; PMCID: PMC8500249.
24. Cogné M, Petit H, Creuzé A, Liguoro D, de Seze M. Are paraspinous intramuscular injections of botulinum toxin a (BoNT-A) efficient in the treatment of chronic low-back pain? A randomised, double-blinded crossover trial. BMC Musculoskelet Disord. 2017 Nov 15;18(1):454. https://doi.org/10.1186/s12891-017-1816-6. PMID: 29141611; PMCID: PMC5688690.
25. De Andrés J, Adsuara VM, Palmisani S, Villanueva V, López-Alarcón MD. A double-blind, controlled, randomized trial to evaluate the efficacy of botulinum toxin for the treatment of lumbar myofascial pain in humans. Reg Anesth Pain Med. 2010 May–June;35(3):255–60. https://doi.org/10.1097/AAP.0b013e3181d23241.
26. Gronseth G, French J. Practice parameters and technology assessments: what they are, what they are not, and why you should care. Neurology. 2008 Nov 11;71(20):1639–43. https://doi.org/10.1212/01.wnl.0000336535.27773.c0.
27. French J, Gronseth G. Lost in a jungle of evidence: we need a compass. Neurology. 2008 Nov 11;71(20):1634–8. https://doi.org/10.1212/01.wnl.0000336533.19610.1b.
28. Yawn BP, Saddier P, Wollan PC, St Sauver JL, Kurland MJ, Sy LS. A population-based study of the incidence and complication rates of herpes zoster before zoster vaccine introduction. Mayo Clin Proc. 2007;82:1341–9.
29. Thyregod HG, Rowbotham MC, Peters M, Possehn J, Berro M, Petersen KL. Natural history of pain following herpes zoster. Pain. 2007 Mar;128(1–2):148–56. https://doi.org/10.1016/j.pain.2006.09.021. Epub 2006 Oct 27. PMID: 17070998; PMCID: PMC1905461.
30. Baron R, Haendler G, Schulte H. Afferent large fiber polyneuropathy predicts the development of postherpetic neuralgia. Pain. 1997 Nov;73(2):231–8. https://doi.org/10.1016/S0304-3959(97)00105-X.
31. Park SY, Kim JY, Kwon JS, Jeon NY, Kim MC, Chong YP, Lee SO, Choi SH, Kim YS, Woo JH, Kim SH. Relationships of varicella zoster virus (VZV)-specific cell-mediated immunity and persistence of VZV DNA in saliva and the development of postherpetic neuralgia in patients with herpes zoster. J Med Virol. 2019 Nov;91(11):1995–2000. https://doi.org/10.1002/jmv.25543. Epub 2019 July 23.
32. Whitley RJ, Weiss H, Gnann JW Jr, Tyring S, Mertz GJ, Pappas PG, Schleupner CJ, Hayden F, Wolf J, Soong SJ. Acyclovir with and without prednisone for the treatment of herpes zoster. A randomized, placebo-controlled trial. The National Institute of Allergy and Infectious Diseases Collaborative Antiviral Study Group. Ann Intern Med. 1996 Sept 1;125(5):376–83. https://doi.org/10.7326/0003-4819-125-5-199609010-00004.
33. Wood MJ, Kay R, Dworkin RH, Soong SJ, Whitley RJ. Oral acyclovir therapy accelerates pain resolution in patients with herpes zoster: a meta-analysis of placebo-controlled trials. Clin Infect Dis. 1996 Feb;22(2):341–7. https://doi.org/10.1093/clinids/22.2.341.
34. Wang J, Xu W, Kong Y, Huang J, Ding Z, Deng M, Guo Q, Zou W. SNAP-25 contributes to neuropathic pain by regulation of VGLuT2 expression in rats. Neuroscience. 2019 Dec 15;423:86–97. https://doi.org/10.1016/j.neuroscience.2019.10.007. Epub 2019 Nov 6. Erratum in: Neuroscience. 2020 June 15;437:256.
35. Hong B, Yao L, Ni L, Wang L, Hu X. Antinociceptive effect of botulinum toxin A involves alterations in AMPA receptor expression and glutamate release in spinal dorsal horn neurons. Neuroscience. 2017 Aug 15;357:197–207. https://doi.org/10.1016/j.neuroscience.2017.06.004. Epub 2017 June 10.

36. Kim DW, Lee SK, Ahnn J. Botulinum toxin as a pain killer: players and actions in Antinociception. Toxins (Basel). 2015 June 30;7(7):2435–53. https://doi.org/10.3390/toxins7072435. PMID: 26134255; PMCID: PMC4516922.
37. Bittencourt da Silva L, Karshenas A, Bach FW, Rasmussen S, Arendt-Nielsen L, Gazerani P. Blockade of glutamate release by botulinum neurotoxin type A in humans: a dermal microdialysis study. Pain Res Manag. 2014 May-June;19(3):126–32. https://doi.org/10.1155/2014/410415. PMID: 24851237; PMCID: PMC4158957.
38. Xiao L, Mackey S, Hui H, Xong D, Zhang Q, Zhang D. Subcutaneous injection of botulinum toxin a is beneficial in postherpetic neuralgia. Pain Med. 2010;11:1827–33.
39. Apalla Z, Sotiriou E, Lallas A, Lazaridou E, Ioannides D. Botulinum toxin A in postherpetic neuralgia: a parallel, randomized, double-blind, single-dose, placebo-controlled trial. Clin J Pain. 2013;29:857–64.
40. Jain P, Jain M, Jain S. Subcutaneous injection of botulinum toxin in patients with post herpetic neuralgia. A preliminary study. J Assoc Physicians India. 2018 July;66(7):48–9.
41. Ding XD, Zhong J, Liu YP, Chen HX. Botulinum as a toxin for treating post-herpetic neuralgia. Iran J Public Health. 2017 May;46(5):608–11. PMID: 28560190; PMCID: PMC5442272.
42. Peng F, Xia TB. Effects of intradermal botulinum toxin injections on herpes zoster related neuralgia. Infect Drug Resist. 2023 Apr 12;16:2159–65. https://doi.org/10.2147/IDR.S401972. PMID: 37077249; PMCID: PMC10106788.
43. Li XL, Zeng X, Zeng S, He HP, Zeng Z, Peng LL, Chen LG. Botulinum toxin A treatment for post-herpetic neuralgia: a systematic review and meta-analysis. Exp Ther Med. 2020 Feb;19(2):1058–64. https://doi.org/10.3892/etm.2019.8301. Epub 2019 Dec 9. PMID: 32010269; PMCID: PMC6966161.
44. Katusic S, Beard CM, Bergstralh E, Kurland LT. Incidence and clinical features of trigeminal neuralgia, Rochester, Minnesota, 1945–1984. Ann Neurol. 1990;27:89–95.
45. Gallay MN, Moser D, Jeanmonod D. MR-guided focused ultrasound central lateral thalamotomy for trigeminal neuralgia. Single center experience. Front Neurol. 2020 Apr 17;11:271. https://doi.org/10.3389/fneur.2020.00271. PMID: 32425870; PMCID: PMC7212452.
46. Wu CJ, Lian YJ, Zhang YK, et al. Botulinum toxin type A for the treatment of trigeminal neuralgia: results from a randomized, double-blind, placebo-controlled trial. Cephalalgia. 2012;32:443–50.
47. Zhang H, Lian Y, Ma Y, et al. Two doses of botulinum toxin type a for the treatment of trigeminal neuralgia: observation of therapeutic effect from a randomized, double-blind, placebo-controlled trial. J Headache Pain. 2014;15(1):65.
48. Barrett AM, Lucero MA, Le T, Robinson RL, Dworkin RH, Chappell AS. Epidemiology, public health burden, and treatment of diabetic neuropathic pain: a review. Pain Med. 2007;8(Suppl 2):S50–62. Review.
49. Stewart WF, Ricci JA, Chee E, Hirsch AG, Brandenburg NA. Lost productive time and costs due to diabetes and diabetic neuropathic pain in the US workforce. J Occup Environ Med. 2007 June;49(6):672–9. https://doi.org/10.1097/JOM.0b013e318065b83a.
50. Preston FG, Riley DR, Azmi S, Alam U. Painful diabetic peripheral neuropathy: practical guidance and challenges for clinical management. Diabetes Metab Syndr Obes. 2023 June 2;16:1595–612. https://doi.org/10.2147/DMSO.S370050. PMID: 37288250; PMCID: PMC10243347.
51. Diabetes Canada Clinical Practice Guidelines Expert Committee, Bril V, Breiner A, Perkins BA, Zochodne D. Neuropathy. Can J Diabetes. 2018 Apr;42(Suppl 1):S217–21. https://doi.org/10.1016/j.jcjd.2017.10.028.
52. Price R, Smith D, Franklin G, Gronseth G, Pignone M, David WS, Armon C, Perkins BA, Bril V, Rae-Grant A, Halperin J, Licking N, O'Brien MD, Wessels SR, MacGregor LC, Fink K, Harkless LB, Colbert L, Callaghan BC. Oral and topical treatment of painful diabetic polyneuropathy: practice guideline update summary: report of the AAN Guideline Subcommittee. Neurology. 2022 Jan 4;98(1):31–43. https://doi.org/10.1212/WNL.0000000000013038.

53. Yuan RY, Sheu JJ, Yu JM, Chen WT, Tseng IJ, Chang HH, Hu CJ. Botulinum toxin for diabetic neuropathic pain: a randomized double-blind crossover trial. Neurology. s2009;72:1473–8.

54. Ghasemi M, Ansari M, Basiri K, et al. The effects of intradermal botulinum toxin type a injections on pain symptoms of patients with diabetic neuropathy. J Res Med Sci. 2014;19:106–11.

55. Salehi H, Moussaei M, Kamiab Z, Vakilian A. The effects of botulinum toxin type A injection on pain symptoms, quality of life, and sleep quality of patients with diabetic neuropathy: a randomized double-blind clinical trial. Iran J Neurol. 2019 July 6;18(3):99–107. PMID: 31749930; PMCID: PMC6858596.

56. Taheri M, Sedaghat M, Solhpour A, Rostami P, Safarpour Lima B. The effect of intradermal botulinum toxin a injections on painful diabetic polyneuropathy. Diabetes Metab Syndr. 2020 Nov–Dec;14(6):1823–8. https://doi.org/10.1016/j.dsx.2020.09.019. Epub 2020 Sept 14.

57. Restivo DA, Casabona A, Frittitta L, Belfiore A, Le Moli R, Gullo D, Vigneri R. Efficacy of botulinum toxin a for treating cramps in diabetic neuropathy. Ann Neurol. 2018 Nov;84(5):674–82. https://doi.org/10.1002/ana.25340. Epub 2018 Oct 16.

58. Kibler WB, Goldberg C, Chandler TJ. Functional biomechanical deficits in running athlitis with plantar fasciitis. Am J Sports Med. 1991;19:63–71.

59. Babcock MS, Foster L, Pasquina P, Jabbari B. Treatment of pain attributed to plantar fasciitis with botulinum toxin A: a short-term, randomized, placebo-controlled, double-blind study. Am J Phys Med Rehabil. 2005;84:649–54.

60. Huang YC, Wei SH, Wang HK, Lieu FK. Ultrasonographic guided botulinum toxin type A treatment for plantar fasciitis: an outcome-based investigation for treating pain and gait changes. J Rehabil Med. 2010;42:136–40.

61. Díaz-Llopis IV, Rodríguez-Ruíz CM, Mulet-Perry S, Mondéjar-Gómez FJ, Climent-Barberá JM, Cholbi-Llobel F. Randomized controlled study of the efficacy of the injection of botulinum toxin type A versus corticosteroids in chronic plantar fasciitis: results at one and six months. Clin Rehabil. 2012;26:594–606.

62. Elizondo-Rodriguez J, Araujo-Lopez Y, Moreno-Gonzalez JA, Cardenas-Estrada E, Mendoza-Lemus O, Acosta-Olivo C. A comparison of botulinum toxin A and intralesional steroids for the treatment of plantar fasciitis: a randomized, double-blinded study. Foot Ankle Int. 2013 Jan;34(1):8–14. https://doi.org/10.1177/1071100712460215.

63. Ahmad J, Ahmad SH, Jones K. Treatment of plantar fasciitis with botulinum toxin. Foot Ankle Int. 2017;38:1–7.

64. Elizondo-Rodríguez J, Simental-Mendía M, Peña-Martínez V, Vilchez-Cavazos F, Tamez-Mata Y, Acosta-Olivo C. Comparison of botulinum toxin A, corticosteroid, and anesthetic injection for plantar fasciitis. Foot Ankle Int. 2021 Mar;42(3):305–13. https://doi.org/10.1177/1071100720961093. Epub 2020 Oct 8.

65. Ranoux D, Attal N, Morain F, Bouhassira D. Botulinum toxin type A induces direct analgesic effects in chronic neuropathic pain. Ann Neurol. 2008 Sept;64(3):274–83. https://doi.org/10.1002/ana.21427. Erratum in: Ann Neurol. 2009 Mar;65(3):359.

66. Attal N, de Andrade DC, Adam F, Ranoux D, Teixeira MJ, Galhardoni R, Raicher I, Üçeyler N, Sommer C, Bouhassira D. Safety and efficacy of repeated injections of botulinum toxin A in peripheral neuropathic pain (BOTNEP): a randomised, double-blind, placebo-controlled trial. Lancet Neurol. 2016 May;15(6):555–65. https://doi.org/10.1016/S1474-4422(16)00017-X. Epub 2016 Mar 2.

67. Han ZA, Song DH, Oh HM, Chung ME. Botulinum toxin type A for neuropathic pain in patients with spinal cord injury. Ann Neurol. 2016 Apr;79(4):569–78. https://doi.org/10.1002/ana.24605. Epub 2016 Feb 16. PMID: 26814620; PMCID: PMC4825405.

68. Chun A, Levy I, Yang A, Delgado A, Tsai CY, Leung E, Taylor K, Kolakowsky-Hayner S, Huang V, Escalon M, Bryce TN. Treatment of at-level spinal cord injury pain with botulinum toxin A. Spinal Cord Ser Cases. 2019 Sept 18;5:77. https://doi.org/10.1038/s41394-019-0221-9. PMID: 31632735; PMCID: PMC6786298.

69. Vacca V, Madaro L, De Angelis F, Proietti D, Cobianchi S, Orsini T, Puri PL, Luvisetto S, Pavone F, Marinelli S. Revealing the therapeutic potential of botulinum neurotoxin type A in counteracting paralysis and neuropathic pain in spinally injured mice. Toxins (Basel). 2020 July 31;12(8):491. doi:https://doi.org/10.3390/toxins12080491. PMID: 32751937; PMCID: PMC7472120.
70. Fishman LM, Anderson C, Rosner B. BOTOX and physical therapy in the treatment of piriformis syndrome. Am J Phys Med Rehabil. 2002;81:936–42.
71. Michel F, Decavel P, Toussirot E, Tatu L, Aleton E, Monnier G, Garbuio P, Parratte B. Piriformis muscle syndrome: diagnostic criteria and treatment of a monocentric series of 250 patients. Ann Phys Rehabil Med. 2013 July;56(5):371–83. https://doi.org/10.1016/j.rehab.2013.04.003. Epub 2013 Apr 25.
72. Elsawy AGS, Ameer AH, Gazar YA, Allam AE, Chan SM, Chen SY, Hou JD, Tai YT, Lin JA, Galluccio F, Nada DW, Esmat A. Efficacy of ultrasound-guided injection of botulinum toxin, ozone, and lidocaine in piriformis syndrome. Healthcare (Basel). 2022 Dec 28;11(1):95. https://doi.org/10.3390/healthcare11010095. PMID: 36611554; PMCID: PMC9818865.

Chapter 6
Botulinum Toxin Therapy
for Complication of Stroke

Abstract Stroke is the most common cause of disability in the US. Many complications of stroke are managed sub-optimally by currently available therapies. This chapter discusses the role of botulinum toxin therapy in management of stroke-related symptoms such as spasticity, muscle spasms, painful postures, abnormal movements (dystonia), bladder dysfunction and drooling.

Keywords Stroke · Botulinum toxin · Botulinum neurotoxin · Spasticity · Muscles spasm · Dystonia · Bladder dysfunction · Drooling

Introduction

Stroke is due to occlusion or rupture of a blood vessel in the brain. Occlusion of a blood vessel acutely deprives a part of the brain from nutrients and oxygen, whereas rupture of a vessel destroys the brain tissue and replaces a part of the brain by a blood clot. Close to 90% of all strokes are caused by occlusion of a blood vessel. Brain's function is highly dependent on its blood supply which provides brain with oxygen. Brain uses oxygen more than any other organ in the body. Brain cells are very sensitive to lack of oxygen which can result in their death within a few minutes. Each year, over 800,000 people in the US suffer from stroke [1]. Stroke is the fourth cause of mortality world -wide and the first cause of adult disability in the US [2].

Acute impairment of brain function or lack of it leads to a variety of neurological deficits. The type of deficit depends on the region of the brain affected by stroke. In small strokes recovery may be quick and sometimes complete. Unfortunately, many strokes result in a sizeable deficit with incomplete recovery despite the best medical treatment.

The most common and often the most disturbing of all mishaps after a stroke is impairment of muscle function. Depending on the severity of the stroke, the aftermath of most strokes is some degree of muscle paralysis. The function of our muscles is based on the nerve signals that they receive from the brain. In human, the brain is extremely well developed and has a larger size per body weight compared

B. Jabbari, *Botulinum Toxin Treatment*,
https://doi.org/10.1007/978-3-031-54471-2_6

to much larger primates. Human brain contains approximately 86 billion nerve cells (neurons) and almost the same number of non-nerve cells (supporting cells-glia) [3]. The most superficial layer of human brain is called cortex. Cortex, which is only 3–4 mm thick, consists of 26 billion nerve cells. Many of these cells are located in the motor region of the cortex which governs the motor function and controls the muscles (Fig. 6.1).

The large nerve cells that are located in the motor region of the cortex send the motor command through their long processes (axons) to another motor cell in the spinal cord and then to the muscle. This is unlike the cells in the sensory system that covey the sensory signals from the skin to the brain. In the sensory system, at least two other sensory cells (one in the spinal cord and one higher up inside the brain) are contacted before the peripheral sensory signal reaches the sensory cortex. Each motor cell has one axon, a long fiber that conveys the message of the cortical nerve cell to motor cells in the spinal cord. The axons of the motor cells in the spinal cord convey the motor message to the muscle. Each axon of spinal cord motor cell when approaching the muscle divides into several branches; each branch connects to one muscle fiber. The point of contact between an axon and a muscle fiber is called neuro-muscular junction. A neuromuscular junction has an axon part and a muscle fiber part with a cleft between the two structures (synaptic cleft) (Fig. 6.2). Since botulinum toxins relieve many muscle-related symptoms through their action on neuromuscular junction, the structure of neuromuscular junction and mechanism of muscle activation is described in more detail below.

The end of each axon (axon terminal) contains many vesicular structures, filled with a chemical called acetylcholine (Fig. 6.2). Acetylcholine is one of many

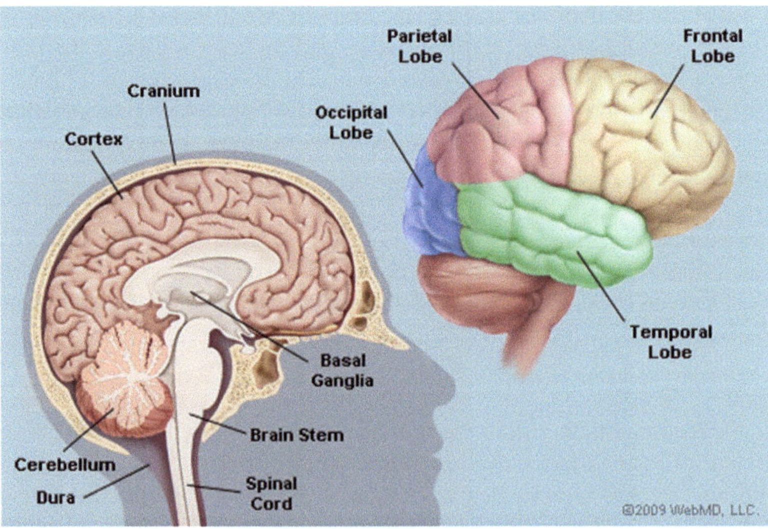

Fig. 6.1 The primary motor area is the most posterior and the primary sensory area is the most anterior part of frontal and parietal lobes, respectively. (Reproduced under free use license PDM 1.0 deed, public domain, courtesy of www.modup Flickr)

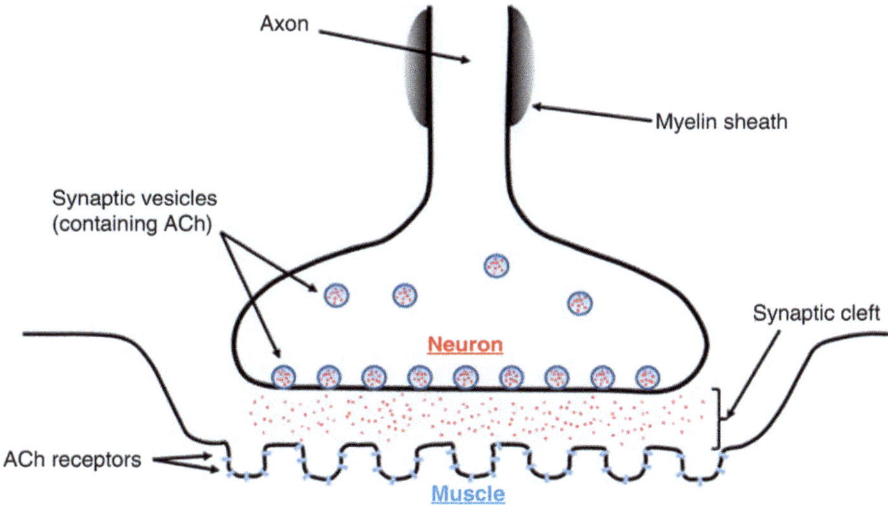

Fig. 6.2 Neuromuscular junction—the end of the motor axon (axon terminal) which faces the muscle fiber contains vesicles that contain acetylcholine (AC). (From Barreda and Zhou 2011. Reproduced under https://creativecommons.org/licenses/by/2.0/)

chemicals that are considered neurotransmitters. This particular neurotransmitter's main function is conveying the nerve message to the muscle. The motor command from a cortical nerve cell travels along the axon to the periphery in form of an electric signal. When the nerve signal from the brain reaches the axon terminal next to the muscle, it activates a set of proteins in the axon terminal. Activation of these proteins ruptures the vesicular structures and releases their content (acetylcholine) into the synaptic cleft [4]. The released acetylcholine attaches itself to muscle receptors (located on the surface of the muscle), excites, activates and contracts the muscle fiber.

In stroke, in addition to paralysis which is the result of loss of nerve cells, degeneration and death of many axons and their terminal connections to muscle fibers results in a cascade of complicated events that leads to significant increase of tone in the weak muscle. This increased tone leads to stiffness of the muscle and causes further functional disability. The increased tone of the muscle which is often associated with increased reflexes is called spasticity.

Spasticity is a major handicap among patients who have suffered from stroke. Between 20% and 40% of patients with stroke develop spasticity within 1–6 weeks after the onset of stroke. Spastic muscles have limited range of motion and lack speed of function and precision. In the lower extremities, spasticity interferes with proper balance and ambulation. The severity of spasticity after stroke increases over time [5].

Why, after stroke the muscles of a weak limb gradually develop increased tone and become spastic has been the subject of extensive research. Brain both excites and inhibits the muscle activity through a set of complex mechanisms. Hence,

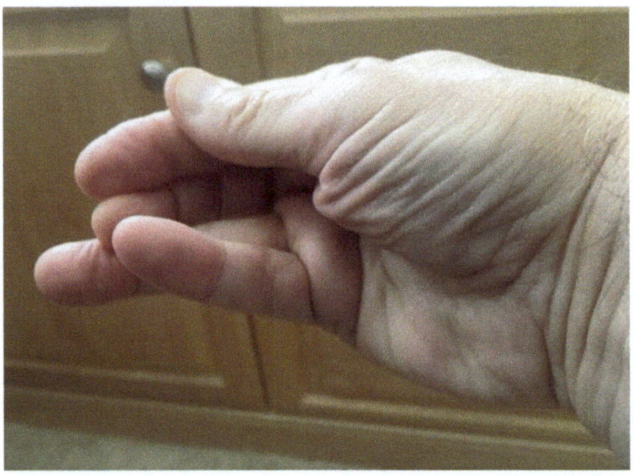

Fig. 6.3 Contracted and spastic muscles leading to contracture and loss of finger function

enhanced excitation or reduced inhibition both can cause abnormally increased muscle tone and muscle spasticity. We have mentioned above the chemical acetylcholine that is present at nerve endings and upon release, excites the muscle. Inhibitory fibers that influence the muscle, work through their own inhibitory chemical (transmitter). Currently, there is strong evidence to support that disruption of these inhibitory fibers, via tissue damage caused by stroke, plays a major role in development of spasticity [6].

Spasticity is not a benign complication of stroke. In addition to impairing balance and interfering with ambulation and promoting fall, spastic muscles can continue to harden and end in a state of continued contraction (contracture) leading to pain and immobility if not properly treated (Fig. 6.3). The muscles affected by contracture are also disfigured and are aesthetically unpleasant for the patient and others to look at.

Treatment of Spasticity

Most stroke specialists advocate aggressive treatment of spasticity as soon as it develops. Specialized physiotherapy such as induced movement therapy, stretching, dynamic elbow-splinting and occupational therapy offer some help and can delay development of contracture to some extent.

A large number of medications are used for reducing the tone in the spastic muscles, among which, baclofen, benzodiazines (valium), tizanidine and dantrolene are the most commonly used. These medications, although partially effective, are beset by undesirable side effects which limit increasing their dose to the required optimal level (Table 6.1).

In severe lower limb spasticity, specially when it is severe, pharmacological treatment is often not very effective. Insertion of baclofen pump can reduce lower

Table 6.1 Medications commonly used for treatment of spasticity [7]

Medication	Dose	Side effects
Valium	2–10 mg, 3–4 times daily	Drowsiness, sedation, impaired balance, drop in blood pressure
Baclofen	5 mg 2 to 3 times daily if needed, increase by 5 mg up to 50–60 mg daily	Drowsiness, nausea, muscle weakness, confusion and in high doses seizures
Tizanidine	2–4 mg daily every 6–8 h. If needed, increase to 12 mg, 3 times daily	Sedation, drop in blood pressure, liver toxicity
Dantroline	25 mg once daily, maximum dose: 100 mg 3 times daily	Drowsiness, weakness, fatigue, liver toxicity

Because of danger of significant toxicity, higher doses of these medications need to be prescribed by experienced physicians and monitors closely

limb spasticity [8]. This is an involved procedure that requires insertion of a small pump surgically into the abdominal wall. A catheter that emerges from the pump delivers a carefully titrated amount of baclofen into the cerebrospinal fluid (flowing inside the spinal canal) of the patient. This treatment requires facilities with experienced surgeons to insert and titrate the dose of baclofen in the pump. Inappropriate titrations can lead to severe side effects such as seizures and depressed level of consciousness. Other non- pharmacological treatments of spasticity include repetitive electrical stimulation of the nerves and magnetic stimulation of the motor cortex with a specially designed magnet [9]. Both procedures have a modest effect and are uncomfortable for the patient.

Botulinum Toxin Treatment of Spasticity

Botulinum toxins inhibit the release of acetylcholine from nerve ending; acetylcholine is an agent that normally activates the muscle and. in abnormal conditions, may intensify the muscle contraction. This unique function makes the botulinum toxins effective therapeutic agents for treatment of hyperactive muscle disorders including spasticity. The commercially available toxin preparations are now used widely for treatment of a variety of neurological disorders [10].

As described earlier in Chap. 3, of the nine recognized serotypes of botulinum toxins, only types A and B are of clinical use due to their long duration of action (3–6 months). This long duration of action after a single injection is an advantage over oral medications which need to be taken daily. Three type A toxins with the trade names of Botox, Xeomin and Dysport are approved by FDA for use in the US for treatment of spasticity. One type B toxin, Myobloc, is approved by FDA and is currently available in the US market. The doses of these toxins are not comparable or interchangeable; in clinical and comparative studies, the following approximations are used:

Each 1 unit of Botox = 1 unit of Xeomin = 2–3 units of Dysport = 40–50 units of Myobloc.

Spasticity not only pertains to stroke but can also be seen after brain and spinal cord trauma, in association with multiple sclerosis and in children with cerebral palsy. Following a large number of animal studies that showed reduction of muscle tone in animal models of spasticity after intramuscular injection of botulinum toxins, significant interest has developed among neuroscientists, neurologists, physiotherapists and pediatricians for investigating the role of botulinum toxins in human spasticity. Early investigations focused on the role of botulinum toxin therapy in upper limb spasticity. These investigations looked at many facets of upper limb spasticity and aimed to answer many questions:

Can injection of Botulinum toxin (Botox, Xeomin, Myobloc, Dysport) into spastic muscles reduce muscle tone in human and improve the patient's quality of life?

Does reduction of spasticity of hand, forearm and shoulder muscles relieve the burden of caregivers and help physical therapy?

In other indications of botulinum toxins therapy such as involuntary, hyperactive muscles of face and neck, improvement lasts 3–4 months after muscle injection(s). Is this the case with spasticity?

Face and neck muscles are commonly injected with botulinum toxins for other FDA approved indications such as cervical dystonia, blepharospasm and hemifacial spasm discussed in Chap. 8 of this book. Because of the size of limb muscles which are considerably larger than face or neck muscles, larger doses of botulinum toxins are needed for injection into spastic limb muscles. Is injection of these higher doses in one session (for Botox up to 500 units or more) safe and devoid of serious side effects?

When spasticity after stroke involves both upper and lower limbs, how high of a total dose of botulinum toxin is safe when both limbs are planned to be injected in one session?

Over the past 20 years, a large number of high quality studies (double-blind, placebo-controlled) have answered these questions.

Spasticity of Upper Limb Muscles After Stroke

Many high quality studies (double-blind, placebo controlled) have been published on the effects of botulinum toxins on spasticity of upper limb muscles; some of these studies include sizeable number (in hundreds) of subjects. The results of these studies and their conclusions have been published in several reviews [11–14]. These studies collectively demonstrate that botulinum toxin injections into the tense and spasticity stricken muscles of stroke subjects, reduces muscle tone, eases physical therapy and improves the patients' quality of life. Most patients are satisfied with botulinum toxin therapy and prefer this mode of treatment over taking large doses of daily medications. Serious side effects in spasticity studies were y rare and the toxin therapy was considered, in general, safe and practical. Based on the positive results of these studies, FDA first approved the use of Botox for treatment of upper limb spasticity in 2010. Subsequently, with availability of further studies, FDA approved the other two type A toxins, Xeomin and Dysport for treatment of upper limb spasticity in 2015.

Botulinum Toxin Treatment for Lower Limb Spasticity

Lower limb spasticity after stroke can be very disabling. Spasticity adds to muscle weakness in stroke patients, limits leg movements and adds to difficulty with ambulation. High quality studies in lower limb spasticity have shown reduction of tone and improvement of quality of life after botulinum toxin therapy. Many studies have clearly demonstrated that botulinum toxin injections into the leg muscles of patients with stroke improve ambulation. Based on availability of these high quality studies, FDA approved the use of Botox and Dysport for lower limb spasticity in adult and children in 2014 and 2017, respectively. In children, cerebral palsy and degenerative disorders of the central nervous system are the most common causes of lower limb spasticity. Dysport was the first botulinum toxin approved for treatment of lower limb spasticity in children (FDA approval, 2016). Botox was approved for spasticity of children by FDA in 2020.

One of the most feared complications of spasticity after stroke is development of muscle contracture. Contracture is loss and shortening of muscle fibers and replacement of muscle by non-elastic connective tissue. Contracture leads to total loss of muscle function and joint deformity. There are now reports from high quality studies that indicate injection of botulinum toxin into the muscles shortly after stroke can delay development of contracture and even prevent it in some patients [15–17]. According to one study, treatment of muscles with botulinum toxin is best effective if it is done within the first 3 months after stroke [18].

Technical Issues in Botulinum Toxin Treatment of Stroke Spasticity

All four of FDA approved botulinum toxins in the market (Botox, Xeomin, Dysport, Myobloc) have shown efficacy in treatment of post stroke spasticity, though the data on Myobloc (type B toxin) is still limited compared to the other three toxins [19]. In case of Botox, Xeomin and Dysport, the powder form of the toxin (provided in a small vial) needs to be mixed with salt water (saline) before injection. Myobloc (type B toxin) is marketed in an already prepared solution form. Injections are often guided by electromyography (EMG), a device that identifies muscles by their electrical activity pattern. Also, location of the muscle can be identified by nerve stimulation. A nerve stimulator stimulates a nerve which is known to serve a certain muscle and, by doing so, identifies the muscle (muscle moves in response to the stimulation). Ultrasound is a more precise way to localize and clearly visualize the muscles [20]. This technique, however, requires a fair amount of expertise and the equipment is considerably more expensive than a small hand held EMG device.

Upper limb spasticity more often involves muscles that flex the joints. For instance, involvement of biceps muscle leads to abnormal flexion of the arm, a position that can interfere with dressing and use of the arm for other activities of daily living. This is often associated with wrist spasticity (flexed wrist) and sometimes with forced flexion of fingers causing "clenched fist." (Fig. 6.4a) The latter two, when severe enough, can make the involved hand non-functional. In the lower limb, abnormal flexion of the knee or foot interferes with standing and ambulation. Flexion of the knee results from spasticity and high tone in the large hamstring muscles located on the back of the thighs. Botulinum toxin injections are usually carried into two to four sites for large muscles (Fig. 6.4a, b).

The units of toxin used per muscle depend on the size of the muscle (Table 6.2). The effect of botulinum toxin injection appears within 3–7 days (muscles loosens) and the peak effect comes in 3–5 weeks. The toxin effect usually lasts for 3–4 months. Reinjections are required every 3–4 months to keep the spastic muscle in the state of reduced tone. It has been shown that with repeated injections, spasticity reduces and patients' satisfaction rate increases. In one study [21], patients satisfaction rate from the initial of 47.4% rose to 66.6% after repeated injections.

In clinical practice, in order to achieve best results, botulinum toxin therapy is often combined with physioerapy. Concurrent pharmacological therapy with antispastic drugs such as baclofen or tizanidine (Table 6.1) may be required in cases of

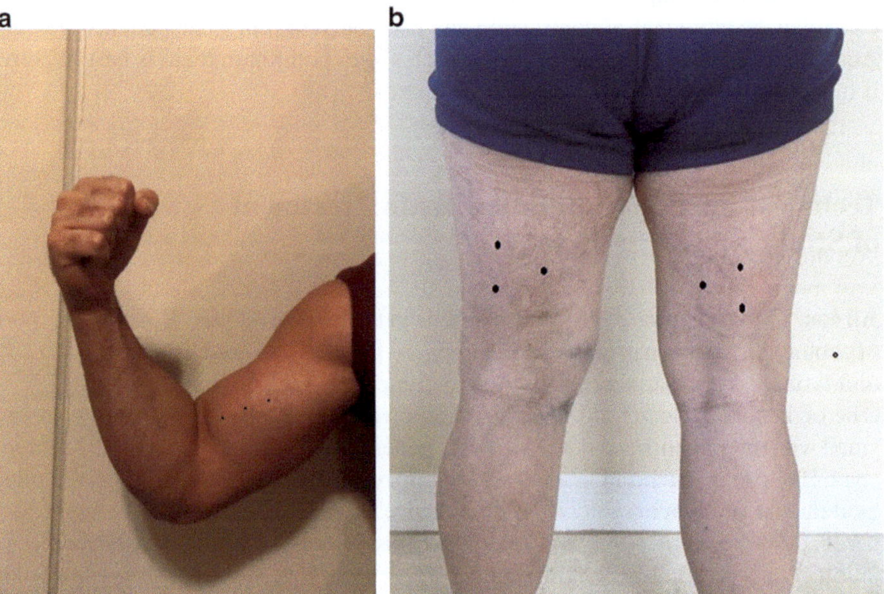

Fig. 6.4 (**a**) Biceps and (**b**) Hamstring

Table 6.2 Approximate doses of Botox or Xeomin with approximately comparable units per muscle, per side for some of the commonly injected muscles in stroke spasticity

Muscle	Dose in units (Botox or Xeomin) per muscle
Biceps	60–100
Triceps	60–100
Wrist flexors	40–50
Hamstring (knee flexor-back of the thigh)	60–200
Quadriceps (knee extensor-front of the thigh)	50–100
Gastrocnemius (foot flexor-back of the leg)	40–80

For Dysport the dose can be multiplied by 2.5–3 times and for Myobloc multiplied by 40–50 times

severe spasticity. Unfortunately, in elderly patients, these medications often cause undesirable side effects, the most disturbing among them are sedation and depressed level of consciousness On the contrary, botulinum toxin injections do not cause sedation or depress the level of consciousness. During the Covid era, restriction of contacts forced some patients who were receiving botulinum toxin therapy for post-stroke spasticity to discontinue treatment. In one study [22], 72.2% and 70.9% of the patients following discontinuation of botulinum toxin therapy, reported significant worsening of spasticity and deterioration of the quality of life, respectively.

In some patients, after stroke, both upper and lower limbs show significant degree of spasticity impairing the patient's quality of life. In such cases, treatment of both limbs with botulinum toxin for spasticity is justified. However, injection of both upper and lower limbs in one session requires larger amount of botulinum toxins especially if large thigh muscles are involved in spasticity. This raises the question of what constitutes a safe amount of toxin to inject in one session.

Currently, FDA recommends not to exceed 600 units of Botox or Zeomin per injection session (2.5–3 times more for Dysport). It has been shown that treatment with 600 units of Botox in one session is safe as side effects are few and insignificant [23]. However, for some years now, investigators have wondered if this upper limit is too restrictive and injecting a larger dose would be safe. Addressing this point, Dr. Wissel and his colleagues have published the results of a combined European-American investigation on 155 patients with spasticity in whom doses of Xeomin (a botulinum toxin A with units similar to Botox) were escalated over several months from 400 to 600 and then, ultimately, to 800 units per session of treatment [24]. They found that increasing the dose was more efficacious in reducing spasticity, but did not increase the percentage or severity of side effects. The main side effects were diarrhea and minor throat infections, noted in 5% of the patients. The higher dose allowed treatment of both upper and lower limbs in one session and improved the patients' quality of life. Although, more studies are needed to justify the high dose toxin therapy in spasticity, publications by expert panels already support the use of higher doses of Botox for certain cases of combined upper and lower limb spasticity [23, 25].

Development of antibodies after repeated botulinum toxin injections, specially when using large doses of the toxin has been a concern to clinicians and researchers alike. The so-called neutralizing antibodies, when they develop, can potentially lead to cessation of the response in some patients. However, research in patients who received repeated injections of Botox has found that these patients developed only a low level of antibodies (0.3%) [26]. Furthermore, it has been shown that in many patients development of neutralizing antibodies do not correspond to development of unresponsiveness (specially in case of type B toxin). In the study of Wissel et al. [24], none of the patients who were treated with high doses of Botulinum toxin-A (800 units) developed antibodies. Furthermore, the use of Xeomin (a type A toxin similar to Botox with comparable unit strength) do not lead to antibody formation due to lack of antigenic proteins. Bakheit et al. [27] also found no antibodies to botulinum toxin after treatment of 27 patients with high doses of the toxin.

Spasticity can have age and gender specific hazards: In women, severe spasticity of lower limbs when involving the adductor muscles (muscles that bring the thighs together) can interfere with urination and sexual function. In children, severe spasticity of adductor muscles can lead to dislocation of the hip and necessitate performance of corrective surgery.

Botulinum Toxin Therapy for Pain Associated with Stroke

Muscle pain is a common complaint in patients who develop spasticity after stroke. Pain is often measured on a scale of 0–10 (visual analogue scale/VAS). A value of over 4 is considered to represent a pain severe enough to interfere with daily activities. In a Canadian study, Dr. Shaikh and his colleagues found that 65% of their patients with post-stroke spasticity had associated muscle pain [28]. The pain was more noticeable during movements. Most patients (80%) believed that their muscle pain was related to their stiff, spastic muscles. Following Botox injections, 62% of the patients reported pain relief within days after injection.

Immobility of the joints after stroke, caused by muscle paralysis, often leads to joint degeneration with subsequent chronic joint pain. As described in Chap. 4, botulinum toxins in addition to acetylcholine, also inhibit the function of a variety of pain transmitters. This inhibition of pain transmitters occurs in the peripheral nervous system as well as in the central nervous system as the molecule of the toxin travels from the site of injection to the spinal cord and influences the sensory cells that convey pain sensation to the brain. Injection of Botox (and other toxins) into the joints has been shown to alleviate joint pain in several kinds of joint problems [29] (Chap. 12 of this book on orthopedic indications). Chronic joint pain after stroke, specially pain in the shoulder joint, has been shown to diminish after botulinum toxin injections into the involved joint.

Botulinum Toxin Therapy of Persistent Drooling After Stroke

In some patients with stroke, excessive drooling becomes an annoying problem. This is because secreted saliva cannot be cleared from the mouth due to the paralysis of the facial muscles (usually on one side). In such patients, reduction in saliva production would be helpful. It has been shown in both animals and human that injection of Botox and other botulinum toxins into the salivary glands (parotid, submaxillary—Fig. 6.5) reduces the production of saliva [30] (Fig. 6.6). This is because the chemical that conveys the nerve signal to the salivary glands and initiates secretion of saliva is acetylcholine; the same chemical that activates the muscle. As was discussed in earlier, botulinum toxins inhibit the release of acetylcholine at the nerve endings.

Parotid gland, the largest of the three salivary glands, is located at the angle of the jaw, a few millimeters under the skin (Fig. 6.6) and is the main target for this treatment. Parotid injections are done with a very small needle, preferably gauge 30. A penetration of 4–5 mm is sufficient. Usually 2–4 sites are injected within the gland, preferably under ultrasound visualization of the gland. However, since ultrasound machines are expensive, many clinicians inject parotid without using the ultrasound machine. Experience of the author of this chapter has shown that even without direct visualization of the gland, the yield of procedure is high and majority of patients express satisfaction after blind injection. Injections take less than a minute and are associated with little discomfort. Numbing the skin is not necessary. Injections need to be repeated every 3–6 months.

Details of saliva secretion, anatomy of salivary glands and effects of botulinum toxins on saliva production are presented in Chap. 14 of this book.

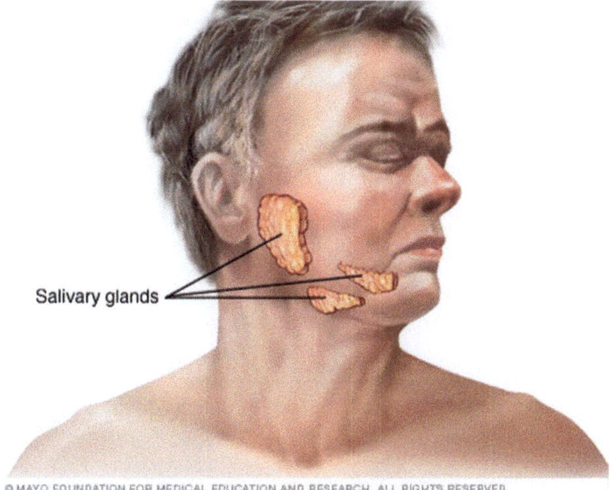

Fig. 6.5 Salivary glands. (Reproduced with permission of Mayo foundation)

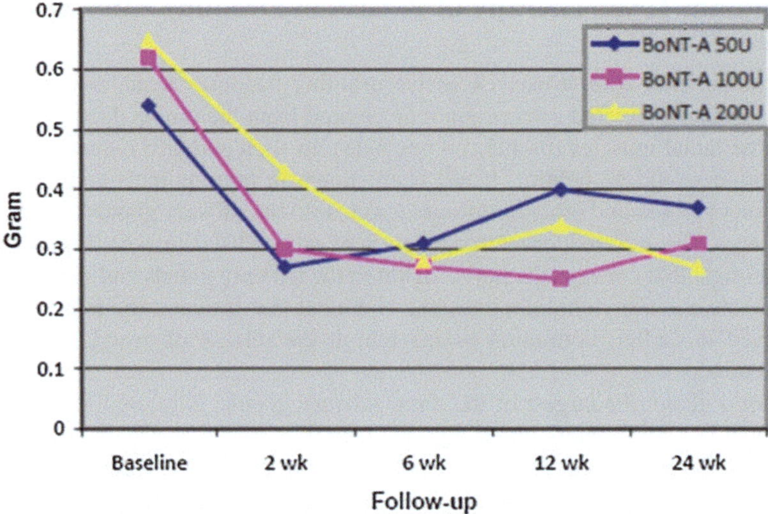

Fig. 6.6 Injection of Dysport (botulinum type A) even in a small dose blocks the secretion of the saliva from the parotid gland. (From Mazlan and co-workers. Courtesy of MDPI publisher Reproduced under (http://creativecommons.org/licenses/by/4.0/))

Movement Disorders After Stroke

A variety of involuntary movement can develop after stroke either due to damage to critical brain areas or due to damage to muscles that receive their nerves from the brain. Many patients with stroke demonstrate weakness of half of the face on the side of limb weakness. The weak eyelids or facial muscles sometimes develop bothersome and persistent involuntary twitches. Injection of small amounts of Botox into these muscles with a fine needle often suppresses the lid or facial movements for 3–4 months.

Dystonia is a movement disorder characterized by twisting and turning, flexion or extension of a joint leading to abnormal postures. Dystonia may develop after stroke affecting the muscles opposite to the side of brain damage. In stroke patients, dystonia is often mixed with spasticity. Dystonia is one of the most responsive movement disorders to botulinum toxin therapy [10].

Conclusion

Introduction of botulinum toxin therapy to clinical medicine has revolutionized the management of stroke related spasticity. Treatment of spastic muscles after stroke with botulinum toxins is effective and has improved the patients' quality of life. Recent data indicates safety of this treatment even with relatively high doses (up to

800 units for Botox or Xeomin). Botulinum toxin therapy also relieves the pain associated with spasticity or chronic joint pain in the paralyzed limb as well as reducing drooling. At the present time treatment of spasticity (after stroke, head and spinal cord injury and in children with cerebral palsy) constitutes one of the largest practices of botulinum toxin therapy in the US and worldwide.

References

1. Benjamin EJ, Blaha MJ, Chiuve SE, Cushman M, Das SR, Deo R, de Ferranti SD, Floyd J, Fornage M, Gillespie C, et al. Heart disease and stroke statistics—2017 update: a report from the American Heart Association. Circulation. 2017;135:e146–603. https://doi.org/10.1161/CIR.000000000000048.
2. Kochanek KD, et al. Deaths: final data for 2009. Natl Vital Stat Rep. 2011;60:1–116.
3. Herculana-houzel S. The human brain in numbers: a linearly scaled up primate brain. Front Hum Neurosci. 2009, Nov 9;3:31. https://doi.org/10.3389/neuro.09.031.2009. eCollection.
4. Söllner T, Rothman JE. Neurotransmission: harnessing fusion machinery at the synapse. Trends Neurosci. 1994 Aug;17(8):344–8. https://doi.org/10.1016/0166-2236(94)90178-3.
5. Welmer AK, Widén Holmqvist L, Sommerfeld DK. Location and severity of spasticity in the first 1-2 weeks and at 3 and 18 months after stroke. Eur J Neurol. 2010 May;17(5):720–5. https://doi.org/10.1111/j.1468-1331.2009.02915.x. Epub 2009 Dec 29.
6. Gracies JM. Pathophysiology of spastic paresis. I: paresis and soft tissue changes. Muscle Nerve. 2005 May;31(5):535–51. https://doi.org/10.1002/mus.20284.
7. Moeini-Naghani I, Hashemi-Zonouz T, Jabbari B. Botulinum toxin treatment of spasticity in adults and children. Semin Neurol. 2016 Feb;36(1):64–72. https://doi.org/10.1055/s-0036-1571847. Epub 2016 Feb 11.
8. Hsieh JC, Penn RD. Intrathecal baclofen in the treatment of adult spasticity. Neurosurg Focus. 2006 Aug 15;21(2):e5. https://doi.org/10.3171/foc.2006.21.2.6.
9. Sharififar S, Shuster JJ, Bishop MD. Adding electrical stimulation during standard rehabilitation after stroke to improve motor function. A systematic review and meta-analysis. Ann Phys Rehabil Med. 2018 Sep;61(5):339–44. https://doi.org/10.1016/j.rehab.2018.06.005. Epub 2018 Jun 26.
10. Jankovic J. Botulinum toxin: state of the art. Mov Disord. 2017;32:1132–8.
11. Kaku M, Simpson DM. Spotlight on botulinum toxin and its potential in the treatment of stroke-related spasticity. Drug Des Devel Ther. 2016;10:1085–99.
12. Moeini-Naghani I, Jabbari B. Botulinum toxin treatment in cerebrovascular disease. In: Jabbari B, editor. Botulinum toxin treatment in clinical medicine. Cham: Springer; 2018. p. 213–30.
13. Wissel J, Ri S. Assessment, goal setting, and botulinum neurotoxin a therapy in the management of post-stroke spastic movement disorder: updated perspectives on best practice. Expert Rev Neurother. 2022 Jan;22(1):27–42. https://doi.org/10.1080/14737175.2021.2021072. Epub 2021 Dec 30.
14. Bonikowski M, Sławek J. Safety and efficacy of botulinum toxin type A preparations in cerebral palsy – an evidence-based review. Neurol Neurochir Pol. 2021;55(2):158–64. https://doi.org/10.5603/PJNNS.a2021.0032. Epub 2021 Apr 16.
15. Lindsay C, Ispoglou S, Helliwell B, Hicklin D, Sturman S, Pandyan A. Can the early use of botulinum toxin in post stroke spasticity reduce contracture development? A randomised controlled trial. Clin Rehabil. 2021 Mar;35(3):399–409. https://doi.org/10.1177/0269215520963855. Epub 2020 Oct 11. PMID: 33040610; PMCID: PMC7944432.
16. Wissel J, Ri S, Kivi A. Early versus late injections of Botulinumtoxin type A in post-stroke spastic movement disorder: a literature review. Toxicon. 2023 Jun 15;229:107150. https://doi.org/10.1016/j.toxicon.2023.107150. Epub 2023 May 3.

17. Baricich A, Wein T, Cinone N, Bertoni M, Picelli A, Chisari C, Molteni F, Santamato A. BoNT-A for post-stroke spasticity: guidance on unmet clinical needs from a Delphi panel approach. Toxins (Basel). 2021 Mar 25;13(4):236. https://doi.org/10.3390/toxins13040236. PMID: 33805988; PMCID: PMC8064476.
18. Picelli A, Santamato A, Cosma M, Baricich A, Chisari C, Millevolte M, Prete CD, Mazzù I, Girardi P, Smania N. Early botulinum toxin type A injection for post-stroke spasticity: a longitudinal cohort study. Toxins (Basel). 2021 May 24;13(6):374. https://doi.org/10.3390/toxins13060374. PMID: 34073918; PMCID: PMC8225105.
19. Gracies JM, Bayle N, Goldberg S, Simpson DM. Botulinum toxin type B in the spastic arm: a randomized, double-blind, placebo-controlled, preliminary study. Arch Phys Med Rehabil. 2014 Jul;95(7):1303–11. https://doi.org/10.1016/j.apmr.2014.03.016. Epub 2014 Apr 4.
20. Alter KE, Karp BI. Ultrasound guidance for botulinum neurotoxin chemodenervation procedures. Toxins (Basel). 2017 Dec 28;10(1):pii: E18. https://doi.org/10.3390/toxins10010018.
21. Kaňovský P, Elovic EP, Munin MC, Hanschmann A, Pulte I, Althaus M, Hiersemenzel R, Marciniak C. Sustained efficacy of incobotulinumtoxina repeated injections for upper-limb post-stroke spasticity: a post hoc analysis. J Rehabil Med. 2021 Jan 5;53(1):jrm00138. https://doi.org/10.2340/16501977-2760. PMID: 33112408; PMCID: PMC8772361.
22. Santamato A, Facciorusso S, Spina S, Cinone N, Avvantaggiato C, Santoro L, Ciritella C, Smania N, Picelli A, Gasperini G, Molteni F, Baricich A, Fiore P. Discontinuation of botulinum neurotoxin type-A treatment during COVID-19 pandemic: an Italian survey in post stroke and traumatic brain injury patients living with spasticity. Eur J Phys Rehabil Med. 2021 Jun;57(3):424–33. https://doi.org/10.23736/S1973-9087.20.06478-3. Epub 2020 Dec 2.
23. Kirshblum S, Solinsky R, Jasey N, Hampton S, Didesch M, Seidel B, Botticello A. Adverse event profiles of high dose botulinum toxin injections for spasticity. PM R. 2020 Apr;12(4):349–55. https://doi.org/10.1002/pmrj.12240. Epub 2019 Oct 1.
24. Wissel J, Bensmail D, Ferreira JJ, et al. Safety and efficacy of incobotulinum toxin A doses up to 800 U in limb spasticity. Neurology. 2017;88:1321–8.
25. Baricich A, Picelli A, Santamato A, Carda S, de Sire A, Smania N, Cisari C, Invernizzi M. Safety profile of high-dose botulinum toxin type A in post-stroke spasticity treatment. Clin Drug Investig. 2018 Nov;38(11):991–1000. https://doi.org/10.1007/s40261-018-0701-x.
26. Jankovic J, Carruthers J, Naumann M, Ogilvie P, Boodhoo T, Attar M, Gupta S, Singh R, Soliman J, Yushmanova I, Brin MF, Shen J. Neutralizing antibody formation with onabotulinumtoxinA (BOTOX®) treatment from global registration studies across multiple indications: a meta-analysis. Toxins (Basel). 2023 May 17;15(5):342. https://doi.org/10.3390/toxins15050342. PMID: 37235376; PMCID: PMC10224273.
27. Bakheit AM, Liptrot A, Newton R, Pickett AM. The effect of total cumulative dose, number of treatment cycles, interval between injections, and length of treatment on the frequency of occurrence of antibodies to botulinum toxin type A in the treatment of muscle spasticity. Int J Rehabil Res. 2012 Mar;35(1):36–9. https://doi.org/10.1097/MRR.0b013e32834df64f.
28. Shaikh A, Phadke CP, Ismail F, et al. Relationship between botulinum toxin, spasticity, and pain: a survey of patient perception. J Neurol Sci. 2016;43:311–5.
29. Castiglione A, Bagnato S, Boccagni C, Romano MC, Galardi G. Efficacy of intra-articular injection of botulinum toxin type A in refractory hemiplegic shoulder pain. Arch Phys Med Rehabil. 2011;92(7):1034–7.
30. Mazlan M, Rajasegaran S, Engkasan JP. A double-blind randomized controlled trial vestigating the most efficacious dose of botulinum toxin-a for sialorrhea treatment in Asian adults with neurological diseases. Toxins (Basel). 2015;7:3758–70.

Chapter 7
Botulinum Toxin Treatment in Multiple Sclerosis

Abstract According to the latest data from the National Multiple Sclerosis Society (2019) nearly one million people live in US with this disease annually. The disease process destroys the nerve fibers in the spinal cord and brain myelin substance resulting in motor and sensory problems. Injection of botulinum toxins into the stiff muscles of patients with multiple sclerosis reduces the muscle tone and improves muscle function. In patients with bladder dysfunction, injection of botulinum toxins into the wall of the bladder decreases abnormal urges to urinate and regulates bladder function. Involuntary and painful muscle spasms in MS patients, can be subdued by injection of botulinum toxin into the affected muscles.

Keywords Multiple sclerosis · Botulinum toxin · Overactive bladder · Neurogenic bladder · Spasticity · Muscle spasms

Introduction

World-wide, multiple sclerosis affects over three million people and is considered the most common cause of disability in the young [1]. In 2019, a study funded by National Multiple Sclerosis Society reported that approximately one million people affected by multiple sclerosis live in US [2]. The people in the north of US living in colder climates, women and whites are more affected than others. The estimated total economic burden of MS in US was $85.4 billion in 2019, with a direct medical cost of $63.3 billion and indirect and nonmedical costs of $22.1 billion. The average per-person annual medical costs was $65,612 [3].

In the late nineteenth century, a famous French neurologist by the name of Charcot was the first to describe, in detail, the symptoms and the pathology of multiple sclerosis. Multiple sclerosis damages both motor and sensory nerve fibers. Motor fibers originate from brain cells and go to the muscles while the sensory fibers convey sensations from skin to the brain. These nerve fibers normally have a protective sheath on their surface that enhances the conduction of electrical signals flowing in them both away and towards the brain. This sheath of tissue that covers

B. Jabbari, *Botulinum Toxin Treatment*,
https://doi.org/10.1007/978-3-031-54471-2_7

the nerves is composed of a specific fat called myelin. Multiple sclerosis is, therefore, considered one of the diseases that specifically destroys myelin and, hence, called a demyelinating disease. Loss of myelin leaves scars in the brain and/or spinal cord and slows the nerve conduction. These scars (plaques) are easily detectable by modern imaging techniques such as Magnetic Resonance Imaging (MRI). Currently, MRI is the most useful diagnostic device used to confirm or support the diagnosis of multiple sclerosis (Fig. 7.1). The scars or plaques (areas of lost myelin) of MS are often multiple and occur at different levels of the central nervous system within the brain and/or spinal cord (multiple sclerosis). One can also use the changes that takes place in the composition of the cerebrospinal fluid (CSF) to confirm the diagnosis of MS. Cerebrospinal fluid is produced in the brain and flows inside the

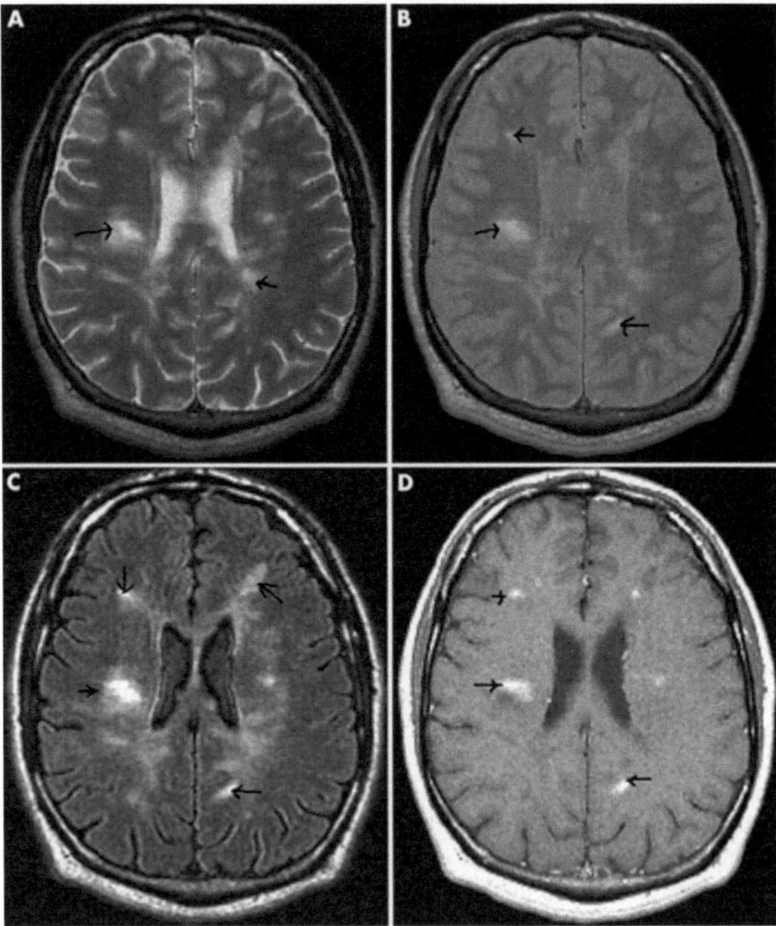

Fig. 7.1 Multiple brain lesions in a patient with multiple sclerosis. The lesions, white patches, marked by arrows in the brain slices on MRI, represent abnormal areas of the brain devoid of myelin. (From Trip and Miller 2005, reproduced with permission from publisher (BMJ group) [4])

spinal canal, all the way from the upper neck to the low back area. To test CSF, a small amount of this fluid is removed for examination by a procedure called spinal tap. For spinal tap, after numbing the skin, a needle is placed at midline between two low backbones (vertebral bodies) in the lumbar area. In most patients with MS, examination of CSF shows an elevation of certain specific proteins (immunoglobulins).

Multiple sclerosis can cause a variety of symptoms depending on the location of the lesions [5]. A large number of patients complain of motor symptoms, such as sudden weakness or even total paralysis of one limb. Others may have sensory symptoms, often described as tingling and numbness affecting some part of the body. Sudden onset of diminished or even total loss of vision in one eye is also a frequent complaint. Symptoms of MS fluctuate in intensity, disappear and reappear over time. In chronic cases, plaques accumulate in the brain or/and spinal cord and lead to permanent loss of function.

The cause of multiple sclerosis is still not fully understood. In current scientific thinking, multiple sclerosis is defined as an "autoimmune disease". Our immune system normally protects us against germs like viruses or bacteria. When body is exposed to foreign invaders, immune system sends a group of fighter cells to attack and destroy the invaders. Usually, the immune system can differentiate between one's own cells and foreign cells. In an autoimmune disease, the immune system mistakenly attacks the cells and organs of one's body. The damage to nervous system in multiple sclerosis is believed to be due to an immune disorder which is associated with an abnormal reaction of lymphocytes (certain blood cells).

In the past two decades, significant strides have been taken to find drugs that work against these immune reactions while aiming to arrest progression of MS and prevent appearance of new lesions in the brain and/or spinal cord. Several newly discovered drugs have succeeded to slow the course of multiple sclerosis and prevent appearance of new lesions in the central nervous system. The most successful of these are drugs known as disease modifying antibodies (DMA). Several of these drugs are now FDA approved; Alemtuzumab, Ofatuzumab and Ublitucimab seems to be the most effective among DMAs. These drugs can slowdown progression of MS and, in many cases, prevent appearance of new lesions in the brain and spinal cord. Unfortunately, DMAs are very expensive costing a sum of $ 34,000 per person per year [3]. Furthermore, despite their effectiveness, still a large number of patients with MS are left with permanent disabilities due to multiple damages sustained within brain and spinal cord over years. Among these disabilities, stiffness of muscles (spasticity) and/or dysfunction of bladder can significantly impair the patients' quality of life. As discussed in Chaps. 6 (stroke and spasticity) and 10 (botulinum toxin therapy in bladder dysfunction), botulinum toxin injections have a significant potential to improve spasticity and bladder dysfunction regardless of the cause.

Botulinum Toxin Treatment of Spasticity in Multiple Sclerosis

In multiple sclerosis, similar to other disease conditions that damage the brain and spinal cord (stroke, trauma), muscles gradually weaken and show increased tone, become stiff and spastic. In many patients with MS, this spasticity can be quite severe and can interfere with the activities of daily living. The spastic muscle often remains contracted resulting in impaired timing and precision of movements. Using fingers and hands for eating, washing, shaving, dressing and any other fine movements becomes exceedingly difficult. In the lower limbs, spasticity adds to weakness and impairs balance. Adductor muscles of the thigh (muscles that bring the thighs together) often show marked spasticity in multiple sclerosis [5]. As a result, sustained contraction of these muscles keeps the thighs stiffly together, a position that impairs normal leg movements and disrupts ambulation. The affected patients complain of poor balance and frequent falls. In women, severe adductor spasticity can lock the thighs together, interfere with sex and disrupt urination.

As time goes by, the spastic muscles become painful to move. The ensuing immobility leads to replacement of muscle fibers by non-elastic tissue, a condition that is termed contracture. Muscles affected by contracture are often shortened and non-functional.

The drugs that treat spasticity including baclofen, tizanidine and valium often have undesirable side effects such a confusion and sedation. In severe cases of spasticity, especially if it predominantly involves the legs, baclofen can be delivered to the body through a baclofen pump. Use of baclofen pump is an involved procedure requiring insertion of a catheter into the spinal canal through which baclofen is continuously delivered into the spinal fluid. The procedure requires collaboration between an expert neurosurgeon, neurologist and a trained nurse who could do careful titration of the drug. Miscalculations can lead to overdosing, leading to serious complications such as suppressed level of consciousness and seizures. Other severe cases of spasticity can be treated by injection of phenol into the nerve that supplies the tight and spastic muscles. Phenol injections are effective but reserved for very severe cases when all other means fail since such injections destroy the nerve permanently. Pharmacological treatments of spasticity are usually combined with physical therapy that includes passive and active exercises. It is believed that 80% of the patients with multiple sclerosis will experience spasticity of muscles some time during their lifetime. In a large US registry of patients with multiple sclerosis, 72% of the patients demonstrated moderate to severe spasticity on examination [6].

Currently, four globally marketed botulinum toxins are approved by FDA for use in the US. Three of these toxins are type A (Botox, Xeomin and Dysport) and one toxin is type B (Myobloc-called Neurobloc in Europe). For detailed description of toxin types and information on toxin characteristics, the reader is referred to Chaps. 2 and 3 of this book. Although the units of these four toxins are not exactly comparable, the following approximations are used in clinical practice and clinical research: 1 unit of Botox = 1 unit of Xeomin=2.5 to 3 units of Dysport = 40–50 units of Myobloc.

Botulinum toxin treatment (with Botox and other toxin brands) provides a reasonable alternative to pharmacotherapy for moderate to severe spasticity of multiple sclerosis. In general, botulinum toxins have less side effects than anti-spasticity drugs. As described in more details in Chaps. 2 and 3 of this book, botulinum toxins decrease the tone of the muscle and relax it via blocking the release of acetylcholine at the junction of nerve to muscle. Acetylcholine is a chemical that upon reaching the muscles allows the electrical nerve signal enter to the muscle and activate it.

In 1990, Dr. Snow, a Canadian investigator and his colleagues reported that injection of Botox into the adductor muscles of the thigh (muscles that bring the thighs together) significantly reduced the spasticity and improved hygiene in seven out of nine patients with multiple sclerosis [7, 8]. A total of 400 units of Botox was divided among three thigh adductor muscles. Following this pioneering observation, several subsequent high quality studies with much larger number of patients (some in hundreds) have supported the value of intramuscular injection of botulinum toxins in reducing spasticity of muscles in multiple sclerosis [9–14]. Furthermore, long-term observations over several years have shown that repeated injections at every 3–4 months are well tolerated and the satisfactory effects continues over months and years of treatment. These studies have also shown the safety of botulinum toxin therapy for treating of MS-related spasticity. Comparative observations have shown that MS-related spasticity is as responsive as any other form of spasticity to the botulinum therapy and the effective dose per muscle in multiple sclerosis is comparable to that used for spasticity caused by medical conditions other than MS such as stroke, spasticity after brain and spinal cord trauma. For this reason, botulinum toxin therapy is now among the first lines of treatment for spasticity in multiple sclerosis.

Technique of Injection

The injection technique for spastic muscles in multiple sclerosis is very similar to what has been described in Chap. 5 for spasticity in stroke. The size of the muscle and the degree of tightness of the muscle determine the dose. The dose is delivered in units. In the upper limbs, for small muscles of the forearm and hand, the dose varies from 5 to 20 units per muscle, whereas, larger muscles (i.e. biceps) may require up to 100 units (for Botox or Xeomin, multiply by 2.5–3 for Dysport and by 40–50 for Myobloc.) Large muscles of lower limb (s) may require larger doses. For instance, severe spasticity of hamstring (the large muscle in the back of the thigh that flexes the knee) may require 150–200 units (Botox). The injecting needle is thin and short for upper limb muscles but longer needles may be required for larger muscles of the lower limb. Injections are delivered at two or three sites into the larger muscles, using anatomical landmarks for identifying nerve-muscle junctions where injections are most effective. For small muscles of the forearm (flexors of fingers or wrist) the muscle may need to be identified by electromyography (recording electrical activity of muscle), nerve stimulation or ultrasound.

Recent studies have shown that larger doses of Botox or Xeomin of up to 800 units, can be injected in one session (into 3–5 muscles), without any serious side effects [15, 16]. Side effects include local pain at the site of injection for a few minutes, minor transient bleeding, and a mild, transient flu like reaction experienced in 5–10% of the patients. It should be remembered that toxin preparation needs to be done by trained personnel and injections should be carried out by experienced injectors familiar with the muscle anatomy and proper technique of injection. Dose miscalculations can lead to serious side effects such as total paralysis and may endanger patient's life. The effect of botulinum toxin injection into spastic muscles becomes evident in 2–5 days and peaks at 2–3 weeks. The muscle relaxing effect of the toxin can last 3–4 months, and then, needs to be repeated for sustainability. This effect is to a large degree, dose dependent considering the size of the muscle and degree of muscle tightness. Long-term data, up to 15 injection cycles (every 3–4 months) are now available and attest to the safety of botulinum toxin therapy in multiple sclerosis [11, 14].

Case Report A 32 years-old female with multiple sclerosis was referred to the Yale Botulinum Toxin Clinic for treatment of severe spasticity of the thigh muscles. For several years, she had suffered from severe tightness of her thigh muscles, the overactivity of which pulled her thighs constantly together. This issue worsened during walking, and impaired her balance. Over years, she had also noticed more difficulty in urination. Oral medications provided modest relief.

On examination, the adductor muscles of the thigh, close to the groin (Fig. 7.2a) very very tight. She was injected with Botox into adductors—150 units/side at two points (Fig. 7.2b). After a week, she reported marked relaxation of her thigh

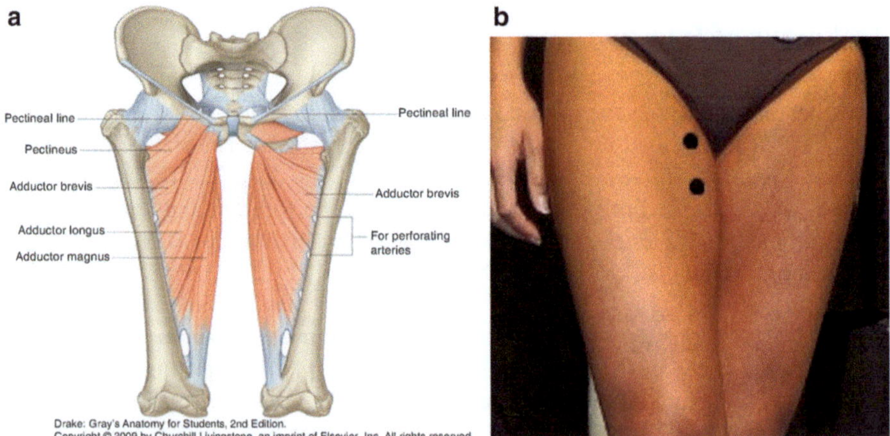

Fig. 7.2 (**a**) Three adductor muscles of the thigh that bring the thighs together; short (brevis), long (longus) and large (magnus) (From Drake Anatomy for students reproduced with permission from Elsevier). (**b**) Common sites of botulinum toxin injection for adductor muscle spasticity

muscles allowing her to stand and walk better with less fear of falling. Moving in bed became easier and she slept better. Movement of the thighs was no longer painful. Hygiene related tasks were carried out with more ease and comfort and her urination improved. The satisfactory effects of Botox lasted for 3 months. Repeated injection 3–4 months sustained relaxation of thigh muscles over a follow up period of 5 years.

Botulinum Toxin Therapy for Bladder Problems in Multiple Sclerosis

Many patients with multiple sclerosis develop a variety of bladder problems as the disease progresses. Bladder, as the organ of urine storage and emptying, functions mainly with three muscles. The major bladder muscle that controls storage and emptying functions of the bladder is called detrusor muscle. This muscle that spreads over nearly all of the bladder wall can expand during urine storage. When the volume of urine in the bladder reaches a certain level, sensory nerves of the bladder signal the bladder centers located in different parts of the brain (there are more than one) to tell the detrusor muscle to contract. Detrusor muscle contraction propels the urine against the hole in the lower part of the bladder through which the urine leaves the bladder. Two circular muscles, called sphincters, control the opening and closing of this hole. The one closer to the inside of the bladder is called inner and the one further out is called outer sphincter. Inner sphincter automatically relaxes after contraction of detrusor muscle. This relaxation is not under conscious control. The outer sphincter is under conscious control and can be relaxed by will, letting the urine out in an appropriate setting. A complex network of nerve cells located in the brain and spinal cord control the bladder function. As spinal cord nerve cells and nerve fibers are major contributors to the innervation of bladder, damage to the spinal cord in multiple sclerosis (with lesions similar to those seen in the brain), (Fig. 7.1) results in erratic and poorly timed contractions of the detrusor muscle with subsequent development of bladder symptoms. These symptoms include frequent urge to urinate and frequent urination as well as bed-wetting at night and urinary incontinence during the day. Poor emptying of the bladder predisposes the patient to development of bladder infections. In more severe cases, the urine can back up toward the kidney and cause kidney damage. This type of bladder dysfunction in MS is called neurogenic bladder i.e. a bladder problem that is related to damage to the nerve supply of the bladder.

According to National Multiple Sclerosis Society, bladder dysfunction occurs in at least 80% of patients with multiple sclerosis during the course of illness [17]. The symptoms of bladder dysfunction in MS include leakage of urine, urinary urgency, frequent urinations at night and urinary incontinence. What happens to the bladder muscle in MS is somewhat similar to what happens to the neuromuscular junction leading to muscle spasticity as described earlier in this chapter. The muscle (in this case detrusor muscle of the bladder), after being weakened by damage to its nerve supply, gradually develops increased tone, and becomes overactive as in other muscles of body with spasticity. Since acetylcholine is also the chemical transmitter (from nerve ending) to the muscular layer of the bladder, injection of botulinum toxins into the bladder wall will subdue the bladder overactivity by reducing the effect of acetylcholine (see Chaps. 2 and 3 on mechanism of botulinum toxins function). The drugs that are used for control of bladder symptoms in MS are anticholinergics—Ditropan, Detrol—also work by reducing or blocking the effects of acetylcholine. The frequent side effects of these drugs such as blurring of vision, impaired memory and dryness of the mouth make them hard to tolerate especially when used for a long period of time.

In 2013, FDA approved the use of Botox for treatment of neurogenic, overactive bladder in multiple sclerosis based on the positive results of two large high quality, multicenter studies (DINGY studies) that investigated close to 700 patients with MS and spinal cord injury [18, 19]. A majority of the patients in these studies had multiple sclerosis. These studies have shown that injection of 200 units of Botox at multiple points into the bladder wall significantly improves the patients' urgency and incontinence as well as their quality of life. Patients also scored highly on a post-treatment satisfaction questionnaire confirming their satisfaction with the treatment.

The main side effect of botulinum toxin injections for bladder symptoms in MS is retention of urine which occurs in 25% of treated patients and may require daily, clean self-catheterization. For many patients with advanced MS, however, this is not problematic since they already have chronic urinary retention and have learned to catheterize themselves for months or years. Nevertheless, patients need to be alerted and trained for this side effect. However, some studies have found that with repeated injections of Botox (every 4–6 months) the incidence of urinary retention improves as time goes by. An analysis of 18 studies on 1553 MS patients in whom bladder dysfunction was treated with Botox injection into the detrusor muscle found sustenance of positive results after repeated injections and a low incidence of side effects [20].

More recently, high quality studies (double-blind and placebo-controlled) with other type A botulinum toxins (Dysport and Xeomin) have also shown efficacy in management of bladder dysfunction due to multiple sclerosis and traumatic spinal cord injury [21, 22]. It is likely that Dysport will soon receive FDA approval for treatment of the type of bladder dysfunction (neurogenic bladder) that occurs in patients with multiple sclerosis.

Injection Technique

Botox is marketed in a powder form stored in small vials. For all indications, it needs to be mixed with normal saline (salt water) before injection. Botox is very heat sensitive so it requires refrigeration. Botox vials marketed as 50, 100 and

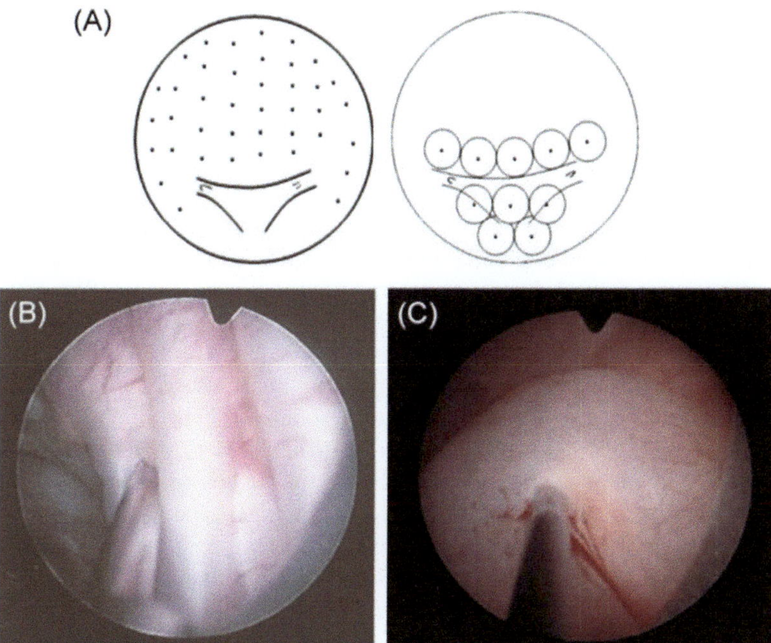

Fig. 7.3 Technique of bladder injection: (**A**) (top left) 30 injections for patients with severe symptoms, (top right) 10 injections for patients with mild symptoms (From Da Silva and coworkers. Toxicon 2015. Reproduced with permission from the publisher Elsevier). (**B and C**) site of injection just under the mucosa of bladder surface

300 units. A total of 200 units is recommended for treatment of overactive bladder in multiple sclerosis. Injections are carried out through a special instrument, cystoscope, that after entering the bladder can visualize inside the bladder via a small light. A hollow needle is attached to the cystoscope through which the injections are performed. The original FDA approved protocol calls for 30 sites of injections sparing the trigone (the lower, triangular par of bladder). Currently, however, different protocols are used at different institutions with the number of injection sites ranging from 20 to 40, including or not including bladder's trigone. Some authors, in patients with mild symptoms, only 10 sites including the tigone that is right in sensory nerves (Fig. 7.3).

Treatment of MS-associated Pain with Botulinum Toxins

Pain is a common symptom in multiple sclerosis. In one study, 63% of the patients with multiple sclerosis complained of chronic pain [13]. Among several types of pain in MS, three types are most frequent: neuropathic, pain associated with spasticity and tonic spasms.

Neuropathic Pain

Neuropathic pain has a burning, searing and jabbing quality; the most severe form of it involves the face in multiple sclerosis. Irritation of damaged nerve fibers that provide sensation to the face is believed to be the cause of facial pain in MS. The trigeminal nerve, the fifth of 12 nerves that exit the brain, provides sensation for the face, inside the mouth, the tongue and the throat. The pain is called trigeminal neuralgia (nerve pain related to the trigeminal nerve). Patients complain of severe bouts of pain lasting for seconds but recurring many times during the day. The most common type of trigeminal neuralgia, however, is seen in older individuals (>50 years of age) due to age related degeneration of this nerve. Trigeminal neuralgia is rare in young individuals. When it occurs in young individuals, one should think of MS. It can be seen in 1–3% of patients with multiple sclerosis [23].

Treatment of trigeminal neuralgia (TN) is difficult. Most patients are not happy with taking daily oral medications. High quality studies (double-blind, placebo-controlled) have shown that injection of Botox and other type A toxin (Chinese type A toxin: Prosigne) with a small and thin needle into skin of the face can alleviate the pain in classic trigeminal neuralgia that occurs in older patients [24–26]. Although no high quality studies are available with botulinum toxins for treatment of TN in multiple sclerosis, a retrospective observation in 31 patients with MS treated with Botox injections disclosed positive results [27]. In this observation, 52% of patients with MS and TN reported relief of facial pain after Botox injections versus 45% of the patients with primary TN (older individuals with no known cause).

How injection of botulinum toxin into and under the skin can help neuropathic pain (TN as an example) has been the subject of many investigations. It is now common knowledge based on both animal and human studies, that BoNTs not only inhibit the function of acetylcholine (nerve-muscle chemical transmitter), but also diminish the effect of a variety of chemicals that are essential for transmission of pain signals from skin to the brain [28–35]. Several of these neurotransmitters, such as substance P, glutamate, and calcitonin gene related peptide (CGRP) are now well known. Though still not approved by FDA for pain disorders (except for chronic migraine), botulinum toxin injection into and under the skin is now used by many clinicians for a variety of neuropathic pains such as pain associated with shingles, pain after limb trauma, heal pain of plantar fasciitis (common among runners) and other pain problems based on the published data from high quality studies [36–40].

Case Report

A 42 year-old women, with history of multiple sclerosis since age 18 with intermittent paralysis, sensory loss and visual symptoms, complained of intermittent severe facial pain. The pain involved the left side of the face and recurred many times daily. The episodes of pain were brief (lasting only seconds) but "brought tears to her eyes." The pain was described as jabbing and burning. She was treated with several

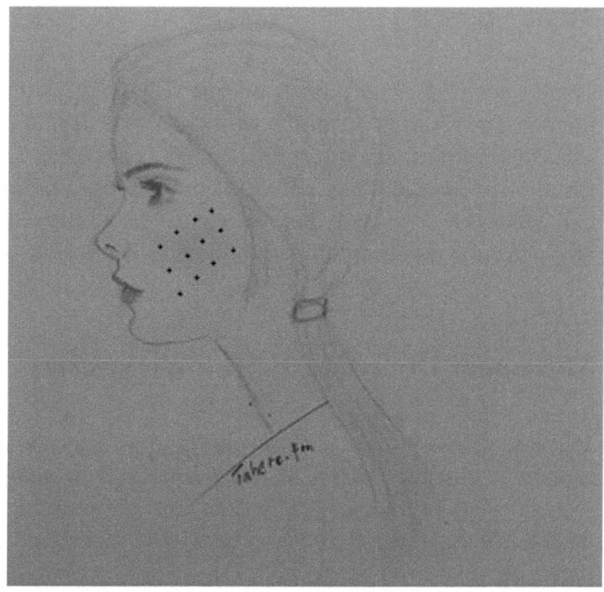

Fig. 7.4 Case report. Injections were carried out using a thin (gauge30), short needle and under the skin. (Drawing courtesy of Dr. Tahereh Mousavi)

medications including the commonly used drugs for trigeminal neuralgia; tegretol and gabapentin—that "did not help much". On the scale of 0 to 10, most of her pain episodes were described as 9 or 10 in severity. The pain occurred as many as 30 times per day. The MRI of her brain showed no abnormality to explain her facial pain. A neurological examination revealed no motor or sensory deficits. The affected area of the face was injected with Botox in a grid-like pattern, using a small thin needle. Injections were under the skin, 2.5 units per site at 12 sites (Fig. 7.4). She reported marked pain relief in a week post injection with the pain intensity dropping to 1–3 on a 0–10 scale. Repeated injections every 4 months had the same positive effect. No side effects were reported.

Pain Associated with Spasticity

As discussed earlier, stiff muscles in patients with multiple sclerosis are often painful. In a study of 1171 adult patients with MS and spasticity, moderate to severe pain was reported in 47% of the patients [41]. Muscle pain associated with spasticity can interfere with rest and sleep deteriorating the patients' quality of life. A literature review of this issue in 2022 assessed the efficacy of botulinum toxin injections for relieving pain associated with spasticity of MS [42]. In this review, seven of eight studies that used standard pain scales such as visual analogue scale (VAS), reported significant pain relief after botulinum toxin injections.

Tonic Spasms

Tonic spasms are intermittent muscle spasms often affecting wrists, feet, toes and fingers. The result is painful twisting of wrists or feet and flexion of toes or fingers. The cause of these painful spasms in MS is not clear, but it is generally attributed to irritation of damaged nerve fibers that travel from brain to muscles. Dr. Restivo and his coworkers reported that these spasms improved significantly when Botox, 80–120 units, was injected into forearm or leg muscles of five affected patients [43].

Movement Disorders in Multiple Sclerosis

Multiple sclerosis can cause involuntary movements of the muscle due to the disruption of muscle control at the brain level. In general, involuntary movements respond well to injection of BoNTs into the muscle through inhibition of nerve-muscle chemical transmitter, acetylcholine (described earlier). Two of these movements are discussed briefly here:

1. Tremor: a special form of tremor, called cerebellar tremor, is sometimes a disabling symptom in multiple sclerosis. Cerebellar tremor, unlike Parkinson tremor increases in amplitude during hand and forearm motion and can interfere with eating and writing. Cerebellum (called by some the little brain) is located below cerebrum—main part of the brain—in the back of the head, and through its extensive connections provides muscle coordination. Multiple sclerosis, via disruption of cerebellar connections, impairs the normal movements and causes a coarse limb tremor. In a double-blind, placebo controlled study of 23 patients with multiple sclerosis related forearm tremor, injection of Botox into the forearm muscles improved the tremor as well as witting of the patients significantly [44]. The drawback was development of some degree of weakness of forearm muscles that ceased within 6 weeks.
2. Facial myokymia (FM): FM is characterized by fine continuous twitching of small muscle fibers of the face seen in some patients with multiple sclerosis. It is due to disruption and irritation of nerve fibers at the base of the brain (brain stem). FM is not painful but a nuisance, esthetically unpleasant and often a cause of social embarrassment. Injection of a small amount of Botox (1 to 2) units (barely under the skin of the face) and into the twitching muscles can reduce or stops the movements for 3–4 months [45, 46].

Treatment of Difficulty with Swallowing (Dysphagia) and Difficulty in Phonation (Dysphonia)

Muscles of swallowing, like other muscles of the body in MS, develop increased tone and stiffness as the disease progresses. This stiffness associated with increased muscle reflexes results in difficulty in swallowing. A well-designed study assessed the effects of Botox injection into the muscles of esophagus (the tube connecting the mouth to the stomach) in 14 patients with MS and difficulty in swallowing. Patients were followed carefully at 1, 4, 6, 12, 16, 18 and 24 months. Difficulty in swallowing improved in all patients following injection of Botox into muscles of the back of the throat that initially had unusually high tones [47].

Dysphonia or spasmodic dysphonia is impaired phonation due to disturbed function of the vocal cords. Most of the affected patients have a shrill voice due to overactivity of the adductor muscles of the vocal cord (muscles that bring the vocal cords together during phonation). Spasmodic dysphonia may occur during the course of a variety of disease conditions including MS. Injection of small amounts of Botox into adductor muscles of vocal cords is an established treatment for management of persistent spasmodic dysphonia [48]. Observations in small number of patients with MS and spasmodic dysphonia have shown that this mode of treatment is also effective in MS-related spasmodic dysphonia [49].

Conclusion

Botulinum toxin therapy is useful for several disturbing symptoms of multiple sclerosis. Treatment of tight and stiff muscles (spasticity) and bladder symptoms (inappropriate urge to urinate, leaking and urinary incontinence) are the two most widely used indications which have shown to improve the patients' quality of life. Emerging data on treatment of facial pain, tonic muscle spasms as well as swallowing and phonation difficulties in MS are also encouraging and expand the utility of BoNT therapy in multiple sclerosis. The role of botulinum toxin therapy in multiple sclerosis is detailed in recent reviews on this subject [50, 51].

References

1. Baccouche I, Bensmail D, Leblong E, Fraudet B, Aymard C, Quintaine V, Pottier S, Lansaman T, Malot C, Gallien P, Levy J. Goal-setting in multiple sclerosis-related spasticity treated with botulinum toxin: the GASEPTOX study. Toxins (Basel). 2022 Aug 24;14(9):582. https://doi.org/10.3390/toxins14090582. PMID: 36136520; PMCID: PMC9504895.
2. Wallin MT, Culpepper WJ, Campbell JD, Nelson LM, Langer-Gould A, Marrie RA, Cutter GR, Kaye WE, Wagner L, Tremlett H, Buka SL, Dilokthornsakul P, Topol B, Chen LH, LaRocca NG; US Multiple Sclerosis Prevalence Workgroup. The prevalence of MS in the

United States: a population-based estimate using health claims data. Neurology. 2019 Mar 5;92(10):e1029–40. https://doi.org/10.1212/WNL.0000000000007035. Epub 2019 Feb 15.

3. Bebo B, Cintina I, LaRocca N, Ritter L, Talente B, Hartung D, Ngorsuraches S, Wallin M, Yang G. The economic burden of multiple sclerosis in the United States: estimate of direct and indirect costs. Neurology. 2022 May 3;98(18):e1810–7. https://doi.org/10.1212/WNL.0000000000200150. Epub 2022 Apr 13. PMID: 35418457; PMCID: PMC9109149.

4. Trip SA, Miller DH. Imaging in multiple sclerosis. J Neurol Neurosurg Psychiatry. 2005 Sept;76 (Suppl 3):iii11–8. https://doi.org/10.1136/jnnp.2005.073213. PMID: 16107385; PMCID: PMC1765701.

5. Flachenecker P, Henze T, Zettl UK. Spasticity in patients with multiple sclerosis—clinical characteristics, treatment and quality of life. Acta Neurol Scand. 2014;129(3):154–62.

6. Rizzo MA, Hadjimichael OC, Preingerova J, Vollmer TL. Prevalence and treatment of spasticity reported by multiple sclerosis patients. Mult Scler. 2004;10:589–95.

7. Snow BJ, Tsui JK, Bhatt MH, et al. Treatment of spasticity with botulinum toxin: a double-blind study. Ann Neurol. 1990;28:512–5.

8. Mahajan ST, Patel PB, Marrie RA. Under treatment of overactive bladder symptoms in patients with multiple sclerosis: an ancillary analysis of the NARCOMS patient registry. J Urol. 2010;183:1432–7.

9. Novarella F, Carotenuto A, Cipullo P, Iodice R, Cassano E, Spiezia AL, Capasso N, Petracca M, Falco F, Iacovazzo C, Servillo G, Lanzillo R, Brescia Morra V, Moccia M. Persistence with botulinum toxin treatment for spasticity symptoms in multiple sclerosis. Toxins (Basel). 2022 Nov 9;14(11):774. https://doi.org/10.3390/toxins14110774. PMID: 36356024; PMCID: PMC9693315.

10. Schnitzler A, Dince C, Freitag A, Iheanacho I, Fahrbach K, Lavoie L, Loze JY, Forestier A, Gasq D. AbobotulinumtoxinA doses in upper and lower limb spasticity: a systematic literature review. Toxins (Basel). 2022 Oct 26;14(11):734. https://doi.org/10.3390/toxins14110734. PMID: 36355984; PMCID: PMC9698883.

11. Bensmail D, Karam P, Forestier A, Loze JY, Lévy J. Trends in botulinum toxin use among patients with multiple sclerosis: a population-based study. Toxins (Basel). 2023 Apr 12;15(4):280. https://doi.org/10.3390/toxins15040280. PMID: 37104218; PMCID: PMC10142089.

12. Ni J, Wang X, Cao N, et al. Is repeat botulinum toxin A injection valuable for neurogenic detrusor overactivity – a systematic review and meta-analysis. Neurourol Urodyn. 2017, July 26; https://doi.org/10.1002/nau.23354. [Epub ahead of print].

13. Foley PL, Vesterinen HM, Laird BJ, Sena ES, Colvin LA, Chandran S, MacLeod MR, Fallon M. Prevalence and natural history of pain in adults with multiple sclerosis: systematic review and meta-analysis. Pain. 2013 May;154:632–42. https://doi.org/10.1016/j.pain.2012.12.002. Epub 2012 Dec 14. PMID: 23318126.

14. Safarpour Y, Jabbari B. Botulinum toxin treatment of pain syndromes – an evidence based review. Toxicon. 2018, Jan 31; https://doi.org/10.1016/j.toxicon.2018.01.017. pii: S0041–0101(18) 30031-X. [Epub ahead of print].

15. Baricich A, Picelli A, Santamato A, Carda S, de Sire A, Smania N, Cisari C, Invernizzi M. Safety profile of high-dose botulinum toxin type A in post-stroke spasticity treatment. Clin Drug Investig. 2018 Nov;38(11):991–1000. https://doi.org/10.1007/s40261-018-0701-x. PMID: 30209743.

16. Wissel J, Bensmail D, Ferreira JJ, Molteni F, Satkunam L, Moraleda S, Rekand T, McGuire J, Scheschonka A, Flatau-Baqué B, Simon O, Rochford ET, Dressler D, Simpson DM; TOWER Study Investigators. Safety and efficacy of incobotulinumtoxinA doses up to 800 U in limb spasticity: The TOWER study. Neurology. 2017 Apr 4;88(14):1321–8. https://doi.org/10.1212/WNL.0000000000003789. Epub 2017 Mar 10. PMID: 28283596; PMCID: PMC5379931.

17. Baldder dysfunction in MS: National MS Society. https://www.nationalmssociety.org › Bladder-Dysfunction

18. Ginsberg D, Gousse A, Keppenne V, Sievert KD, Thompson C, Lam W, Brin MF, Jenkins B, Haag-Molkenteller C. Phase 3 efficacy and tolerability study of onabotulinumtoxinA for

urinary incontinence from neurogenic detrusor overactivity. J Urol. 2012 June;187(6):2131–9. https://doi.org/10.1016/j.juro.2012.01.125. Epub 2012 Apr 12. PMID: 22503020.

19. Cruz F, Herschorn S, Aliotta P, Brin M, Thompson C, Lam W, Daniell G, Heesakkers J, Haag-Molkenteller C. Efficacy and safety of onabotulinumtoxinA in patients with urinary incontinence due to neurogenic detrusor overactivity: a randomised, double-blind, placebo-controlled trial. Eur Urol. 2011 Oct;60(4):742–50. https://doi.org/10.1016/j.eururo.2011.07.002. Epub 2011 July 13. PMID: 21798658.

20. Ni J, Wang X, Cao N, Si J, Gu B. Is repeat botulinum toxin A injection valuable for neurogenic detrusor overactivity—a systematic review and meta-analysis. Neurourol Urodyn. 2018 Feb;37(2):542–53. https://doi.org/10.1002/nau.23354. Epub 2017 July 26. PMID: 28745818.

21. Giannantoni A, Gubbiotti M, Rubilotta E, Balzarro M, Antonelli A, Bini V. IncobotulinumtoxinA versus onabotulinumtoxinA intradetrusor injections in patients with neurogenic detrusor overactivity incontinence: a double-blind, randomized, non-inferiority trial. Minerva Urol Nephrol. 2022 Oct;74(5):625–35. https://doi.org/10.23736/S2724-6051.21.04227-2. Epub 2021 Mar 26. PMID: 33769020.

22. Kennelly M, Cruz F, Herschorn S, Abrams P, Onem K, Solomonov VK, Del Rosario Figueroa Coz E, Manu-Marin A, Giannantoni A, Thompson C, Vilain C, Volteau M, Denys P, Dysport CONTENT Program Group. Efficacy and safety of abobotulinumtoxinA in patients with neurogenic detrusor overactivity incontinence performing regular clean intermittent catheterization: pooled results from two phase 3 randomized studies (CONTENT1 and CONTENT2). Eur Urol. 2022 Aug;82(2):223–32. https://doi.org/10.1016/j.eururo.2022.03.010. Epub 2022 Apr 7. PMID: 35400537.

23. Gupta K, Burchiel KJ. Atypical facial pain in multiple sclerosis caused by spinal cord seizures: a case report and review of the literature. J Med Case Rep. 2016 Apr 20;10:101. https://doi.org/10.1186/s13256-016-0891-x. PMID: 27095098; PMCID: PMC4837532.

24. Wu CJ, Lian YJ, Zheng YK, et al. Botulinum toxin type A for the treatment of trigeminal neuralgia: results from a randomized, double-blind, placebo-controlled trial. Cephalalgia. 2012;32:443–50.

25. Zhang H, Lian Y, Ma Y, Chen Y, He C, Xie N, Wu C. Two doses of botulinum toxin type A for the treatment of trigeminal neuralgia: observation of therapeutic effect from a randomized, double-blind, placebo-controlled trial. J Headache Pain. 2014 Sept 27;15(1):65. https://doi.org/10.1186/1129-2377-15-65. PMID: 25263254; PMCID: PMC4194456.

26. Zúñiga C, Piedimonte F, Díaz S, Micheli F. Acute treatment of trigeminal neuralgia with onabotulinum toxin A. Clin Neuropharmacol 2013 Sept–Oct;36(5):146–50. https://doi.org/10.1097/WNF.0b013e31829cb60e. PMID: 24045604.

27. Asan F, Gündüz A, Tütüncü M, Uygunoğlu U, Savrun FK, Saip S, Siva A. Treatment of multiple sclerosis-related trigeminal neuralgia with onabotulinumtoxinA. Headache. 2022 Nov;62(10):1322–8. https://doi.org/10.1111/head.14414. Epub 2022 Nov 27. PMID: 36437599.

28. Cui M, Khanijou S, Rubino J, et al. Subcutaneous administration of botulinum toxin A reduces formalin-induced pain. Pain. 2004;107:125–33.

29. Marino MJ, Terashima T, Steinauer JJ, et al. Botulinum toxin B in the sensory afferent: transmitter release, spinal activation, and pain behavior. Pain. 2014;155:674–84.

30. Hou YP, Zhang YP, Song YF, Zhu CM, Wang YC, Xie GL. Botulinum toxin type A inhibits rat pyloric myoelectrical activity and substance P release in vivo. Can J Physiol Pharmacol. 2007 Feb;85(2):209–14. https://doi.org/10.1139/y07-018. PMID: 17487262.

31. Lucioni A, Bales GT, Lotan TL, McGehee DS, Cook SP, Rapp DE. Botulinum toxin type A inhibits sensory neuropeptide release in rat bladder models of acute injury and chronic inflammation. BJU Int. 2008;101:366–70.

32. Meng J, Wang J, Lawrence G, Dolly JO. Synaptobrevin I mediates exocytosis of CGRP from sensory neurons and inhibition by botulinum toxins reflects their anti-nociceptive potential. J Cell Sci. 2007;120:2864–74.

33. Meng J, Ovsepian SV, Wang J, Pickering M, Sasse A, Aoki KR, Lawrence GW, Dolly JO. Activation of TRPV1 mediates calcitonin gene-related peptide release, which excites trigeminal sensory neurons and is attenuated by a retargeted botulinum toxin with anti-nociceptive potential. J Neurosci. 2009;29:4981–92.
34. Matak I, Tékus V, Bölcskei K, Lacković Z, Helyes Z. Involvement of substance P in the anti-nociceptive effect of botulinum toxin type A: evidence from knockout mice. Neuroscience. 2017 Sept 1;358:137–45. https://doi.org/10.1016/j.neuroscience.2017.06.040. Epub 2017 July 1. PMID: 28673722.
35. Tang M, Meng J, Wang J. New engineered-botulinum toxins inhibit the release of pain-related mediators. Int J Mol Sci. 2019. Dec 30;21(1):262. https://doi.org/10.3390/ijms21010262. PMID: 31906003; PMCID: PMC6981458.
36. Yuan RY, Sheu JJ, Yu JM, Chen WT, Tseng IJ, Chang HH, Hu CJ. Botulinum toxin for diabetic neuropathic pain: a randomized double-blind crossover trial. Neurology. 2009;72:1473–8.
37. Li XL, Zeng X, Zeng S, He HP, Zeng Z, Peng LL, Chen LG. Botulinum toxin A treatment for post-herpetic neuralgia: a systematic review and meta-analysis. Exp Ther Med. 2020 Feb;19(2):1058–64. https://doi.org/10.3892/etm.2019.8301. Epub 2019 Dec 9. PMID: 32010269; PMCID: PMC6966161.
38. Babcock MS, Foster L, Pasquina P, Jabbari B. Treatment of pain attributed to plantar fasciitis with botulinum toxin A: a short-term, randomized, placebo-controlled, double-blind study. Am J Phys Med Rehabil. 2005;84:649–54.
39. Foster L, Clapp L, Erickson M, Jabbari B. Botulinum toxin A and chronic low back pain: a randomized, double-blind study. Neurology. 2001;56:1290–3.
40. Ranoux D, Attal N, Morain F, Bouhassira D. Botulinum toxin type A induces direct analgesic effects in chronic neuropathic pain. Ann Neurol. 2008 Sept;64(3):274–83. https://doi.org/10.1002/ana.21427. Erratum in: Ann Neurol 2009 Mar;65(3):359. PMID: 18546285.
41. Newsome SD, Thrower B, Hendin B, Danese S, Patterson J, Chinnapongse R. Symptom burden, management and treatment goals of people with MS spasticity: results from SEEN-MSS, a large-scale, self-reported survey. Mult Scler Relat Disord. 2022 Dec;68:104376. https://doi.org/10.1016/j.msard.2022.104376. Epub 2022 Oct 26. PMID: 36544321.
42. Jabbari B. Botulinum toxin treatment of pain disorders. 2nd ed. New York: Springer; 2022.
43. Restivo DA, Tinazzi M, Patti F, Palmeri A, Maimone D. Botulinum toxin treatment of painful tonic spasms in multiple sclerosis. Neurology. 2003 Sept 9;61(5):719–20. https://doi.org/10.1212/01.wnl.0000080081.74117.e4. PMID: 12963779.
44. Van Der Walt A, Sung S, Spelman T, Marriott M, Kolbe S, Mitchell P, Evans A, Butzkueven H. A double-blind, randomized, controlled study of botulinum toxin type A in MS-related tremor. Neurology. 2012 July 3;79(1):92–9. https://doi.org/10.1212/WNL.0b013e31825dcdd9. PMID: 22753445.
45. Sedano MJ, Trejo JM, Macarrón JL, Polo JM, Berciano J, Calleja J. Continuous facial myokymia in multiple sclerosis: treatment with botulinum toxin. Eur Neurol. 2000;43(3):137–40. https://doi.org/10.1159/000008152. PMID: 10765052.
46. Habek M, Adamec I, Gabelić T, Brinar VV. Treatment of facial myokymia in multiple sclerosis with botulinum toxin. Acta Neurol Belg. 2012 Dec;112(4):423–4. https://doi.org/10.1007/s13760-012-0092-3. Epub 2012 Jun 5. PMID: 22669610.
47. Restivo DA, Marchese-Ragona R, Patti F, Solaro C, Maimone D, Zappalá G, Pavone A. Botulinum toxin improves dysphagia associated with multiple sclerosis. Eur J Neurol. 2011 Mar;18(3):486–90. https://doi.org/10.1111/j.1468-1331.2010.03189.x. Epub 2010 Aug 22. PMID: 20731706.
48. Blitzer A. Spasmodic dysphonia and botulinum toxin: experience from the largest treatment series. Eur J Neurol. 2010 July;17(Suppl 1):28–30. https://doi.org/10.1111/j.1468-1331.2010.03047.x. PMID: 20590805.
49. Di Stadio A, Bernitsas E, Restivo DA, Alfonsi E, Marchese-Ragona R. Spasmodic dysphonia in multiple sclerosis treatment with botulin toxin A: a pilot study. J Voice 2019 July;33(4):550–3. https://doi.org/10.1016/j.jvoice.2018.01.002. Epub 2018 Apr 9. PMID: 29650331.

50. Safarpour Y, Mousavi T, Jabbari B. Botulinum toxin treatment in multiple sclerosis – a review. Curr Treat Options Neurol. 2017 Aug 17;19(10):33. https://doi.org/10.1007/s11940-017-0470-5. PMID: 28819801.
51. Safarpour Y, Jabbari B. Botulinum toxin treatment in multiple sclerosis. In: Jabbari B, editor. Botulinum toxin treatment in clinical medicine. Cham: Springer; 2018.

Chapter 8
Treatment of Involuntary Movements (Dystonia, Tremor, Tic)

Abstract Botulinum toxins, after injection into the muscle, block the release of acetylcholine from the neuromuscular junction. Acetylcholine is a chemical neurotransmitter that, upon release from nerve endings, activates the muscles. In disease conditions characterized by presence of overactive muscles with involuntary movements (dystonias, tremors, tics), injection of the botulinum toxin into the affected muscles decreases the involuntary movements substantially and improves the patients' quality of life.

Keywords Botulinum toxin · Botulinum neurotoxin · Dystonia · Cervical dystonia · Oromandibular dystonia · Tremor · Tic

Introduction

Abnormal involuntary movements are seen during the course of a large number of neurological disorders. Dystonia, tremor and tics are the three most common forms of these abnormal movements. These involuntary movements, when severe and disabling, limit the function of the limbs and impair the patients' quality of life. Current treatments of dystonia and tremor are partially effective but often fall short of patients' satisfaction. In addition, in many patients, side effects of the drugs limits their use. Over the past 35 years, injection of botulinum toxins into the muscles affected by dystonias and tremor has dramatically improved the quality of life in many of these patients.

Dystonia

Dystonia is a neurological movement disorder characterized by involuntary (unintended) muscle contractions that cause slow repetitive movements or abnormal postures that can sometimes be painful. There are several different forms of dystonia that may affect only one muscle, groups of muscles, or muscles throughout the body. The affected areas and severity of symptoms varies from person to person" [1]. Dystonic movements have a twisting and turning character causing abnormal posture in the face, neck and affected body parts [2]. Dystonia is probably the most common form of movement disorder and is seen in a variety of disease conditions. A large number of dystonic problems are genetic and start in early childhood (primary dystonias). These, genetically determined dystonias start focally—usually in 1 ft, but gradually spread to other parts of the body and, at one point, become generalized. With the passage of time, dystonia gets worse and results in limb(s) that are fixed in abnormal posture(s). Patients affected by genetically determined dystonias may have additional symptoms such as weakness of the limbs, walking problems and/or mental deficits.

Focal dystonias with no or low genetic patterns affect one part of the body and usually remain confined to that part (i.e. blepharospasm, musicians' dystonia). Most focal dystonias start later in life, usually after age 40. Focal dystonia can affect the face, neck, upper or lower limb. Currently, botulinum toxins are among the first line of management for focal dystonias. Blepharospasm, a focal dystonia of the eyelid muscles, was one of the two movement disorders for which FDA approved botulinum toxin therapy in 1989 (see Chaps 2 and 3 of this book).

Focal Dystonias

Focal Dystonias of the Face Region

The two most frequent dystonias of the face which respond to botulinum toxin therapy are blepharospasm and mouth-jaw (oromandibular) dystonias.

Blepharospasm

Blepharospasm is uncontrolled, tonic contraction of the muscles that close the eyelids (orbicularis oculi/OO muscles) (Fig. 8.1a). Spasm of these thin muscles, which are barely under the skin, forces the eyes to close (Fig. 8.1b).

Blepharospasm is almost always bilateral and affects both eyes. The eyelid spasms are frequent and can occur hundreds of times per day. Many patients are unable to drive a motor vehicle due to impaired vision. In over 90% of patients with blepharospasm, a cause cannot be found (essential blepharospasm). Genetic predisposition is believed to play a role in many of such patients, but culprit genes have not been identified. In rare cases, blepharospasm can be caused by stroke or a brain tumor. Belpharospasm is an uncommon disorder. Approximately 2000 new cases of blepharospasm are diagnosed each year in the United States. Women are affected more often than men with a ratio of 2.8/1 [4].

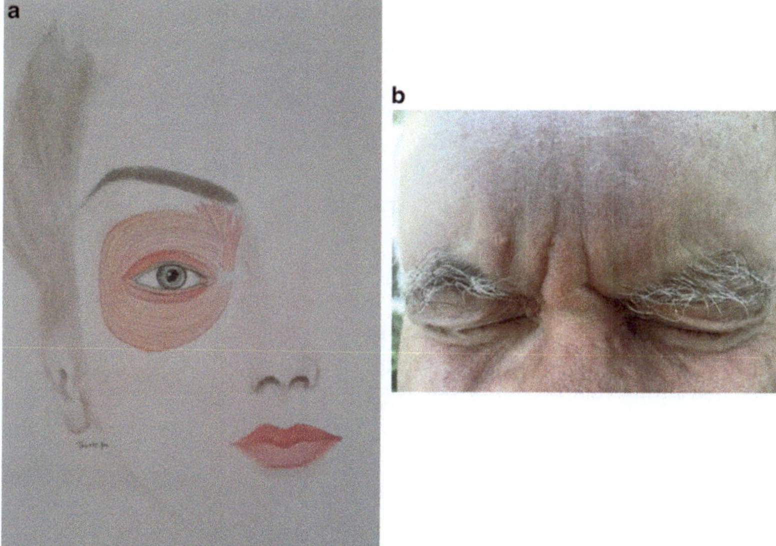

Fig. 8.1 (a) Orbilularis oculi muscle presented in red color. The muscle has a palpebral part that is attached to the lid and an orbital part that is further out and circles the eye. (b) Belpharospasm causing forced eye closure

The onset of blepharospasm is usually after age 40. Blepharospasm should be differentiated from facial tics involving the eyelids, psychogenic eye closures, and a condition called apraxia of eyelid opening. The latter, most often seen in elderly with dementias and Parkinson's disease, is due to failure of cerebral cortex to exert proper activation of eye muscles.

Treatment of blepharospasm was disappointing before the introduction of botulinum toxin injections. The commonly used drugs for treatment of blepharspasm are from a group of drugs called anticholinergics. Artane, the most widely used of these drugs in blepharospasm, is provided in 2 and 5 mg tablets. Treatment of blepharospasm with Artane requires slow dose escalation starting with 1 mg/day and gradually working up to the effective dose. Most patients respond when the dosage reaches 10–20 mg/day, but some patients require higher doses. Side effects that include blurred vision, severe dryness of the mouth and confusion/hallucinations are especially troublesome in elderly.

Botulinum Toxin Therapy in Blepharospasm

Introduction of botulinum toxins revolutionalized the management of blepharospasm. The toxin is prepared by diluting the powdered preparation (provided in a small vial) in a small amount of salt water (saline); it is then injected with a very thin needle around each eye. Injections are performed close to the eye and introduced barely under the skin into the orbicularis oculi (OO) muscle. Usually five to six locations around each eye are injected (Fig. 8.2). Initial sites of injection can be later modified in subsequent injections.

The author of this book uses a similar scheme as in Fig. 8.2 but with a minor change for the initial injection; it includes an additional injection with small amount of the toxin between sites 5 & 6 (Fig. 8.2), but with no injection at site 2, unless the area is clearly active (moving) during inspection.

Over 90% of the patients with blepharospasm respond well to botulinum toxin injections [3]. While some patients note the result within 2–3 days, the peak effect becomes apparent within 10–14 days and the effect lasts for 3–4 months. Injections cause mild discomfort. In experienced hands, side effects are uncommon and minor; the patient may experience seconds of pain in the area of injection and minor local bleeding. Drooping of upper eye lid, seen in a small number of patients, can be avoided by not injecting at midline close to the upper lid (in proximity of the muscle that lifts the upper eyelid) and rather inject higher on the lower edge of the eyebrow with a small amount of toxin (in case of Botox, not to exceed 2–2.5 units).

We usually start with 2.5 units of Botox at 6 locations (locations 1, 3, 4, 5, 6 in Fig. 8.2 and an extra one between the locations 5 and 6). In many patients, this approach suffices to stop the lid spasms (twitches) or markedly reduce them. Later, when the injector becomes more familiar with the patient's facial response to the injections, the dose may be increased in one or more of the above-mentioned locations to 3–5 units/site. Other type A marketed and FDA approved botulinum toxins (Xeomin, Dysport) are also effective in management of blepharospasm (see Chap. 2 for description FDA marketed botulinum toxins in the US). In case of Dysport the dose need to be 2.5 to 3 times larger than Botox or Xeomin (see Chap. 2). In severe cases of blepharospasm, the injections may include an additional injection into the

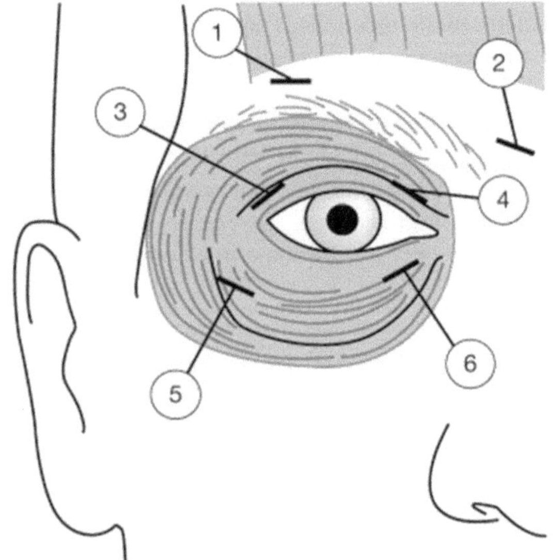

Fig. 8.2 Sites of initial botulinum toxin injection for treatment of blepharospasm advocated in a large multicenter study. Injections are around both eyes. (From Troung and co-workers 2012. Reproduced with permission from the publisher. Elsevier [5])

upper cheek muscles and/or into the muscles that bring the eyebrows together. The latter muscle (corrugator) is located above the medial part of each eyebrow (site 2, Fig. 8.2). Treatment of blepharospasm with botulinum toxins has now a track record of over 30 years and is associated with a high degree of patient satisfaction. Over time, some adjustment of the dose may be required, but the dose escalation is usually minor. The treatment is for life since the condition recurs after 3–4 months. The clinical efficacy of Botulinum toxin injections in blepharospasm is supported by several high quality, double-blind, placebo-controlled studies [6–10]. Comparative studies have shown no significant difference between FDA approved type A botulinum toxins (Botox and Xeomin) regarding efficacy, patient satisfaction and side effects in blepharospasm [11]. Likewise, there was no difference regarding these measures between Botox and Asian Toxins (Chinese type A toxin: Prosigne, Korean type A: Meditox) [12, 13]. Sustained efficacy with repeated injections of Xeomin (every 3–4 months) has been reported in a carefully crafted study, with some patients followed for up to 69 weeks [14]. The author of this book has noticed sustained efficacy for 10 years or more in many patients with blepharospasm.

Dystonia of the Mouth and Jaw Muscles

Trembling and twitching of the lips, twisting and protrusion of the tongue, locking of the jaw (jaw closure dystonia) and forced jaw opening (jaw opening dystonia) are a group of involuntary movements that can be caused by certain groups of drugs—neuroleptics—used for treatment of psychosis and severe depression. Although the new generation of neuroleptics have fewer of these side effects, these involuntary movements still occur and challenge the psychiatrists. Since these abnormal movements often occur with a delay, the term of tardive (late) dyskinesia (abnormal movement) is used to designate the abnormal movements in this setting. Neuroleptic drugs are not the only drugs that cause tardive dyskinesia, but they are the prime drug culprits for this form of dyskinesia/dystonias. Dystonias of the tongue, face, lips and jaws may also develop during the course of degenerative diseases that involve deep brain structures (basal ganglia). Many of these disorders resemble Parkinson's disease, but have other symptoms in addition to slowness of movements, rigidity and tremor. For some of these disorders, a defective gene has been already discovered.

Treatment of involuntary, face and jaw movements caused by brain disease or drugs (tardive dyskinesia) is difficult. Valium, Baclofen, Artane, Gabapentine and Tetrabenazine are partially effective, but the effect is usually modest and not sustained. In some lucky patients, the drug induced movements may go away by themselves after weeks or months; once started, however, the movements continue for years or even persist for life in many patients.

Botulinum Toxin Treatment

Injection of botulinum toxin into the muscles involved by involuntary jaw movements results in at least moderate, sustained relief and satisfaction in two thirds of the patients [15]. A majority of the affected patients with jaw dystonia are females [15]. Luckily, muscles of jaw closure or jaw opening are well known and can be easily identified by examination. The masseter muscle, located at the angle of the jaw and the temporalis muscle located at the temple, are the main muscles that close and lock the jaw (Fig. 8.3a). Both muscles can be easily seen under the skin and activated by asking the patients to clinch their teeth. Furthermore, in patients with jaw closure dystonia, these muscles are enlarged due to their frequent and prolonged contractions. An initial dose of 30 and 40 units (in case of Botox or Xeomin) per muscle/per side may be injected into 2–4 sites for temporalis and masseter muscles, respectively (Fig. 8.3b). In severe cases, the dose for subsequent injections may be increased to 50 and 80 units into temporalis and masseter muscle, respectively, if necessary. The effect of Botox injection usually lasts 3–4 months.

Jaw opening dystonia (JOD) also responds well to botulinum toxin therapy, although fewer patients do as well as JCD. This may be due to the fact that muscles for jaw opening are located deeper and are harder to reach. External pterygoid (EPT) muscle that opens the jaw, sometimes can be injected in front of the ear after asking the patient to open the jaw widely. This will contract the muscle and the contracted muscle can be palpated and injected through the covering skin. Sometimes, however, deeper EPT muscle is not easy to palpate and its identification requires using electromyography (EMG) that records the electrical activity of the muscle. The contracted muscle makes noise in EMG. Some injectors prefer to inject this muscle through the open mouth.

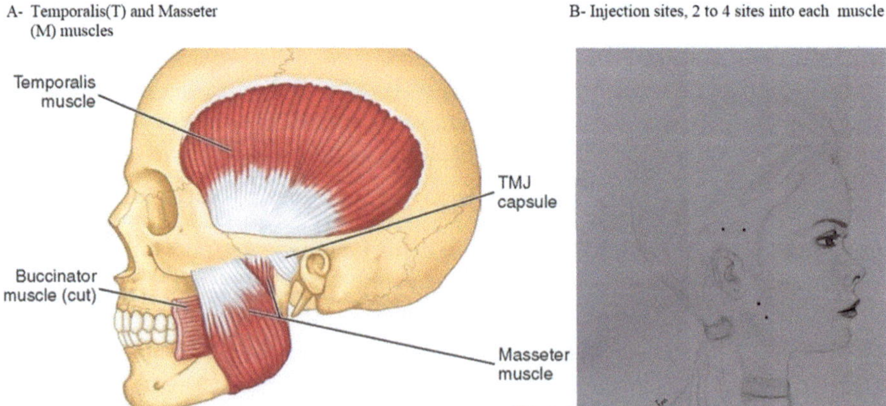

Fig. 8.3 The site of botulinum injection for Jaw Closure Dystonia (JCD). (**a**) Temporalis (T) and Masseter (M) muscles, (**b**) injection sites, two to four sites into each muscle. (Reproduced with permission from Mayo Foundation. Drawing Courtesy of Dr. Tahereh Mousavi)

In tongue dystonia [16], often a complication of anti-psychotic drug use is an involuntary turning and rolling tongue movement that interferes with speaking and eating. Most affected patients are extremely disturbed by their difficulty in eating and speaking. In the author's experience, between half to two thirds of patients with tongue dystonia respond to Botox injection into the tongue. Tongue injections require significant amount of expertise and need to be performed by physicians with substantial knowledge in management of difficult dystonias. Overdosing the tongue can cause tongue paralysis and worsen patient's eating and speaking problems. The author starts with a small dose of 5 units injected into each side of the tongue; doses higher than 7.5 units per side are not recommended. Tongue injection is not FDA approved.

In a recently published multicenter study [17], the clinical features and the response of the patients to botulinum toxins was described in 2000 patients with oromandibular dystonia (OMD) (jaw opening and jaw closure, perioral movements, tongue dystonia). Presence of OMD showed significant association with impaired quality of life regardless of the severity of the disease. Social anxiety was found to be more than three times common than depression. In the patient cohorts injected in expert centers, botulinum toxin injections improved symptom severity by more than 50% in 80% of the subjects, regardless of the cause of OMD.

Hemifacial Spasm (HFS)

Hemifacial spasm is characterized by involuntary movements involving half of the face. Although hemifacial spasm is not a dystonia (movements are faster and jerkier), it is mentioned here due to its facial location and exquisite sensitivity and remarkable response to botulinum toxin therapy. The movements of HFS are observed below the eye, as well as in the lower facial muscles. The movements below the eye involve the OO muscle (see above -blepharospasm) and, when severe, tend to close the eye. The lower face movements present with twitches in the lower part of the cheek, chin and lips. Frequent hemifacial spasms can become the source of serious social embarrassment (especially in ladies).

Hemifacial spasm is more common than blepharospasm, affecting 14.5 and 7.4 of women and men in a 100,000 population, respectively [18]. Unlike blepharospasm in that, more than 80% of the cases are essential (has no known cause), in approximately 80% of the patients with hemifacial spasm, the cause is known and is related to an abnormal blood vessel that presses against the facial nerve as it emerges from the lower part of the brain (brain stem). Chronic pressure against the nerve (for years), leads to the hyperexcitability of the nerve which consequently makes the facial muscles twitch. The condition is not usually dangerous since the culprit blood vessel rarely ruptures. In a small number of patients, less than 5%, hemifacial spasm can be the result of a brain tumor in the lower part of the brain. It is for this reason that in new cases of hemifacial spasm performing CT scan or MRI is indicated.

Oral medications such as benzodiazepines (clonopin and valium), baclofen and gabapentin have minimal effect on hemifacial spasm. Before the introduction of botulinum toxins, many patients required brain surgery during which the surgeon separated the culprit vessel from the facial nerve-releasing the pressure on the nerve. However, HFS surgery could leave the patient with major deficits such as paralysis of the face, loss of hearing and poor balance while walking. Currently, due to efficacy of botulinum toxin therapy surgery is reserved for very recalcitrant cases. The surgical utilization rate in North America for hemifacial spasm is currently around 10% [19].

In 1989, FDA approved the use of Botox for treatment of hemifacial spasm in the US despite lack of multicenter high quality studies (one of the first two approved movement disorders for which Botox was approved; the other condition was blepharospasm). The published data shows that between 76 and 100% of the patients demonstrate over 75% improvement with reduction of facial movements after botulinum toxin therapy [20, 21]. Injections are carried by a small, short needle (gauge 27.5 or 30 with ½ in. length) around the eye in a manner similar that used for blepharospasm and also into the check and lower face muscles starting with a small dose of 1.25 to 2.5 units (in case of Botox or Xeomin) per site [22] (Fig. 8.4). The dose can be adjusted every 3–4 months when reinjection is required. The main side effect of botulinum toxin injection for HFS is weakness of facial muscles that could last for weeks. The lower face muscles are particularly sensitive to botulinum toxin,

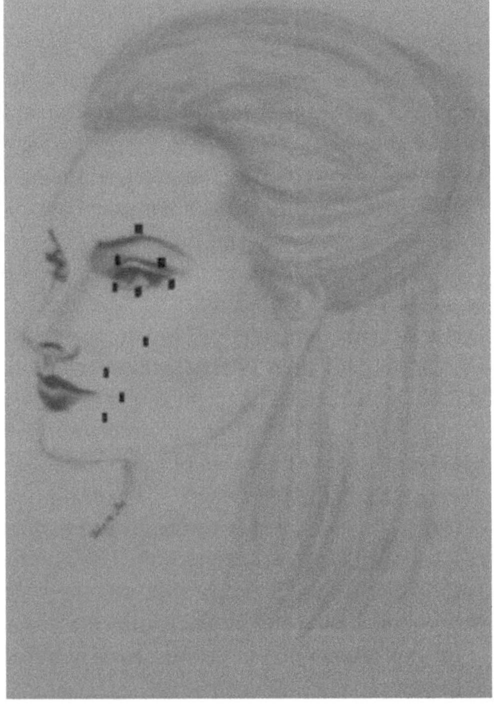

Fig. 8.4 Author's preferred scheme of initial injections for blepharospasm (around the eyes) and hemifacial spasm (face). The dose around the eye is 2.5 units/site, and in the lower face around the mouth, it is 1.5 units/site (for Botox and Xeomin). Injection into the cheek is performed only if the movements involve the cheek. (Drawing, courtesy of Dr. Tahere Mousavi)

hence, the initial dose used for lower face, especially around the lips, should be small (1–1.25 unit/site). The issue of facial weakness needs to be discussed with the patient prior to injections for HFS. In practice, some patients may prefer to not have lower face injections, at least, during the first session. Long-term experience with botulinum toxin injections for HFS indicates continued efficacy and low incidence of side effects. Some dose adjustments may be necessary over time. Sustained results require repeat injections every 3–4 months. There are now patients with HFS on record, who have been receiving botulinum toxin injections, every 3–4 months for over 20 years. Since the rate of response is very high (<90%), unresponsiveness to botulinum toxin therapy should raise the possibility of other disorders such as facial tics or psychogenic facial movements. Experience of the past 20 years has confirmed that injection of all FDA approved type A toxins (Botox, Xeomin, Dysport, Daxxify) into the appropriate facial muscles effectively reduces the involuntary facial movements in HFS and results in patient satisfaction.

This chapter's author over a time span of 25 years has performed thousands of botulinum toxin injections for hemifacial spasm and blepharospasm. His experience matches the information on efficacy and safety of botulinum toxin therapy on these to movement disorders as described in the above-cited literature. The patients' satisfaction rate is high and side effects (infrequent minor bleeding and local pain at the time of injection) are minor and tolerable. The number of injections are acceptable by the patients (Fig. 8.4).

Cervical Dystonia (CD): Dystonia of Neck Muscles

This is one of the most common forms of focal and segmental dystonia that responds very well to botulinum toxin therapy. In this condition, affected patients gradually develop increased tone and contraction of certain neck muscles leading to forced rotation of the neck to one side (torticollis) or neck tilt toward the shoulder (laterocollis). A less common form of CD is when the neck is pulled back (retrocollis) or when the neck is bent forward (anterocollis) (Fig. 8.5). Cervical dystonia is often associated with neck pain. Sometimes neck pain is more distressing to the patient than neck tilt or neck rotation (posture and cosmetic issues). Several neck muscles and some shoulder muscles contribute to the abnormal neck posture (Table 8.1).

The mean age for onset of symptoms in CD is 49 years and there is a strong female predominance (74%) [23]. Up to 70% of the patients with CD suffer from chronic neck pain [24] which is often more bothersome to the patients than either rotation or tilting of the neck. If untreated, the pain gradually intensifies and the intermittent and abnormal neck posture becomes fixed making the neck rigid and immobile. Chronic cervical dystonia is often associated with poor quality of life and a significant degree of disability [25].

Before introduction of botulinum toxin therapy, CD was treated mainly with a group of drugs that block the function of a chemical called acetylcholine (anticholinergics). Acetylcholine is released at the nerve ending at the point where nerve

A - Torticollis and retrocollis   B - antercollis and laterocollis

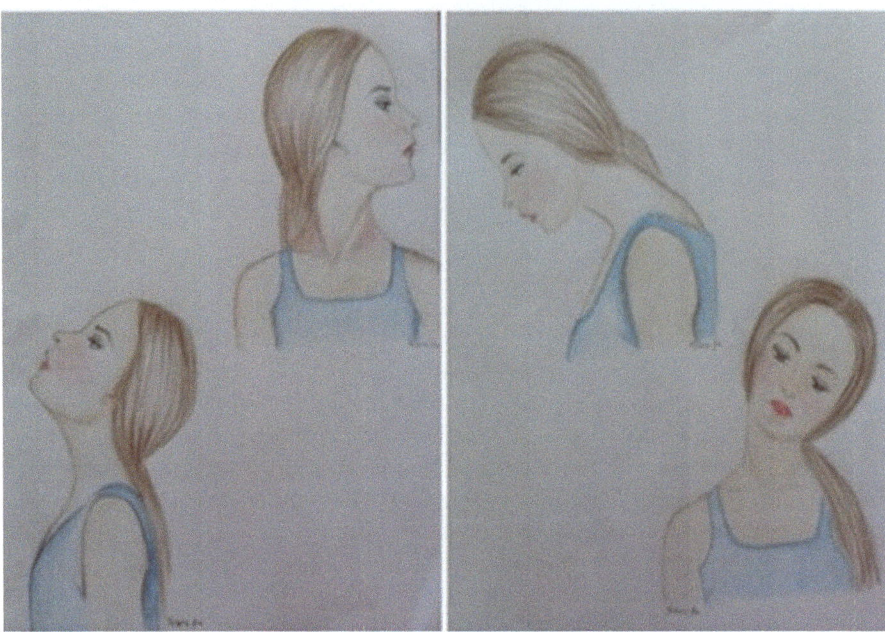

Fig. 8.5 Of the four types of cervical dystonia illustrated below, torticollis (neck rotation) is the most common accounting for nearly half of the patients. (Drawing, courtesy of Dr. Tahere Mousavi)

Table 8.1 Some of the commonly injected muscles in cervical dystonia and their function

Muscle	Location	Function
Stenocleidomastoid (SCM)	Front of the neck	Turns the neck to the opposite side, tilts the neck to the same side, bends the neck
Splenius capitis (SC)	Back of the neck	Rotates and tilts the neck to the same side
Scalenius anterior (SCA)	Front the neck	Tilts the head to the same side
Trapezius (Tr)	Shoulder	Elevates the shoulder
Levator scapulae (LS)	Upper back extending to the front of the neck	Elevates the scapula
		Tilts the head to the same side

contacts with the muscle. These drugs block the effect of acetylcholine, hence, resulting in relaxation of contracted neck muscles and improvement of the neck posture. However, anticholinergic drugs are hard to tolerate by older people due side effects of dryness of the mouth, blurring of vision and mental confusion. Other drugs such as baclofen, clonopin and valium are also used alone or in combination for treatment of CD but they may require a dose escalation to be effective. Too often, this limits their use in CD due to excessive sedation.

The efficacy of Botox in treatment of cervical dystonia was first suggested by Dr. Tsui and his colleagues from Canada in a small pilot study of 12 patients in 1985

[26]. Encouraged by this observations, over the subsequent 25 years, several high quality studies (double-blind, placebo-controlled and conducted in a large number of patients) was published that confirmed the efficacy of both type A and Type B toxins in cervical dystonia [8, 27–31]. This led to FDA approval of four type A marketed botulinum toxins (Botox, Xeomin, Dysport and Daxxify) and the type B toxin (Myobloc) for treatment of cervical dystonia.

Currently, botulinum toxin has become the treatment of choice for management of CD due to its much fewer side effects compared to oral medications. In patients that have been on oral medications for some time, injection of botulinum toxins into neck muscles can allow the patients to reduce the daily dose of medications, and in many patients it allow them to stop the use of oral medications safely. Moreover, several studies have shown that improvement of neck posture is associated with marked improvement of the associated neck pain in CD [32].

The effectiveness of botulinum toxin therapy in CD is sustained after repeated injections of botulinum toxins [33]. There are patients on record who have been receiving botulinum toxin injections for cervical dystonia, every 3–6 months for over 20 years [33]. Careful assessments of quality of life have shown that patients' quality of life show notable improvement along with improvements of head and neck posture and neck pain [34].

Technical Issues A good knowledge of location and function of neck muscles is required in order to succeed with botulinum toxin therapy in cervical dystonia. Some physicians use merely their knowledge of anatomy (anatomic landmarks) for injecting botulinum toxins into the neck muscles, while others perform the injections under the guidance of electromyography. Electromyography identifies muscles by their electrical activity via a needle which probes into the muscles. A smaller number of physicians use the ultrasound which directly visualizes the muscle and confirms that the tip of the injecting needle is in the right muscle.

Like all other indications of botulinum toxin therapy, it is wise to start with a small dose and gradually increase the dose (if necessary) to an effective or more effective dose level. For torticollis (rotation type of CD), one could start first by injecting the main neck rotator muscles. If the neck is rotated to the right side, two sets of neck rotators are overactive, one on the right side located in the back of the neck (splenius—Fig. 8.6) rotating the head to the right (same side); the other rotator is on the left side of the neck (sternocleidomastoid muscle—SCM) located in front of the neck, rotating the head to the right side (opposite side). In case of Botox or Xeomin (with almost comparable units), the author of this chapter usually starts with a dose of 60 units per each muscle injected into three sites (Fig. 8.6). If there is shoulder elevation, trapezius muscle (T) is injected with the same dose. Doses up to 500 units (of Botox) may be required for patients with severe cervical dystonia, but usually not during the first session. In some patients, however, the problem is more complex, and obtaining a satisfactory response requires injection of a larger number of muscles. Many muscles in the neck have more than one function (rotation, tilt, etc.), the knowledge of these various functions is essential for proper treatment of cervical dystonia.

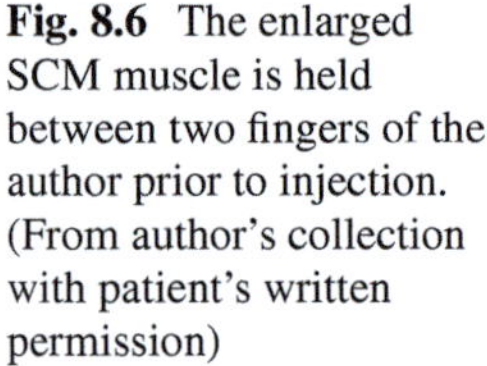

Fig. 8.6 The enlarged SCM muscle is held between two fingers of the author prior to injection. (From author's collection with patient's written permission)

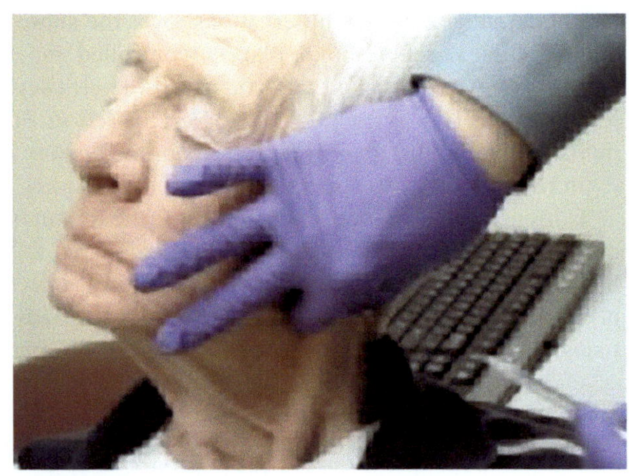

Case Report

A 72 year-old man with history of torticollis (rotational cervical dystonia) for 20 years was referred for to the Yale University Botulinum Toxin Clinic for evaluation and treatment. The patient stated that his problem had begun slowly with difficulty in turning his head to the right side. Over months and years, the neck gradually started to turn to the left and for the past 2 years, it had become very stiff and fixed to the left side. Attempting to turn the neck to the right was painful. There was also a head tilt to the left side (most common combination in CD—rotation and tilt). Patient also complained of a fair amount of neck pain which had been bothering him for years. He felt his balance was not good and his quality of life was greatly diminished. Driving was "almost impossible." On examination, the patient had fixed rotation of the head to the left with mild head tilt to the left. The right SCM muscle was very large and contracted (Fig. 8.6). He was injected with a total of 280 units of Botox (Table 8.2).

One week after Botox injection, he demonstrated marked improvement of his neck posture and the ability to rotate his neck to the right side without discomfort. Over the subsequent weeks, he reported notable decrease in his neck pain and believed his quality of life had substantially improved. Over a follow up period of almost 10 years, patient received repeat Botox injections into his neck muscles every 3–4 months. He reported no side effects.

Side effects after botulinum toxin injections for cervical dystonia are usually minor and limited to seconds or minutes of pain at the site of injection and/or minor transient local bleeding. About 30% of patients may develop some difficulty in swallowing which is usually subtle and is usually not reported by the patients unless asked for. Nevertheless, more serious cases of swallowing difficulty may develop after BoNT therapy for CD; rarely requiring hospitalization. Such cases, however, usually occur when large doses of toxin are injected into SCM muscles located in front of the neck on both sides and/or when the injecting needle is not properly

Table 8.2 Name of the muscle, muscle function, side of injection, dose and number of injections. In this patient with very severe cervical dystonia the doses for SCM and SC muscles are larger than that usually used for the first injection

Name of muscle	Muscle function and the side injected	Side of injection	Total dose	Number of sites injected
Sternocleidomastoid (SCM)	Rotates head and neck to the opposite side	Right	100 u (Botox)	Divided into 4 sites along the length of the muscle—25 u/site
Splenus Capitis (SC)	Tilts the head and neck to the same side	Left	80 u (Botox)	Divided into 2 sites. 40 u/site
Trapezius	Elevates the shoulder—right side	Right	60 units (Botox)	Divided into 3 sites. 30 u/site
Evator scapulae (LS)	Elevates the upper back bone, scapula Tilts the head to the same side—left side	Left	40 units (Botox)	Divided into two sites 20 u/site

placed in SCM, but rather misplaced close to the esophagus—the tube that connects the throat to stomach.

In some patients' SCM is hard to find if the injector performs injections when the patient is sitting up. Having the patient lie down with the head raised helps to better identify SCM bulk and its borders. Performing injections under electromyography guidance or ultrasound, helps more accurate identification of the neck muscles and proper placement of the injecting needles. Between 60% and 70% of the patients, with cervical dystonia express satisfaction with botulinum toxin therapy after the first injection session. This percentage increases with repeat injections.

In non-responders, attempts should be made to better identify and localize of the muscles. Unresponsiveness after several attempts should raise the possibility of other diagnoses including a psychogenic condition resembling CD. In rare cases, unresponsiveness may be due to the development of antibodies against the botulinum toxin in the blood. Individuals who have been vaccinated against botulinum toxin may not respond to BoNT therapy. With earlier preparations of Botox (before 1997), repeated and closely spaced injections (especially with large doses) antibodies against Botox could be detected in 25–30% of the patients and between 5% and 10% of such patients became non-responsive to subsequent treatment. With the new Botox preparations (introduced to the market in 1997) that contain lower levels of antigenic proteins, antibody formation is uncommon (close to 1%) and reported non-responsiveness is below 1% [36]. A recent report on 5876 patients treated with Botox at different centers found neutralizing antibodies (the types that may lead to clinical non-responsiveness) only in 0.3% of the patient at the completion of study [37]. Even among those few with neutralizing antibodies, less than one third demonstrated clinical non-responsiveness (5 of 16 patients). Another form of botulinum toxin type A, Xeomin (with units comparable to Botox and currently widely used in clinical practice), almost never produces unresponsiveness due to presence of negligible immunogenic proteins in its molecule [38].

Comparative studies have shown that all FDA approved botulinum toxins are effective in cervical dystonia and render a comparable efficacy in this disorder [35, 39].

Focal Limb Dystonias After Limb Trauma, Stroke and Cerebral Palsy

After head injury and stroke, many patients develop dystonia in the affected weak limbs along with increased muscle tone (spasticity). Children with spastic cerebral palsy also demonstrate dystonic hand and finger features associated with increased muscle tone in the involved limbs. The use of botulinum toxins for treatment of these secondary dystonias is described in more detail in other chapters of this book.

Task Specific Dystonias

Task specific dystonias are a group of focal dystonias that usually present in the hand and forearm muscles after performing any specific fine motor movement repetitively. There is a wide range of tasks that upon months or years of repetition can cause focal hand dystonia; those tasks include typing, playing musical instruments such as piano, guitar and writing. In sports, "golfers yip" is a kind of task specific dystonia affecting the hand in golfers. Foot dystonia of runners is an example of task specific dystonia in the lower limb. In runner's dystonia, the foot, the knee or the hip may demonstrate involuntary twisting and turning postures after prolonged running.

In the hand/finger dystonia, the most common form of TSD, dystonic postures occur after months or years of performing the same specific act. The wrist and fingers can flex or extend involuntarily and interfere with the patient's performance.

Treatment of task specific dystonia (TSD) can start with behavior modification. The results of oral medications are disappointing. In a review of literature in 2016, Drs. Lungu and Ahmad concluded that botulinum toxin therapy reduces dystonic hand and finger postures and improves the patient's performance in task specific dystonia [40]. Injections into small forearm muscles are performed under electromyographic (EMG) or ultrasound (US) guidance. The latter is able to show individual forearm muscles and has more accuracy than EMG in TSD. In practice, although effective, BoNT therapy does not completely eliminate the TSD; in case of musicians, dystonia, rarely, the initial level of performance is attainable. Based on Drs. Lungu and Ahmad's literature review [40], for writers' cramp, the total applied initial dose for Botox and Dysport is 24 and 82 units, respectively (each unit of Botox is approximately 2.5–3 units of dysport). This dose is applied to multiple forearm muscles identified by EMG or ultrasound. In established patients and after several injection sessions, the dose may be increased by 40–45% [40].

Case Report from Author's Experience

A 52 year-old music professor complained of difficulty with playing guitar for the past 3 years. He noted that after playing for a few minutes, the index finger of the right hand pulled ups and away from the other fingers impairing the quality of his music. Sometimes, the middle finger would do the same thing, although to a lesser extent. He complained also of a constant pain at the middle of his forearm "as if a knott were there". Otherwise, the patient was in good health. He had played guitar since his early teens and has been a music instructor (guitar) for the past 20 years. He denied any history of trauma to that forearm. His condition has been getting worse gradually.

While playing guitar during clinic, the right hand's index and middle fingers of the patient involuntarily pulled up and took a dystonic posture (Fig. 8.7). He complained of increased tightness of his forearm. We injected 5 units of Botox into the extensor of the index finger, (extensor indicis—Fig. 8.8) under EMG guidance. The procedure of identifying and injecting the muscle took 10–12 min; he tolerated the procedure well.

Two weeks after the injection, the patient visited the clinic and expressed deep satisfaction with the results. The pain in the forearm was gone and the index finger no longer pulled up; there were no side effects. He noted a 26-point increase in his performance scale rising from 100 to 126 points. The patient returned to the clinic 6 month later for a repeat treatment. A repeat injection of Botox with the same dose produced the same positive effect.

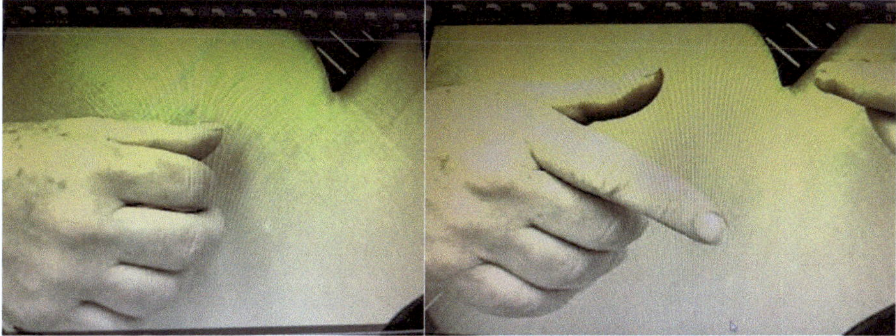

Fig. 8.7 (**a**): 30 s into playing and (**b**) 60 s into playing

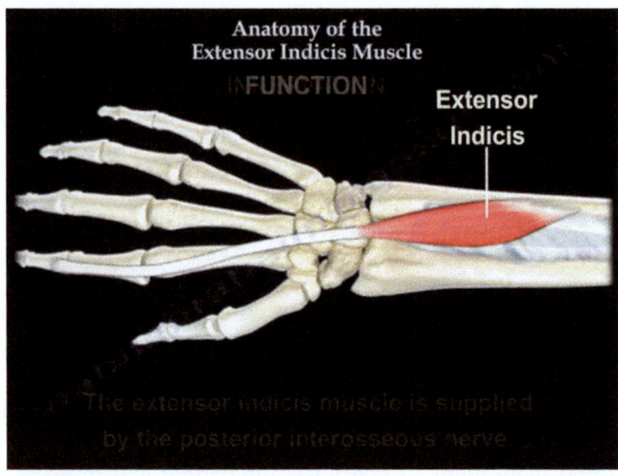

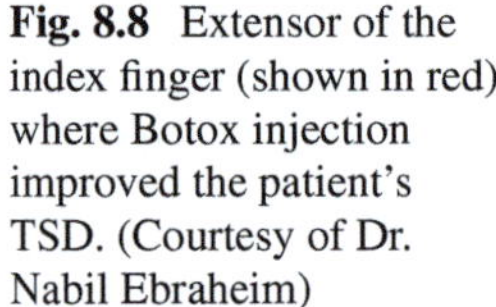

Fig. 8.8 Extensor of the index finger (shown in red) where Botox injection improved the patient's TSD. (Courtesy of Dr. Nabil Ebraheim)

The cause of task specific dystonia is not yet established. Current data suggests that the disorder may be at the brain level. In human brain, excitatory and inhibitory mechanisms are constantly at work and check each other in order to keep optimum balance between the two. Using advanced physiological techniques, investigators have shown that cortical inhibition time (cortical silence period) is significantly prolonged and the amount of inhibitory neurotransmitter (a chemical called GABA) is significantly less than normal in the brain of individuals with task specific disorders [41, 42].

Generalized Dystonia

As briefly described earlier, generalized dystonia starts usually in childhood and many affected children have a genetic predisposition. It is possible to help patients with generalized dystonia by injecting botulinum toxins into selected, more severely affected muscles. The method and dose of these local injections in adults are not different from what is used for focal dystonias. In children the dose needs to be adjusted per weight.

Tremor

Tremor is an involuntary movement that is due to rhythmic oscillation of muscles in a body part. The muscle oscillations usually alternate between two sets of muscles that have opposite functions; For example muscles that bend or extend the wrist. High quality studies (comparing botulinum toxin with placebo injection) have shown significant reduction of two types of tremors after botulinum toxin injection—Parkinson tremor and essential tremor.

Parkinson Tremor

Parkinson disease (PD) affects 1% of US population over 60 years of age [43]. Men are affected slightly more than women. The three cardinal symptoms of Parkinson disease consist of slowness of movements (bradykinesia), muscle rigidity and hand tremor. Tremor of Parkinson's disease has the highest amplitude when the hand and forearm are at rest. In many patients with PD, this resting tremor interferes with sleeping. Approximately half of patients with PD have action tremor—a tremor that gets worse with moving the limb [44]. Such tremors interfere with writing, playing musical instruments, shaving and other activities that require fine motor control.

Parkinson disease is due to loss of dopamine in the brain and other parts of the nervous system. Dopamine is essential for maintaining both the speed of movement and healthy tone of muscles. Most drugs that are used for treatment of Parkinson's disease either replenish the lost dopamine or enhance the effect of remaining dopamine. These drugs improve slow movement and muscle stiffness (rigidity), but are less effective on Parkinson's tremor. A surgical procedure called "deep brain stimulation" can markedly improve Parkinson's tremor by electrical stimulation of deep brain structures (basal ganglia). However, the procedure requires inserting a metal wire inside the brain and embedding a stimulator box in the muscles of the chest wall. There are also potential complications with this surgery such as infection, minor bleeding inside the brain and malfunction of the stimulator.

Botulinum Toxin Treatment of Parkinson Tremor

In 1991, Trosch and Pulmann first reported that 5 patients with Parkinson tremor expressed satisfaction after injecting Botox into their forearm muscles [45]. The mechanism of tremor improvement—as improvement in other movement disorders—was speculated to be related to inhibition of acetylcholine release from nerve endings by Botox. In a later study [46], authors reported excellent response of jaw tremor to botulinum toxin injection in three patients with PD. In this study, patients received 30–100 units of dysport (Type A botulinum toxin) into each masseter muscle. Subsequent publications also supported the positive role of botulinum toxin therapy for Parkinson tremor [47], although weakness of the hand and fingers lasting for a few weeks (a side effect seen in 30% of patients) remains a drawback of this treatment.

Over the past 10 years (since 2013) investigators aimed to develop an injection plan that would significantly reduce intensity and frequency of hand and finger weakness after botulinum toxin injections for Parkinson tremor.

In a 3-year study that lasted from 2012 to 2014, the author of his chapter and his colleagues at Yale University, conducted a study with Xeomin (a type A toxin like Botox) injection into forearm muscle of patients with Parkinson tremor [48].

Thirty-three patients were enrolled in the study and 30 patients completed the study. The study was placebo controlled i.e. the effect of Xeomin injections were compared with placebo (salt water injection). It also had a flexible design i.e. in each patient, different sets of muscles were injected based on the pattern of muscles' activity seen in electromyography. Electromyography screens the electrical activity of the muscle by a special instrument. In each patient 8–12 muscles in the forearm that are often involved in finger or hand tremor were screened by EMG first. Only those muscles that showed increased electrical activity by EMG were injected. The magnitude and frequency of patients' hand tremor was measured by standard tremor—scales at baseline and at 4 and 8 weeks after injection. A global impression of change assessed also the Patients' perception regarding changes (or lack of it) in hand tremor after injections. The study was a "cross over study"—the substance (placebo or Xeomin) was alternated at 3 months (second injection). For example, if a patient had received Xeomin the first time, the second injection was placebo and vice versa. The study was double-blind meaning that both the injectors and patients were not aware of what was injected (Xeomin or placebo). A nurse not involved in injections or rating of the response prepared the Xeomin or saline in a small syringe and kept a record in a password protected computer.

At the conclusion of this study, the results strongly favored Xeomin injections for treatment of Parkinson tremor. Rating assessment, both at 4 and 8 weeks after injection, demonstrated that tremor improvement was significant in the Xeomin group compared to the placebo group. Patients who had received Xeomin also demonstrated improved quality of life and were much happier with injections than those who had received placebo injections. Subtle decreased hand strength, measured by ergometer only but not perceptible by the patient, was noted in 37% of Xeomin and 22% of placebo group (not a statistically significant difference). Hand weakness, perceptible to the patient, was reported by 7% of patients in the Xeomin group considerably less than what had been reported in prior studies of tremor (30–40%) [49, 50]. The authors concluded that a flexible pattern of injection that covers more muscles with smaller doses is effective in reducing the amplitude of PD without causing notable hand weakness in a high percentage of patients.

Over the past 10 years, the researcher from the Western University in Canada have also developed a system of botulinum toxin injection for tremor that results in low incidence of finger and hand weakness after the toxin injection. In their protocol, muscle selection for injection was guided through four transducers attached to four joints of the forearm and hand. Their result with botulinum toxin treatment of PD tremor is comparable with results of the Yale protocol i.e. efficacy associated with low incidence of finger and hand weakness [51]. Their device, however, is not commercially available. Details of the two above-mentioned techniques (Yale in US and Western University in Canada) and comparison of their results have been published in a recent review article [52].

Essential Tremor

Essential tremor is a common genetic disorder characterized by a 4–8/s forearm tremor observed mainly when the hands are in action (moving or stretched). This is the opposite of Parkinson's tremor which is usually observed at rest. Approximately half of the patients have a history of a similar type of tremor in their close relatives (unlike PD tremor). Severe essential tremors can significantly interfere with the activities of daily living and handicap the patient. Beta blockers (propranolol and others), primidone and topiramate are effective in reducing essential tremor, but the efficacy often wears off after chronic use. Deep brain stimulation (see under Parkinson tremor) is very effective, but requires brain surgery.

Three high quality studies (comparing the effect of toxin with placebo) have investigated the utility of botulinum toxin injection into the forearm muscles of patients with essential tremor. In 1996, Dr. Jankovic and his colleagues at Baylor Medical College in Houston [49] injected 50 and 100 units of Botox into the forearm muscles (wrist flexors) of 25 patients with severe essential tremor. After 4 weeks, 75% of the patients demonstrated improvement of their tremor by 2 grades (on scale of 0–10). However, between 30% and 40% of the patients reported disabling weakness of fingers. These positive results were duplicated in another placebo-controlled study of 123 patients with essential tremor using the same technique and dosage of Botox [50]. Unfortunately, still a sizeable number of patients (approximately 30%) developed notable weakness of their fingers. The investigators of both studies attributed weakness of fingers after Botox injection to applying a fixed dose injection approach and to the sensitivity of finger extensor muscles to Botox.

Between years 2013 to 2016, the author of this chapter and his colleagues at the Yale University, New Haven, CT conducted a third double-blinded, placebo-controlled study on essential tremor [53]. Thirty-three patients participated and 28 completed the study. The methodology was exactly as their previous study of botulinum toxin therapy in PD tremor (described earlier). Culprit muscles were identified by a special EMG unit registering the sound of increased electrical activity during tremor. Patients received injections of either 80–120 units (total) of Xeomin (a type A toxin similar to Botox), or a placebo (salt water) into 6–8 forearm and two arm (biceps and triceps) muscles. The injecting doctor was blinded to what patient received (Xeomin or placebo) and the patients did not know whether what they received was toxin or salt water. Standard scales were used to assess the intensity of tremor and quality of life at baseline and every 4 weeks after injection. After 4 months, the patients received a second injection alternating placebo for Xeomin or vice versa, depending on what the patient had received initially. The assessments were carried out for the next 14 months, at monthly intervals.

Statistically significant improvement of tremor was noted after Xeomin injections along with improvement of quality of life. Patients also expressed their satisfaction with Xeomin injections (not placebo) on a patient satisfaction scale. One patient (4%) developed notable finger weakness which lasted for 2 months. Using a flexible injection scheme and smaller amount of toxin into forearm finger extensor muscles, this study demonstrated efficacy of Xeomin in reducing ET tremor along with low incidence of finger weakness (4% versus 30–40% reported in previous studies).

Over the past 10 years, researchers from Western University of Canada, have conducted open label studies (not-blinded) assessing the efficacy of botulinum toxin injections in essential tremor. Using the kinetic approach (identifying tremoring muscles with joint-attached transducers), they reported similar efficacy and low incidence of finger and hand weakness [54, 55].

Tics

Tics are involuntary, rapid and repetitive movements that, at times, can be stopped momentarily by will. Most tics are simple motor tics associated with no sensory or other symptoms. A more complex type of tic, presents with associated glottal sound, and sometimes vocalization (saying words or sentences) in addition to the motor manifestations. Vocalizations may include profanity (coprolalia). This condition bears the name of the French physician (Tourette) who provided the first detailed description of this type of tic; it is hence called Tourette syndrome. Almost all tics start in childhood and gradually improve after age 30 years (some totally disappear). However, when present and especially if they are frequent and complex, in addition to social embarrassment, they deteriorate the patients' quality of life. Many patients with tics have premonitory signs (different sensations) or an urge to move before the emergence of tic episodes.

Treatment of tics may start with behavioral modification, for which, several programs are currently available. Pharmacological treatment of tics basically uses three groups of drugs; dopamine blockers, dopamine depleters such as flufenazine or tetrabenazine and clonidine, an alpha 2 enhancer. Dopamine is a protein that is present in abundance in deep brain structures (basal ganglia). Dopamine deficiency (in Parkinson's disease) or enhanced activity of dopamine (tics) are major players in manifestation of motor disorders. Some patients with disabling tics and failure to respond to oral medications have responded to electrical stimulation of brain's deep structures (deep brain stimulation-DBS) [56].

Dr. Jankovic and his colleagues at the Baylor College of Medicine (Houston, Texas) were first to demonstrate in 10 patients that injection of Botox into the muscles involved in repetitive involuntary movements of tics can reduce the frequency and severity of the motor tics [57]. Subsequently, in a larger study of 35 patients with tics, Botox was compared to placebo (saline injections) and authors came to the same conclusion [58]. In this study, approximately 40% of patients with recalcitrant tics, not responding to oral medications, demonstrated marked mitigation of tic movements after Botox injections into the moving muscles (arm, shoulder, neck). In another study, injection of very small doses of Dysport (approximately 2.5 units of Dysport equals 1 unit of Botox) into the vocal cord muscles of patients with tics and vocalization (vocal tics) resulted in total resolution of vocal tics in 50% of the 22 patients studied. In this study, in a majority of patients, the voice became soft for several weeks after toxin injection but patients did not think it changed their quality of life.

During the so-called malignant tics, repetitive and erratic tic movements can cause serious injury such as biting the tongue, lacerating the face or poking the eyes [58]. Botulinum toxin injection into the hand or arm of patients with malignant, fast targeting tic movements can reduce the urge to move the limb and, by weakening the limb buy time for preventing or recovery from the injury. The author of this chapter treated a 19-year-old male for repetitive flinging movements of the left hand and arm targeting his own left eye leading to corneal laceration. Treatment with a variety of medications for his severe motor tics caused sedation but did not succeed to stop the movements. His parents and his treating physician were worried that he would eventually lose the left eye. Injection of Botox, a total of 200 units in different arm and forearm muscles of the left upper limb, weakened the left arm and forearm, stopped the urge to move as well as stopping the movements themselves. Three months later after the effect of Botox wore off, tics returned with less intensity and were managed with medications.

Conclusion

Botulinum toxin therapy is approved by FDA for treatment of blepharospasm, hemifacial spasm and cervical dystonia in US. Because of its efficacy and safety, it is now considered the first line of treatment for these conditions. In task specific dystonias (musicians' dystonia, writers' dystonia), oromandibular dystonias (jaw opening, jaw closure), Parkinson and Essential tremor the results are also encouraging and botulinum toxin therapy is practiced by experts in the different medical centers around the word. Botulinum toxin injections are also effective in patients with troublesome focal motor tics and patients suffering from phonic tics resulting in unpleasant guttural sounds [59].

References

1. Definition provided by the National Institutes of neurological disorders and Stroke (NIH).
2. Hallett M. Blepharospasm: recent advances. Neurology. 2002;59:1306–12.
3. Nutt JG, Meunter MD, Aranson A, et al. Epidemiology of focal and generalized dystonia in Rochester, Minnesota. Mov Disord. 1988;3:188–94.
4. Illowsky-Karp B, Alter K. Botulinum treatment of blepharospasm, orofacial/oromandibular dystonia, and hemifacial spasm. Semin Neurol. 2016;36:84–91.
5. Truong D, Comella C, Fernandez HH, et al. Efficacy and safety of purified botulinum toxin type A (dysport) for the treatment of benign essential blepharospasm: a randomized, placebo-controlled phase II trial. Parkinsonism Relat Disord. 2008;14:407–14.

6. Jankovic J. Blepharospasm and oromandibular-laryngeal-cervical dystonia: a controlled trial of botulinum A toxin therapy. Adv Neurol. 1988;50:583–91. PMID: 3041763

7. Park YC, Lim JK, Lee DK, Yi SD. Botulinum a toxin treatment of hemifacial spasm and blepharospasm. J Korean Med Sci. 1993 Oct;8(5):334–40. https://doi.org/10.3346/jkms.1993.8.5.334. PMID: 8305141; PMCID: PMC3053713.

8. Jankovic J, Comella C, Hanschmann A, Grafe S. Efficacy and safety of incobotulinumtoxinA (NT 201, Xeomin) in the treatment of blepharospasm – A randomized trial. Mov Disord. 2011 July;26(8):1521–8. https://doi.org/10.1002/mds.23658. Epub 2011 Apr 22. PMID: 21520284.

9. Roggenkämper P, Jost WH, Bihari K, Comes G, Grafe S, NT 201 Blepharospasm Study Team. Efficacy and safety of a new botulinum toxin type A free of complexing proteins in the treatment of blepharospasm. J Neural Transm (Vienna). 2006 Mar;113(3):303–12. https://doi.org/10.1007/s00702-005-0323-3. Epub 2005 June 15. PMID: 15959841.

10. Truong D, Comella C, Fernandez HH, Ondo WG, Dysport Benign Essential Blepharospasm Study Group. Efficacy and safety of purified botulinum toxin type A (Dysport) for the treatment of benign essential blepharospasm: a randomized, placebo-controlled, phase II trial. Parkinsonism Relat Disord. 2008;14(5):407–14. https://doi.org/10.1016/j.parkreldis.2007.11.003. Epub 2008 Mar 5. PMID: 18325821.

11. Wabbels B, Reichel G, Fulford-Smith A, Wright N, Roggenkämper P. Double-blind, randomised, parallel group pilot study comparing two botulinum toxin type A products for the treatment of blepharospasm. J Neural Transm (Vienna). 2011 Feb;118(2):233–9. https://doi.org/10.1007/s00702-010-0529-x. Epub 2010 Dec 16. PMID: 21161715.

12. Yoon JS, Kim JC, Lee SY. Double-blind, randomized, comparative study of Meditoxin versus Botox in the treatment of essential blepharospasm. Korean J Ophthalmol. 2009 Sept;23(3):137–41. https://doi.org/10.3341/kjo.2009.23.3.137. Epub 2009 Sept 8. PMID: 19794937; PMCID: PMC2739960.

13. Rieder CR, Schestatsky P, Socal MP, Monte TL, Fricke D, Costa J, Picon PD. A double-blind, randomized, crossover study of Prosigne versus Botox in patients with blepharospasm and hemifacial spasm. Clin Neuropharmacol 2007 Jan–Feb;30(1):39–42. https://doi.org/10.1097/01.WNF.0000236771.77021.3C. PMID: 17272968.

14. Truong DD, Gollomp SM, Jankovic J, LeWitt PA, Marx M, Hanschmann A, Fernandez HH, Xeomin US Blepharospasm Study Group. Sustained efficacy and safety of repeated incobotulinumtoxinA (Xeomin®) injections in blepharospasm. J Neural Transm (Vienna). 2013 Sept;120(9):1345–53. https://doi.org/10.1007/s00702-013-0998-9. Epub 2013 Feb 23. PMID: 23435927; PMCID: PMC3751217.

15. Sinclair CF, Gurey LE, Blitzer A. Oromandibular dystonia: long-term management with botulinum toxin. Laryngoscope. 2013 Dec;123(12):3078–83. https://doi.org/10.1002/lary.23265. Epub 2013 Oct 5. PMID: 24122897.

16. Blitzer A, Brin MF, Fahn S. Botulinum toxin injections for lingual dystonia. Laryngoscope. 1991 July;101(7 Pt 1):799. https://doi.org/10.1288/00005537-199107000-00024. PMID: 2062167.

17. Scorr LM, Factor SA, Parra SP, Kaye R, Paniello RC, Norris SA, Perlmutter JS, Bäumer T, Usnich T, Berman BD, Mailly M, Roze E, Vidailhet M, Jankovic J, LeDoux MS, Barbano R, Chang FCF, Fung VSC, Pirio Richardson S, Blitzer A, Jinnah HA. Oromandibular dystonia: a clinical examination of 2,020 cases. Front Neurol. 2021 Sept 16;12:700714. https://doi.org/10.3389/fneur.2021.700714. PMID: 34603182; PMCID: PMC8481678.

18. Colosimo C, Bologna M, Lamberti S, et al. A comparative study of primary and secondary hemifacial spasm. Arch Neurol. 2006;63:441–4.

19. Kaufmann AM. Hemifacial spasm: a neurosurgical perspective. J Neurosurg. 2023 July 7:1–8. https://doi.org/10.3171/2023.5.JNS221898. Epub ahead of print. PMID: 37439481.

20. Ababneh OH, Cetinkaya A, Kulwin DR. Long-term efficacy and safety of botulinum toxin A injections to treat blepharospasm and hemifacial spasm. Clin Experiment Ophthalmol. 2014 Apr;42(3):254–61. https://doi.org/10.1111/ceo.12165. Epub 2013 Aug 4. PMID: 23844601.

21. Hallett M, Albanese A, Dressler D, Segal KR, Simpson DM, Truong D, Jankovic J. Evidence-based review and assessment of botulinum neurotoxin for the treatment of movement disorders. Toxicon. 2013 June 1;67:94–114. https://doi.org/10.1016/j.toxicon.2012.12.004. Epub 2013 Feb 4. PMID: 23380701.

22. Karp BI, Alter K. Botulinum toxin treatment of blepharospasm, orofacial/oromandibular dystonia, and hemifacial spasm. Semin Neurol. 2016 Feb;36(1):84–91. https://doi.org/10.1055/s-0036-1571952. Epub 2016 Feb 11. PMID: 26866500.

23. Jankovic J, Adler CH, Charles D. Primary results from cercical dystonia patient egistry for observation of onabotulinum toxin A efficacy (CD Probe). J Neurol Sci. 2015;349:84–93.

24. Avenali M, De Icco R, Tinazzi M, Defazio G, Tronconi L, Sandrini G, Tassorelli C. Pain in focal dystonias – a focused review to address an important component of the disease. Parkinsonism Relat Disord 2018 Sept;54:17–24. https://doi.org/10.1016/j.parkreldis.2018.04.030. Epub 2018 Apr 27. PMID: 29724604.

25. Camfield L, Ben-Shlomo Y, Warner TT, Epidemiological Study of Dystonia in Europe Collaborative Group. Impact of cervical dystonia on quality of life. Mov Disord. 2002 July;17(4):838–41. https://doi.org/10.1002/mds.10127. PMID: 12210891.

26. Tsui JK, Eisen A, Mak E, Carruthers J, Scott A, Calne DB. A pilot study on the use of botulinum toxin in spasmodic torticollis. Can J Neurol Sci. 1985 Nov;12(4):314–6. https://doi.org/10.1017/s031716710003540x. PMID: 4084867.

27. Marsh WA, Monroe DM, Brin MF, Gallagher CJ. Systematic review and meta-analysis of the duration of clinical effect of onabotulinumtoxinA in cervical dystonia. BMC Neurol. 2014 Apr 27;14:91. https://doi.org/10.1186/1471-2377-14-91. PMID: 24767576; PMCID: PMC4013807.

28. Poewe W, Deuschl G, Nebe A, Feifel E, Wissel J, Benecke R, Kessler KR, Ceballos-Baumann AO, Ohly A, Oertel W, Künig G. What is the optimal dose of botulinum toxin A in the treatment of cervical dystonia? Results of a double blind, placebo controlled, dose ranging study using Dysport. German Dystonia Study Group. J Neurol Neurosurg Psychiatry. 1998 Jan;64(1):13–7. https://doi.org/10.1136/jnnp.64.1.13. PMID: 9436721; PMCID: PMC2169893.

29. Truong D, Duane DD, Jankovic J, Singer C, Seeberger LC, Comella CL, Lew MF, Rodnitzky RL, Danisi FO, Sutton JP, Charles PD, Hauser RA, Sheean GL. Efficacy and safety of botulinum type A toxin (Dysport) in cervical dystonia: results of the first US randomized, double-blind, placebo-controlled study. Mov Disord. 2005 July;20(7):783–91. https://doi.org/10.1002/mds.20403. PMID: 15736159.

30. Evidente VG, Truong D, Jankovic J, Comella CL, Grafe S, Hanschmann A. IncobotulinumtoxinA (Xeomin®) injected for blepharospasm or cervical dystonia according to patient needs is well tolerated. J Neurol Sci. 2014 Nov 15;346(1–2):116–20. https://doi.org/10.1016/j.jns.2014.08.004. Epub 2014 Aug 10. PMID: 25186131.

31. Lew MF, Adornato BT, Duane DD, Dykstra DD, Factor SA, Massey JM, Brin MF, Jankovic J, Rodnitzky RL, Singer C, Swenson MR, Tarsy D, Murray JJ, Koller M, Wallace JD. Botulinum toxin type B: a double-blind, placebo-controlled, safety and efficacy study in cervical dystonia. Neurology. 1997 Sept;49(3):701–7. https://doi.org/10.1212/wnl.49.3.701. PMID: 9305326.

32. Bledsoe IO, Comella CL. Botulinum toxin treatment of cervical dystonia. Semin Neurol. 2016;36:47–53.

33. Jankovic J. Botulinum toxin therapy for cervical dystonia. Neurotox Res 2006 Apr;9(2–3):145–8. https://doi.org/10.1007/BF03033933. PMID: 16785112.

34. Mordin M, Masaquel C, Abbott C, Copley-Merriman C. Factors affecting the health-related quality of life of patients with cervical dystonia and impact of treatment with abobotulinumtoxinA (Dysport): results from a randomised, double-blind, placebo-controlled study. BMJ Open. 2014 Oct 16;4(10):e005150. https://doi.org/10.1136/bmjopen-2014-005150. PMID: 25324317; PMCID: PMC4201999.

35. Yun JY, Kim JW, Kim HT, Chung SJ, Kim JM, Cho JW, Lee JY, Lee HN, You S, Oh E, Jeong H, Kim YE, Kim HJ, Lee WY, Jeon BS. Dysport and Botox at a ratio of 2.5:1 units in cervical dystonia: a double-blind, randomized study. Mov Disord. 2015 Feb;30(2):206–13. https://doi.org/10.1002/mds.26085. Epub 2014 Dec 5. PMID: 25476727; PMCID: PMC4359015.

36. Brin MF, Comella CL, Jankovic J. Long-term treatment with botulinum toxin type A in cervical dystonia has low immunogenicity by mouse protection assay. Mov Disord. 2008;23:1353–60.
37. Jankovic J, Carruthers J, Naumann M, Ogilvie P, Boodhoo T, Attar M, Gupta S, Singh R, Soliman J, Yushmanova I, Brin MF, Shen J. Neutralizing antibody formation with onabotulinumtoxinA (BOTOX®) treatment from global registration studies across multiple indications: a meta-analysis. Toxins (Basel). 2023 May 17;15(5):342. https://doi.org/10.3390/toxins15050342. PMID: 37235376; PMCID: PMC10224273.
38. Dressler D. Five-year experience with incobotulinumtoxinA (Xeomin®): the first botulinum toxin drug free of complexing proteins. Eur J Neurol. 2012 Mar;19(3):385–9. https://doi.org/10.1111/j.1468-1331.2011.03559.x. Epub 2011 Oct 28. PMID: 22035051.
39. Duarte GS, Castelão M, Rodrigues FB, Marques RE, Ferreira J, Sampaio C, Moore AP, Costa J. Botulinum toxin type A versus botulinum toxin type B for cervical dystonia. Cochrane Database Syst Rev. 2016 Oct 26;10(10):CD004314. https://doi.org/10.1002/14651858.CD004314.pub3. PMID: 27782297; PMCID: PMC6461154.
40. Lungo C, Ahmad OF. Update on the use of botulinum toxin therapy for focal and task specific dystonias. Semin Neurol. 2016;36:41–6.
41. Levy LM, Hallett M. Impaired brain GABA in focal dystonia. Ann Neurol. 2002 Jan;51(1):93–101. PMID: 11782988.
42. Merchant SHI, Wu T, Hallett M. Diagnostic neurophysiologic biomarkers for task-specific dystonia. Mov Disord Clin Pract. 2022 Apr 14;9(4):468–472. https://doi.org/10.1002/mdc3.13448. PMID: 35586528; PMCID: PMC9092748.
43. Jindal P, Jankovic J. Botulinum toxin treatment in Parkinson' disease and atypical Parkinsonian disorders. In: Jabbari B, editor. Botulinum toxin treatment in clinical medicine. A disease-oriented approach. Cham: Springer; 2018. p. 23–58.
44. Louis ED, Frucht SJ. Prevalence of essential tremor in patients with Parkinson's disease vs. Parkinson-plus syndromes. Mov Disord. 2007 July 30;22(10):1402–7. https://doi.org/10.1002/mds.21383. PMID: 17516475.
45. Trosch RM, Pullman SL. Botulinum toxin A injections for the treatment of hand tremors. Mov Disord. 1994 Nov;9(6):601–9. https://doi.org/10.1002/mds.870090604. PMID: 7845399.
46. Schneider SA, Edwards MJ, Cordivari C, Macleod WN, Bhatia KP. Botulinum toxin A may be efficacious as treatment for jaw tremor in Parkinson's disease. Mov Disord. 2006 Oct;21(10):1722–4. https://doi.org/10.1002/mds.21019. PMID: 16817198.
47. Sheffield JK, Jankovic J. Botulinum toxin in the treatment of tremors, dystonias, sialorrhea and other symptoms associated with Parkinson's disease. Expert Rev Neurother. 2007 June;7(6):637–47. https://doi.org/10.1586/14737175.7.6.637. PMID: 17563247.
48. Mittal SO, Machado D, Richardson D, Dubey D, Jabbari B. Botulinum toxin in Parkinson disease tremor: a randomized, double-blind, placebo-controlled study with a customized injection approach. Mayo Clin Proc. 2017;92:1359–67.
49. Jankovic J, Schwartz K, Clemence W, Aswad A, Mordaunt J. A randomized, double-blind, placebo-controlled study to evaluate botulinum toxin type A in essential hand tremor. Mov Disord. 1996 May;11(3):250–6. https://doi.org/10.1002/mds.870110306. PMID: 8723140.
50. Brin MF, Lyons KE, Doucette J, Adler CH, Caviness JN, Comella CL, Dubinsky RM, Friedman JH, Manyam BV, Matsumoto JY, Pullman SL, Rajput AH, Sethi KD, Tanner C, Koller WC. A randomized, double masked, controlled trial of botulinum toxin type A in essential hand tremor. Neurology. 2001 June 12;56(11):1523–8. https://doi.org/10.1212/wnl.56.11.1523. PMID: 11402109.
51. Samotus O, Lee J, Jog M. Standardized algorithm for muscle selection and dosing of botulinum toxin for Parkinson tremor using kinematic analysis. Ther Adv Neurol Disord. 2020 Sept 23;13:1756286420954083. https://doi.org/10.1177/1756286420954083. PMID: 33014139; PMCID: PMC7517980.
52. Mittal SO, Jog M, Lee J, Jabbari B. Novel botulinum toxin injection protocols for Parkinson tremor and essential tremor – the Yale technique and sensor-based kinematics procedure for safe and effective treatment. Tremor Other Hyperkinet Mov (N Y). 2020 Dec 31;10:61. https://doi.org/10.5334/tohm.582. PMID: 33442486; PMCID: PMC7774361.

53. Mittal SO, Machado D, Richardson D, Dubey D, Jabbari B. Botulinum toxin in essential hand tremor – a randomized double-blind placebo-controlled study with customized injection approach. Parkinsonism Relat Disord 2018 Nov;56:65–9. https://doi.org/10.1016/j.parkreldis.2018.06.019. Epub 2018 June 12. PMID: 29929813.
54. Samotus O, Rahimi F, Lee J, Jog M. Functional ability improved in essential tremor by incobotulinumtoxinA injections using kinematically determined biomechanical patterns – a new future. PLoS One. 2016 Apr 21;11(4):e0153739. https://doi.org/10.1371/journal.pone.0153739. PMID: 27101283; PMCID: PMC4839603.
55. Samotus O, Kumar N, Rizek P, Jog M. Botulinum toxin type A injections as monotherapy for upper limb essential tremor using kinematics. Can J Neurol Sci. 2018 Jan;45(1):11–22. https://doi.org/10.1017/cjn.2017.260. Epub 2017 Nov 21. PMID: 29157315.
56. Bajwa RJ, de Lotbinière AJ, King RA, Jabbari B, Quatrano S, Kunze K, Scahill L, Leckman JF. Deep brain stimulation in Tourette's syndrome. Mov Disord. 2007 July 15;22(9):1346–50. https://doi.org/10.1002/mds.21398. PMID: 17580320.
57. Jankovic J. Botulinum toxin in the treatment of dystonic tics. Mov Disord. 1994 May;9(3):347–9. https://doi.org/10.1002/mds.870090315. PMID: 8041378.
58. Marras C, Andrews D, Sime E, Lang AE. Botulinum toxin in simple motor tics. A randomized, double blind, controlled clinical trial. Neurology. 2001;56:605–10.
59. Jankovic J. Treatment of tics associated with Tourette syndrome. J Neural Transm (Vienna). 2020 May;127(5):843–50. https://doi.org/10.1007/s00702-019-02105-w. Epub 2020 Jan 18. PMID: 31955299.

Chapter 9
Botulinum Toxin Treatment in Children

Abstract Over the past 35 years, botulinum toxin therapy in adults has been established as a major mode of treatment for a variety of medical conditions. Several of these conditions including involuntary movements, spasticity, chronic migraine, excessive sweating/drooling, and bladder dysfunction have received FDA approval for use in the US. In this chapter, major indications of botulinum toxin therapy in childhood including stiffness of muscles with increased reflexes (spasticity), involuntary movements, strabismus (crossed eyes) and excessive sweating/drooling will be addressed.

Keywords Botulinum toxin · Botulinum neurotoxin · Children · Spasticity · Dystonia · Strabismus · Sialorrhea

Introduction

The first childhood medical disorder that was researched and received approval from FDA (1989) for botulinum toxin therapy was strabismus (crossed eyes)—a predominantly childhood ailment (see Chap. 1 on history of botulinum toxin therapy). Approval for other potential indications in childhood lagged behind the adult indications for sometimes due to safety concerns. Currently, botulinum toxin therapy in children has been approved by FDA for spasticity associated with cerebral palsy, stroke, brain and spinal cord trauma as well as involuntary movement disorders (dystonia), sialorrhea(excessive drooling) and excessive sweating (hyperhidrosis). Other conditions such as bladder dysfunction and chronic migraine, in which botulinum toxin therapy has been approved for adult are now actively under investigation for childhood application.

As discussed in the first three chapters of this book, only two of eight serotypes of botulinum toxins (types A and B) are currently in medical use. Five type A toxins—Botox, Xeomin, Dysport, Jeuveau and Daxxify -and one type B toxin (Myobloc) have FDA approval for use in the US. Jeuveau is currently approved only for aesthetic use. The units of these marketed formulations are not truly comparable, but an approximation is often used in medical research and practice: 1unit of Botox = 1 unit of Xeomin = 2.5 units of Dysport = 40–50 units of Myobloc.

The pharmacological characteristics, modes of preparation for clinical use and other issues differentiating these toxin formulations are discussed in Chaps. 2 and 3 of this book. Safety issues in botulin toxin therapy with particular emphasis among children, are addressed in Chap. 17 of this book.

Botulinum Toxin Therapy in Childhood Spasticity

Childhood spasticity is probably the condition for which botulinum toxin therapy is most widely used among children today. Spasticity is increased muscle tone leading to muscle stiffness, decreased range of joint movements and progressive immobility. Spasticity is associated with increased reflexes [1–4]. It is caused by damage to the central nervous system (brain or spinal cord). The most common causes of spasticity in children include cerebral palsy, trauma to the brain and spinal cord, as well as hereditary/genetic disorders that result in alteration of brain tissue and impairment of brain or spinal cord function. Untreated spasticity leads to muscle contracture a condition characterized by shortened and non-functioning muscles. In the advanced cases of spasticity, the joints also become non-functional and immobile. The spastic muscles and involved joints are often painful.

Treatment of spasticity includes both physical therapy and medicinal approach. Subtle and mild spasticity can improve with physical therapy and stretch exercises alone. Moderate or severe spasticity requires more aggressive approach to improve range of motion across the joint (s) and prevent immobility. In these cases, physical therapy is often combined with pharmacological therapy. Among different anti-spasticity drugs, benzodiazepines (Valium), Baclofen and Tizanidine are the most widely used medications for treatment of spasticity [5, 6]. Although partially effective, the side effects of these drugs often prevent dose escalation to the level that can produce the optimal desirable results. Valium can cause drowsiness, sedation, balance problems and drop in blood pressure. Nausea, confusion, muscle weakness and drowsiness are common side effects of Baclofen. Tizanidine (Zanaflex) can cause sedation, drop in blood pressure and liver toxicity. Very severe cases of spasticity, especially when involving the legs and impairing ambulation are sometimes treated with baclofen pump. Treatment with baclofen pump is an involved procedure that requires implanting a small pump into the abdominal wall that drips baclofen solution directly into the spinal fluid via an inserted tube. It requires availability of an experienced surgeon as well as a trained and dedicated nurse for insertion of the pump and titration of the baclofen dose for continuous infusion. Incorrect titration can lead to baclofen toxicity with serious side effects (seizures, coma).

Intramuscular injection of Botulinum toxins relaxes the muscles by blocking the release of acetylcholine. Acetylcholine is released from nerve endings to activate the muscle [8]. It is this function that makes BoNT injection a desirable commodity for relieving the troublesome effects of spasticity such as stiff muscles, limitation of movements across the joints as well as muscle and joint pain. Detailed description of how botulinum toxins exert this effect on the neuromuscular junction is provided in Chaps. 2 and 3 of this book. This antispasticity function is shared among four FDA-approved marketed botulinum toxins (Dysport, Botox, Xeomin, Myobloc) in US. Daxxify is effectiv3e against cervical dystonia (see Chap. 8) but its effect on spasticity has not been thoroughly studied.

Cerebral Palsy (CP)

The term cerebral palsy describes a medical condition in which children, from a very young age, develop neurological problems following brain damage. In a majority of these children, the damage happens during the first 2 years of life when the immature brain is very sensitive to the lack of oxygen. Birth difficulties and birth trauma are the leading causes of cerebral palsy [7, 9, 10].

The prevalence of cerebral palsy is 1.5–3 per 1000 live births worldwide [11]. Cerebral palsy has two common forms of clinical presentation. The more common of the two, is weak and stiff limbs (spasticity). In some children abnormal involuntary movements are the prominent clinical feature of CP. Cognition is impaired in a large number of children with CP, but some children may have near normal or even normal mentation. The spastic form of cerebral palsy (commonest form), leads to limitation in range of motion of the limbs across the joints and pain in the joints and muscles. Progressive shortening of the muscles may lead to immobility. Since with current medical managements, the life expectancy of children with CP is comparable with children without CP (near normal), CP is a major cause of impaired motor function and gait in adults with CP. Treatment of spasticity in CP requires medications as described earlier in this chapter combined with physical therapy. For most children, however, these treatments are mostly palliative with no or little observable return of motor function.

In 1993, Dr. Andrew Koman and his coworkers were the first to show that injection of Botox into the spastic muscles of children with cerebral palsy can improve and reduce muscle tone and help delay the corrective surgery to more appropriate age when the child is older [12]. In this open label study (no comparison with placebo), a majority of the 27 children who were poorly responsive to conventional pharmacotherapy demonstrated improvement in motor function after Botox injection. Since then, several high quality, blinded (both injector and patient), placebo–controlled studies have confirmed that spasticity of children with CP responds well to botulinum toxin injections with ultimate improvement in quality of life similar to treatment results in adults [13–18].

Based on the above mentioned literature, FDA approved the type A toxin Dysport (each unit of Dysport is 2.5–3 units of Botox) for treatment of children's lower limb spasticity in 2016. In 2019, FDA also approved Botox for the same indication in children. In 2020, Xeomin, another type A botulinum toxin, was approved by FDA for use in children of 2 years and older affected by spasticity.

Case Report-Author's Patient

A 16 year-old girl, with diagnosis of cerebral palsy, weakness and stiffness of all limbs was referred to Botulinum Toxin Clinic at Walter Reed Army Medical Center in Washington DC for treatment of painful and stiff muscles. She had developed severe problems with her movements during infancy. She could never walk and never developed normal speech. At age 12, she was wheel chair bound. Her Weight was 160 pounds.

Neurological examination showed a pleasant Caucasian girl who smiled frequently during examination. She had little speech output. Her cognition was impaired, but she was able to communicate with opening or closing her eyes and could attempt to perform simple commands. There was marked stiffness and spasticity of all limbs with diffusely increased reflexes. Both elbows and knees were flexed. The left hand showed flexed, clinched and immobile fingers with no function. The right hand also had clinched fingers but less for forceful than the left side. After several attempts, she could finally take an object (pen or pencil) between her right index and middle fingers, but was unable to hold it for long or transfer it to the left hand.

After obtaining consent from the child and her parents, Botox was injected into the flexor of the wrist and fingers into both forearms and hand muscles. The total dose per side was 60 units. She reported loosening of her hand and forearm muscles after a week. An examination, 4 weeks after Botox injection, showed marked reduction of tone in the finger and hand muscles on both sides. The left hand was now open. She could move fingers in both hands at will. When given a pen and a cup, she slowly grabbed the pen with the right hand and was able to transfer it to the left hand. Both the child and her family expressed much satisfaction with her response to the Botox treatment. Repeat injections, every 3–4 months, produced the same effect. She reported no side effects after Botox injections.

Aside from cerebral palsy, trauma to the brain or spinal cord as well as genetic and hereditary diseases also are major causes of spasticity in children. Spasticity caused by these conditions also responds to botulinum toxin therapy [19, 20].

Technical Issues

In most CP children with spasticity, due to the diffuse nature of the spasticity, the injector needs to be selective and treat the most affected muscles. In this regard parents' and child's view need to be taken into consideration. Due to safety issues, the total dose per injection should not exceed the safe levels reported in the literature. Currently, for Botox, a total dose 10–15 units/kg of body weight is considered safe by most injectors. Although the units among the toxins are not truly comparable, the following formula can be used for dose comparison among the various toxin formulations: 1Botox unit = 2.5 Dysport = 40 myobloc, the first three being type A toxins.

The FDA recommended dosage for Dysport (first botulinum toxin approved for lower limb spasticity in children) is 30unit/kg for one leg or 60 units/kg for both legs or up to a total dose of 1000 units (approximately 300–350 units of Botox in older children), whichever is lower. Botox is also now approved for treatment of lower limb spasticity in children. Xeomin, another botulinum toxin type a is approved for treatment of upper extremity in children over 2 years of age.

Injections for spasticity are usually done without generalized anesthesia. A numbing cream (for instance Emla cream) can be applied to the skin an hour prior to toxin injections if necessary. In the upper limb spasticity, flexor muscles of the arm, wrist and fingers are mostly affected. Overflexion of these muscles due to increased tone leads to flexed elbow, flexed wrist and if finger flexors are severely affected, a clinched hand with all fingers flexed (Fig. 9.1).

In the lower limbs, adductors of the thigh (muscles that bring the thighs together), flexors of the knee (hamstring muscles in the back of the thigh) and flexors of the foot (gastrocnemius and soleus—Fig. 9.2b) are the most commonly affected muscles. Involvement of these two latter muscles pushes the front part of the foot down and pulls the heal up, giving the foot the appearance of a foot in a high heal shoe (equinus position- Fig. 9.2a). This is a common problem among children with CP and spasticity interfering with walking and standing.

For injections, the calf muscles are easily approached from the surface of the calf using anatomical landmarks. Ancillary techniques can be used for better localization of the muscles such as electromyography (recording electrical activity of the muscle- EMG), nerve stimulation (to identify the desired muscle by stimulating its nerve) and the ultrasound technique. Ultrasound has the advantage of directly showing the muscle and the position of the tip of injecting needle into the muscle as well as causing no pain (unlike EMG).

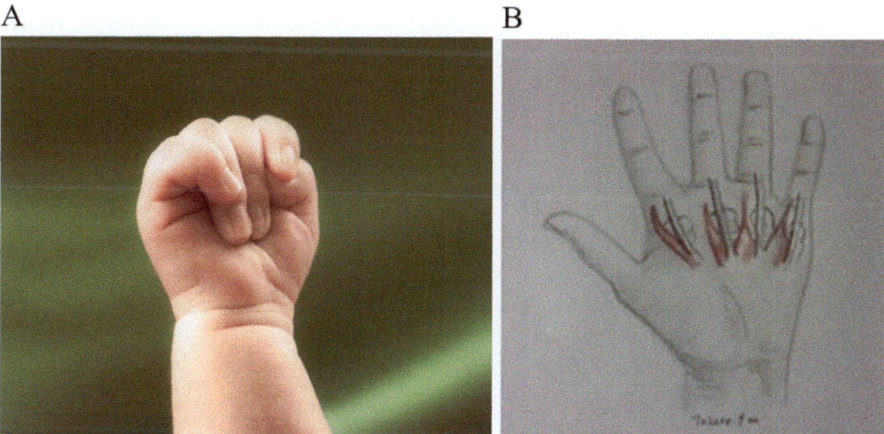

Fig. 9.1 (**a**) Clinched fist. ("Designed by Freepik" www.freepik.com) (**b**) lumbrical muscles. Contraction of lumbrical muscles along with finger flexors of the forearm contributes to the position of clinched fist. (Drawing courtesy of Dr. Tahere Mousavi)

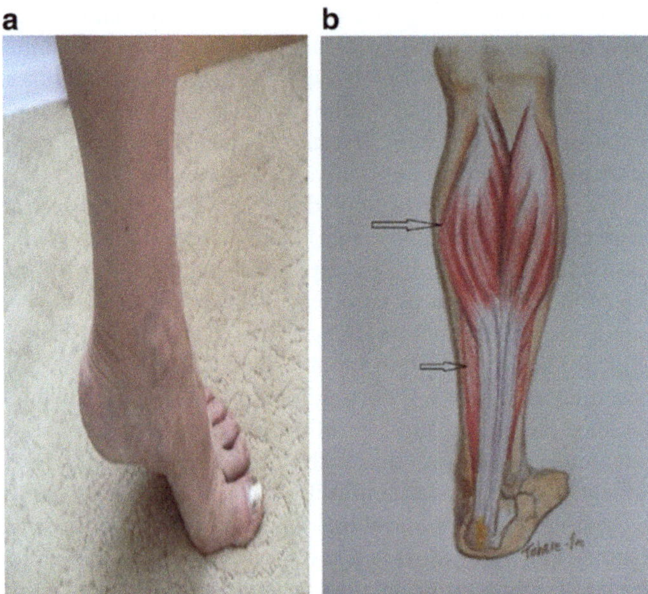

Fig. 9.2 (**a**) Equinus foot position (like horse foot) (**b**) Gastrocnemius (*upper arrow*) and soleus (*lower arrow*) muscles of the calf the spasticity and high tone of which results in Equinus foot position. (Drawing courtesy of Tahere Mousavi M.D.)

In equinous deformity, injection of botulinum toxin into the hamstring and soeus muscles results in relaxation of culprit muscles and correction of the faulty position [21]. It is important to start this treatment early before development of contractures (replacement of muscle by connective tissue which is devoid of muscle function).

Botox, Dysport and Xeomin need to be diluted with normal saline before injection. Myobloc, a type B toxin is provided in a prepared solution form. Botox, Dysport and Myobloc need refrigeration, while Xeomin does not. Details of toxin preparation are provided in Chap. 3 of this book. In experienced hands, injections are performed with a short thin needle and can be completed in a within few minutes. School age children often appreciate the positive effects of botulinum toxin therapy which results in improvement of their gait and posture.

Botulinum Toxin Therapy for Prevention of Hip Dislocation in Spasticity

In young children, spasticity of muscles around the hip joint gradually pushes the head of the long thigh bone outward, away from the hip joint (subluxation). In one study of 98 children with CP, continuous lateral hip migration occurred in 86% during growth and resulted in subluxation in 11.4% [22]. In young children, hip joint subluxation is painful and can interfere with sitting and walking. Corrective surgeries are not always helpful. Botox injection into the severely spastic muscles of the thighs around the hip joints has been used to reduce the rate of hip dislocation in young children with cerebral palsy [23].

Botulinum Toxin for Treatment of Movement Disorders in Children with Cerebral Palsy

Alleviation of involuntary movements is another major indication of BoNT therapy in childhood. Cerebral palsy and childhood diseases related to genetic or hereditary disorders can affect nerve cells deep in the brain (basal ganglia) and cause a variety of involuntary movements. Among these movements, one movement—dystonia- is particularly responsive to BoNT therapy. Dystonia is described as involuntary twisting and twitching movement of a limb or a part of it due to dysfunction of basal ganglia, a part of brain that controls and coordinates movements. Dystonic movements of the hand and finger disrupt the performance of daily tasks and impair the child's quality of life. As drugs used to alleviate dystonia are often associated with side effects, injection of botulinum toxin into the muscles involved in dystonic movements is now considered the first line of treatment for many such conditions in both adults and children.

In children, three disease conditions produce dystonia more often than others:

1. As mentioned earlier, in one type of cerebral palsy, abnormal movements are more prominent than spasticity. In children with this type of CP, dystonia of neck muscles pulls, turns and twists the neck and causes neck and shoulder pain in addition to social embarrassment (cervical dystonia). BoNT injection into shoulder and neck muscles suppresses dystonic posture and neck movements and relieves pain [24].
2. Genetic disorders in which dystonia is the main clinical feature are referred to as primary dystonias. To date, more than 40 different types of primary dystonias have been described and, in more than half, the gene(s) has been identified. Although these early onset dystonias are generalized (affecting all limbs), botulinum toxin injection can be focused on the muscles that are more severely involved (arm, leg, neck) and provide relief.
3. A group of drugs called neuroleptics (example: haldol) used for treating depression or schizophrenia are capable of producing persistent abnormal, involuntary movement. Sine these movements (side effects) can develop late during treatment with these drugs they are called tardive (delayed) dyskinesia (abnormal movement). Such dyskinesias may develop in the face, limbs or both. The movements can be persistent focal muscle twitches or take the form of dystonic movements (as described earlier). These movements respond well to injection of botulinum toxin into the quivering or dystonic muscles. A more detailed description of botulinum toxin treatment in dystonia is given in Chap. 8.

Tic Movements

Tic is an involuntary, abnormal movement characterized by rapid onset, short duration (seconds) and repetitive nature, often preceded by an urge to move. Motor tics can be simple (just movement) or have more complex manifestations. In Tourette syndrome/TS (named after a French physician), motor tics are associated with guttural sounds and involuntary vocalization. Repetitive, frequent motor tics involving shoulder and neck muscles are exhausting and sometimes painful. Tics have their onset in childhood. Frequent tics of Tourette's syndrome (TS) can be disabling in teenagers.

Dr. Jankovic and his group from Baylor college of medicine were first to show that shoulder and neck tics can be greatly reduced after injecting Botox into the affected muscles [25]. Botox injections also reduced the urge to move in these patients. Others have shown that injecting Botox into the vocal cord muscles (with minscule doses of 1–2 units) in older children with TS can reduce vocalization (more detail on botulinum toxin therapy for tic disorders is described in Chap. 8).

Indications for Use of Botulinum Toxin in Eye–Related Problems in Children

In several disease conditions, one or more muscles that move the eyes develop abnormal hyperactivity and increased tone. This overactive, hypertonic muscle (s) can interfere with normal eye movements and cause symptoms such as double vision (diplopia), blurred vision and headache. Since the chemical neurotransmitter released at the nerve endings that activate eye muscles is acetylcholine (same chemical as that of other body muscles), injection of BoNTs into the affected eye muscle can improve patients' symptoms by inhibiting the release of this neurotransmitter. Before discussing botulinum toxin therapy in children with strabismus (crossed eyes), providing a brief knowledge of eye- muscle anatomy would be helpful:

Each eye has six muscles that control movements of the eyeballs in different directions. Two of these muscles move the eyes straight up or down; they are called rectus (straight) muscles. For example, the right superior rectus muscle, moves the right or left eye straight up and the right inferior rectus moves the eye straight down. There are two oblique muscles that also move the eye obliquely up or obliquely down toward the midline. There is one medial rectus muscle per eye that moves the eye straight toward the nose and one lateral rectus muscle per each eye that moves the eyeball straight laterally (toward the ear) (Fig. 9.3). The nerve supply for eye muscles comes from the so called cranial nerves. There are 12 nerves that after emerging from the brain provide innervation to the eyes, head and face muscles. The fourth cranial nerve innervates the oblique muscles, the sixth cranial nerve innervates the lateral rectus muscles and the rest of the eye muscles (superior and inferior rectus and medial rectus) get their nerve supply from the third cranial nerve.

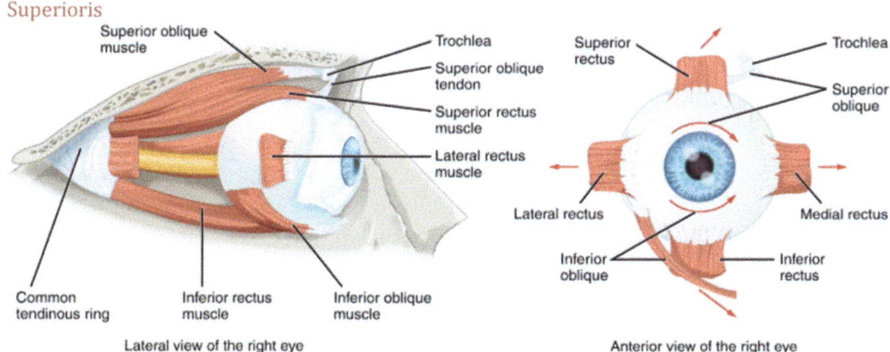

Fig. 9.3 Muscles that move the eye in different directions. (Courtesy of Ludwig and Czyz [26] and Stat Perls publishing, 2018 and OpenStax. Reproduced under creative commons licence CC by 3)

These muscles are yoked, meaning that the two muscles with opposite functions closely work with each other. For example, lateral rectus muscle of one eye and medial rectus of the other eye work together to align the axis of the two eyes in lateral and medial directions of gaze so that a single image from the two eyes is conveyed to the brain.

A separate single and small muscle, attached to the upper lid at the midpoint above each eye, moves the upper lid up and helps to open the eyes. It is called lifter of the upper lid (levator palpebrae superioris).

Strabismus

The word strabismus means squint in Greek. In medical terms, it means malaligned eyes (crossed eyes). It results from hyperactivity of one or more eye muscles leading to impaired alignment of the two eyes. When one eye deviates medially toward the nose, strabismus is called esotropia (crossed eyes). Exotropia refers to divergent strabismus when one eye deviates laterally.

Strabismus can develop in infancy, childhood or in adulthood. When it develops in infancy or early childhood (most cases), the cause is often unknown; in many older children and adults, strabismus develops after trauma to the eyes or local infections. Esotropic strabismus (crossed eyes) occurs in 1% of normally born children. In infants with strabismus, the danger is loss of vision (amblyopia) in the affected eye since brain suppresses the image that comes from that eye. The recommended management for infants with strabismus is patching one eye at a time (alternate patching) until the child grows older and can have corrective surgery or botulinum toxin injections. Surgery via cutting the fibers of the hyperactive muscle—for example, medial rectus in the case of esotropia (eye turned in medially toward the nose) had been the main approach until late 1980s. After 1989, botulinum toxin injection provided an alternative to surgery. In older children and adults, common complaints of strabismus are double vision, headaches and blurred vision.

The neurotransmitter, a chemical that is released by the nerves near the eye muscles and activates them—same as other muscles of the body, is acetylcholine. As mentioned earlier in this chapter and in more detail in Chap. 2 of this book, botulinum toxins block the release of acetylcholine at nerve endings. Alan Scott, an ophthalmologist in California, first introduced botulinum toxin injections for treatment of strabismus (Chap. 1, history of botulinum toxin therapy) . After decades of research on monkeys' eyes, Dr. Scott showed that injecting Botox into the hyperactive eye muscles of the patients with strabismus can relax the injected muscle, correct eye alignment and alleviate the symptoms of strabismus [27]. In 1989, FDA approved injection of Botox into the eye muscles for treatment of strabismus. Strabismus was one of the first three FDA approvals for botulinum toxin therapy in the US—the other two were spasm of the eyelids (blepharospasm) and hemifacial spasm (twitching of half of the face—both predominantly adult ailments.

Currently, it is believed that botulinum toxin therapy and surgery have comparable efficacy in correcting strabismus. Botulinum toxin therapy has three advantages over surgery:

1. Duration of anesthesia is shorter
2. The local pain after botulinum toxin injection is subtle and short lived
3. The procedure is considerably shorter than surgery

The main disadvantage is the need for meticulous titration, as overdosing can lead to too much weakening of the injected muscles causing further problems such as drooping of the eyelid and persistent double vision, albeit all disappear after a few months.

Since the original observation of Dr. Scott, and his group, other researchers have shown the efficacy of botulinum toxin treatment in alleviating strabismus related symptoms in several studies [28–30]. In England, Dysport, another type A botulinum toxin, is used more often than Botox for treatment of strabismus. The results of Dysport therapy for strabismus have been reported to be as effective as Botox and, in some reports even more promising. In general, esotropia (eyes turned in) responds better than exotropia (eyes turned out). In children, one injection often produces long-term effects, whereas in adults, similar to other movement disorders treated with botulinum toxins, repeated injections are necessary. Children younger than 2 years are not usually injected since in some children, strabismus may resolve spontaneously up to that age. Recent studies are focused on long-term results of surgery compared with botulinum toxin therapy and/ or possible benefits from combined therapy (surgery and botulinum toxin injections). Some debate still continues in academic circles on the issue that what is the preferable procedure—surgery or botulinum toxin injections. Currently, three high quality protocols are ongoing to answer this question [31].

Technique of Injection

Currently, three methods are applied for injection of Botox or Dysport into the eye muscles for improving crossed eyes. In most cases, a short-term 10–15 min inhalation anesthesia is required. Some practitioners inject Botox or Dysport with a fine needle through the surface of the eye (conjunctiva) directly, using only anatomical guidelines. This has the drawback of sometimes missing the culprit muscle and causing spread of the toxin to unwanted eye muscles. The results can be development of double vision and drooping of eyelids. An alternative way preferred by many ophthalmologists, is starting with a small (2 mm) incision on the surface of the eye through which (inspection) the muscle of choice is identified and injected. Injections are carried out with a very fine needle (gauge 30). The third method is injecting the eye muscle after confirmation by electromyography (EMG). Electromyography is a procedure that records the electrical activity of the muscle. Special hollow EMG needles are available in the market that allow EMG recording as well as injection of the BoNT into the muscle via the hollow core of the same needle. The drawback is additional time spent for electromyographic identification and availability of an expert electromyographer during the procedure.

The dose of the injected toxin) into the eye muscles is small, only a few units (usually 2–3), compared to the much larger doses used for dystonias or spasticity.

Promoting Healing of Damaged Cornea

Trauma and infection when damage the cornea, if not managed properly, can leave a scar in the cornea leading to permanent loss of vision. Blinking and exposure to air can further irritate the damaged area and delay or prevent healing. Injection of a small amount of botulinum toxin in the muscle that moves the eyelid up and initiates the "blink" movement can paralyze this muscle (levator of the upper lid) and close the eye for 2–3 months. This will prevent constant eye irritation through blinking and air exposure and facilitate healing of the damaged area [32].

Treatment of Excessive Drooling (Sialorrhea) in Cerebral Palsy

Children and adults with severe cerebral palsy may develop excessive drooling that impairs their quality of life. Injection of botulinum toxins (Botox, Dysport, Zeomin, Myobloc) into the glands that secrete saliva (mostly parotid and submaxillary glands) can reduce saliva production and drooling. Both glands are easily approachable from the surface. The parotid gland is located over the angle of the jaw- barely under the skin. The submaxillary gland is located under the arch of the jaw, a few

Fig. 9.4 Parotid and submaxillary glands are the main glands that secret saliva. Parotid gland is in front of the ear and at the angle of the Jaw. Submaxillary gland is under the jaw. Sublingual gland (under the tongue) is a minor contributor. (Printed with permission from Mayo Foundation)

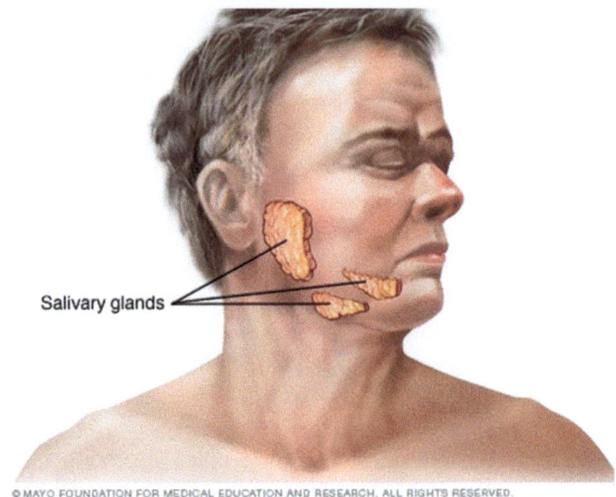

centimeters medial to the jaw's angle [Fig. 9.4]. Many injectors use just anatomical landmarks for injection. Since the skin is sensitive, it needs to be numbed in children by a numbing cream, or spray or both prior to injection. Injections are performed with a very thin, and small needle (½ inch, 30 gauge) and quickly into two sites per gland. Some injectors prefer to inject four sites for the parotid gland. . Using ultrasound technique is a more precise way to perform injections into these glands since ultrasound shows the gland and the needle entering it and even the volume of injected material into the gland.

Side effects are pain during injection, minor self-limited bleeding and, in rare cases, transient swallowing problems. The latter is more of a problem when injecting into the submaxillary gland, since missing it can spread the toxin close to the esophagus- the tube that connects the mouth to the stomach. For submaxillary gland, injections under ultrasound are highly advisable. For more detailed description of botulinum toxin injections for drooling and anatomical information related to the salivary glands the reader is referred to Chap. 14 of this book. Recent literature indicate that injection of botulinum toxins into the salivary gland of children is highly effective to reduce disabling drooling of children with cerebral palsy [33].

Ghazavi and co-workers [34] recently reported on the results of botulinum toxin injections into the parotid and submaxillary glands in 12 children with cerebral palsy. Each gland was injected with 0.5 units of Botox/Kg of body weight (10 units for a child weighing 20 Kg). Injections reduced excessive drooling in all children. Two thirds of parents were pleased with the results. Two of 12 children developed a mild transient swallowing problem as a side effect. Recently, a meta-analysis of literature on this issue derived from 24 studies concluded that botulinum toxin treatment of drooling in children is effective and safe with no serious side effects [35]. Authors recommended not to exceed a total injected dose of 4 units per Kg body weight (in case of Botox) per session.

Conclusion

Botulinum toxin therapy can improve a variety of symptoms in children. High quality studies have demonstrated efficacy of botulinum toxin therapy in spasticity of different causes (CP, neurodegeneration, trauma), involuntary movements (dystonia, tics) and crossed eyes (strabismus) as well as excessive drooling in children. These studies have shown that botulinum toxin therapy for these indications also improves the quality of life of children. Long-term studies of botulinum toxin therapy in children with spasticity and strabismus have demonstrated sustained efficacy with repeated treatments. Injections for these indications in children is generally safe if performed by experienced injectors adhering to recommended dosage guidelines. More on the safety issues with botulinum toxin therapy among children and adults are reviewed and discussed in Chap. 17 of this book.

References

1. Lance JW. The control of muscle tone, reflexes, and movement: Robert Wartenberg lecture. Neurology. 1980 Dec;30(12):1303–13. https://doi.org/10.1212/wnl.30.12.1303. PMID: 7192811.
2. Gracies JM. Pathophysiology of spastic paresis. I: paresis and soft tissue changes. Muscle Nerve. 2005 May;31(5):535–51. https://doi.org/10.1002/mus.20284. PMID: 15714510.
3. Gracies JM. Pathophysiology of spastic paresis. II; emergence of muscle over activity. Muscle Nerve. 2005;31(5):552–71.
4. Young RR, Delwaide PJ. Drug therapy: spasticity (first of two parts). N Engl J Med. 1981 Jan 1;304(1):28–33. https://doi.org/10.1056/NEJM198101013040107. PMID: 6448959.
5. Alshahrani AM. Oral Antispasticity drugs and non-progressive neurological diseases: a meta-analysis on safety and efficacy. J Pharm Bioallied Sci. 2023 Jan–Mar;15(1):1–8. https://doi.org/10.4103/jpbs.jpbs_556_22. Epub 2023 Apr 14. PMID: 37313540. PMCID: PMC10259735.
6. Dario A, Tomei G. A benefit-risk assessment of baclofen in severe spinal spasticity. Drug Saf. 2004;27(11):799–818. https://doi.org/10.2165/00002018-200427110-00004. PMID: 15350152.
7. Colver A, Fairhurst C, Pharoah P. Cerebral palsy. Lancet. 2014;383(9924):1240–9.
8. Barnes M. Botulinum toxin—mechanisms of action and clinical use in spasticity. J Rehabil Med. 2003 May;41(Suppl):56–9. https://doi.org/10.1080/16501960310010151. PMID: 12817658.
9. Rosenbaum P, Paneth N, Leviton A, Goldstein M, Bax M, Damiano D, Dan B, Jacobsson B. A report: the definition and classification of cerebral palsy April 2006. Dev Med Child Neurol Suppl. 2007 Feb;109:8–14. Erratum in: Dev Med Child Neurol. 2007 Jun;49(6):480. PMID: 17370477.
10. Sadowska M, Sarecka-Hujar B, Kopyta I. Cerebral palsy: current opinions on definition, epidemiology, risk factors, classification and treatment options. Neuropsychiatr Dis Treat. 2020 June 12;16:1505–18. https://doi.org/10.2147/NDT.S235165. PMID: 32606703. PMCID: PMC7297454.
11. Surveillance of Cerebral Palsy in Europe. Surveillance of cerebral palsy in Europe: a collaboration of cerebral palsy surveys and registers. Surveillance of Cerebral Palsy in Europe (SCPE). Dev Med Child Neurol. 2000 Dec;42(12):816–24. https://doi.org/10.1017/s0012162200001511. PMID: 11132255.

12. Koman LA, Mooney JF 3rd, Smith B, et al. Management of cerebral palsy with botulinum–a toxin: preliminary investigation. Pediatr Orthop. 1993;13:489–95.

13. Copeland L, Edwards P, Thorley M, Donaghey S, Gascoigne-Pees L, Kentish M, Cert G, Lindsley J, McLennan K, Sakzewski L, Boyd RN. Botulinum toxin A for nonambulatory children with cerebral palsy: a double blind randomized controlled trial. J Pediatr. 2014 July;165(1):140–6.e4. https://doi.org/10.1016/j.jpeds.2014.01.050. Epub 2014 Mar 12. PMID: 24630348.

14. Delgado MR, Tilton A, Carranza-Del Río J, Dursun N, Bonikowski M, Aydin R, Maciag-Tymecka I, Oleszek J, Dabrowski E, Grandoulier AS, Picaut P; Dysport in PUL study group Efficacy and safety of abobotulinumtoxinA for upper limb spasticity in children with cerebral palsy: a randomized repeat-treatment study. Dev Med Child Neurol. 2021 May;63(5):592–600. https://doi.org/10.1111/dmcn.14733. Epub 2020 Nov 18. PMID: 33206382; PMCID: PMC8048784.

15. Heinen F, Kanovský P, Schroeder AS, Chambers HG, Dabrowski E, Geister TL, Hanschmann A, Martinez-Torres FJ, Pulte I, Banach M, Gaebler-Spira D. IncobotulinumtoxinA for the treatment of lower-limb spasticity in children and adolescents with cerebral palsy: a phase 3 study. J Pediatr Rehabil Med. 2021;14(2):183–97. https://doi.org/10.3233/PRM-210040. Erratum in: J Pediatr Rehabil Med. 2022;15(2):407–9. PMID: 34092664; PMCID: PMC8673523.

16. Dabrowski E, Chambers HG, Gaebler-Spira D, Banach M, Kaňovský P, Dersch H, Althaus M, Geister TL, Heinen F. IncobotulinumtoxinA efficacy/safety in upper-limb spasticity in pediatric cerebral palsy: randomized controlled trial. Pediatr Neurol. 2021 Oct;123:10–20. https://doi.org/10.1016/j.pediatrneurol.2021.05.014. Epub 2021 May 21. PMID: 34339951.

17. Dimitrova R, Kim H, Meilahn J, Chambers HG, Racette BA, Bonikowski M, Park ES, McCusker E, Liu C, Brin MF. Efficacy and safety of onabotulinumtoxinA with standardized physiotherapy for the treatment of pediatric lower limb spasticity: a randomized, placebo-controlled, phase III clinical trial. NeuroRehabilitation. 2022;50(1):33–46. https://doi.org/10.3233/NRE-210070. PMID: 34957954; PMCID: PMC8925123.

18. Oleszek J, Tilton A, Carranza Del Rio J, Dursun N, Bonikowski M, Dabrowski E, Page S, Regnault B, Thompson C, Delgado MR. Muscle selection and dosing in a phase 3, pivotal study of AbobotulinumtoxinA injection in upper limb muscles in children with cerebral palsy. Front Neurol. 2021 Oct 29;12:728615. https://doi.org/10.3389/fneur.2021.728615. PMID: 34803878. PMCID: PMC8603760.

19. Akbar M, Abel R, Seyler TM, Bedke J, Haferkamp A, Gerner HJ, Möhring K. Repeated botulinum–a toxin injections in the treatment of myelodysplastic children and patients with spinal cord injuries with neurogenic bladder dysfunction. BJU Int. 2007 Sept;100(3):639–45. https://doi.org/10.1111/j.1464-410X.2007.06977.x. Epub 2007 May 26. Erratum in: BJU Int. 2007 Sep;100(3):719. Bedke, Jens [added]; Haferkamp, Axel [added]. PMID: 17532858.

20. van Rhijn J, Molenaers G, Ceulemans B. Botulinum toxin type A in the treatment of children and adolescents with an acquired brain injury. Brain Inj. 2005 May;19(5):331–5. https://doi.org/10.1080/02699050400013675. PMID: 16094780.

21. Hong BY, Chang HJ, Lee SJ, et al. Efficacy of repeated botulinum toxin type a injections for spastic equinus in children with cerebral palsy–a secondary analysis of the randomized clinical trial. Toxins (Basel). 2017 Aug 21;9(8)

22. Pascale Leone SI. Use of of botulinum toxin in the preventive and palliative treatment of the hips in children with infantile cerebral palsy. Rev Neurol. 2003;37:80–2.

23. Lee Y, Lee S, Jang J, Lim J, Ryu JS. Effect of botulinum toxin injection on the progression of hip dislocation in patients with spastic cerebral palsy: a pilot study. Toxins (Basel). 2021 Dec 6;13(12):872. https://doi.org/10.3390/toxins13120872. PMID: 34941710; PMCID: PMC8707328.

24. Koukouni V, Martino D, Arabia G, Quinn NP, Bhatia KP. The entity of young onset primary cervical dystonia. Mov Disord. 2007 Apr 30;22:843–7.

25. Kwak A, Hanna PACH, Jankovic J. Botulinum toxin in the treatment of tics. Arch Neurol. 2000;57:1190–3.

26. Ludwig PE, Czyz CN. Anatomy, head, eye muscles. StatPearls [Internet]. Treasure Island (FL): StatPearls Publishing;2017 Dec 11; 2018 Jan. PMID:29262013.
27. Scott AB, Fahn S, Brin MF. Treatment of strabismus and blepharospasm with Botox (onabotulinumtoxinA): development, insights, and impact. Medicine (Baltimore). 2023 Jul 1;102(S1):e32374. https://doi.org/10.1097/MD.0000000000032374. PMID: 37499080; PMCID: PMC10374181.
28. Crouch ER. Use of botulinum toxin in strabismus. Curr Opin Ophthalmol. 2006;17:435–40.
29. Basar E, Arici C. Use of botulinum neurotoxin in ophthalmology. Turk J Ophthalmol. 2016;46(6):282–90.
30. Niyaz L, Yeter V, Beldagli C. Success rates of botulinum toxin in different types of strabismus and dose effect. Can J Ophthalmol. 2023 Jun;58(3):239–44. https://doi.org/10.1016/j.jcjo.2021.12.002. Epub 2022 Jan 14. PMID: 35038409.
31. Bort-Martí AR, Rowe FJ, Ruiz Sifre L, Ng SM, Bort-Martí S, Ruiz Garcia V. Botulinum toxin for the treatment of strabismus. Cochrane Database Syst Rev. 2023 Mar 14;3(3):CD006499. https://doi.org/10.1002/14651858.CD006499.pub5. PMID: 36916692; PMCID: PMC10012406.
32. Mackie IA. Successful management of three consecutive cases of recurrent corneal erosion with botulinum toxin injections. Eye (Lond). 2004 Jul;18(7):734–7. https://doi.org/10.1038/sj.eye.6701307. PMID: 14765101.
33. Mahadevan M, Gruber M, Bilish D. Botulinum toxin injections for chronic Sialorrhoea in children are effective regardless of the degree of neurological dysfunction: a single tertiary institution experience. Int J Pediatr Otorhinolaryngol. 2016 Sep;88:142–5. https://doi.org/10.1016/j.ijporl.2016.06.031. Epub 2016 Jun 11.
34. Ghazavi M, Rezaii S, Ghasemi M, Azin N, Reisi M. Botox injection in treatment of sialorrhea in children with cerebral palsy. Am J Neurodegener Dis. 2023 Jun 15;12(3):97–102. PMID: 37457841; PMCID: PMC10349299.
35. Hung SA, Liao CL, Lin WP, Hsu JC, Guo YH, Lin YC. Botulinum toxin injections for treatment of drooling in children with cerebral palsy: a systematic review and meta-analysis. Children (Basel). 2021 Nov 25;8(12):1089. https://doi.org/10.3390/children8121089. PMID: 34943284. PMCID: PMC8700360.

Chapter 10
Botulinum Toxin Treatment of Bladder and Pelvic Disorders

Abstract Botulinum toxins blocks the release of neurotransmitters at nerve-muscle junction. Neurotransmitters are chemicals that convey the message of the nerve to the muscle and activate the muscle. In human, the main neurotransmitter of nerve-muscle junction is acetylcholine that activates all skeletal muscles as well as visceral muscles such as those present in the bladder. Clinical research and experience over the past 30 years have proved the efficacy of botulinum toxin injection into the bladder wall in improving bladder overactivity problems. The symptoms of bladder dysfunction, overactivity, urinary urgency and incontinence impairs the patients' quality of life. Botulinum toxins are also effective in relieving pelvic pain in both genders due to their blocking effect on pain neurotransmitters (substance P, glutamate and CGRP).

Keywords Botulinum toxin · Botulinum neurotoxin · Bladder overactivity · Urinary urgency · Incontinence of urine · Pelvic pain

Introduction

Bladder functions through the action of its muscles and nerves. Bladder muscles, like any other muscle in the body, respond to nerve signals that come from the brain and spinal cord. Botulinum toxins block the release of neurotransmitters at nerve-muscle junction. Neurotransmitters are secreted at the nerve endings and their role is activating the muscle. In human, the main neurotransmitter of nerve-muscle junction is acetylcholine that activates all skeletal muscles as well as visceral muscles such as those present in the bladder. Clinical research and experience over the past 25 years have proven the efficacy of botulinum toxin injection into the bladder wall in improving bladder overactivity problems. The bladder overactivity problems are either due to damage to the bladder nerves seen in spinal cord injury and multiple sclerosis or they may have unknown causes. The former is called neurogenic detrusor overactivity (NDO). Detrusor muscle is the main bladder muscle that participates in bladder filling and emptying. The conditions of unknown cause are simply

© The Author(s), under exclusive license to Springer Nature Switzerland AG 2024

B. Jabbari, *Botulinum Toxin Treatment*,

https://doi.org/10.1007/978-3-031-54471-2_10

designated as over active bladder (OAB) or idiopathic (cause unknown) overactive bladder (IOB).

Botulinum toxins are also effective in relieving pelvic pain in both genders due to their blocking effect on the pain neurotransmitters. Limited data indicate that pain generated by inflammation of the bladder (interstitial cystitis) also responds to injection of botulinum toxins into the bladder wall.

Botulinum Toxins

Botulinum toxin is produced by a form of bacteria called clostridium botulinum and ingestion of a large amount of the toxins produced by these bacteria leads to the serious illness of botulism. The history of botulinum toxin's discovery as a therapeutic agent when prepared in an injectable and safe form is presented in detail in Chap. 1. There are eight serological types of the toxin (A to G and X). Different types of type A and type B toxin are described in detail in Chap. 3.

Because of the powerful effect of botulinum toxins on nerve- muscle junction (see Chap. 2 for details), over the past 30 years, botulinum toxins have become first line drugs for treatment of several hyperactive movement disorders. Botulinum toxins are now approved by FDA for treatment of blepharospasm (forced and repeated eye closures due to overactivity of eyelid muscles), hemifacial spasm (involuntary spasm of the facial muscles on one side) and cervical dystonia (a hyperactive condition causing neck jerks and abnormal neck postures) [1, 2]. In addition, through the same mode of action (blocking the release of acetylcholine release at nerve-muscle junction), botulinum toxins' role has now been established as a major mode of treatment for improving and reducing increased muscle tone and muscle spasm (spasticity) which occur after stroke or after brain or spinal cord injury [3–5].

The above-mentioned positive results with botulinum toxin therapy in a variety of clinical muscle overactivity disorders have encouraged neurologists and urologists to look into the potential use of botulinum toxins for management of bladder dysfunction related to the overactivity of bladder's detrusor muscle.

Physiology of Bladder Function and the Role of Detrusor Muscle

In healthy subjects, human kidneys generate 800–2000 milliliters of urine per 24 h. The urine that is generated by the kidneys is carried to the bladder by two tubes called ureters (Fig. 10.1).

The ureters connect the kidneys to the bladder where they insert into the posterior aspect of the lower and narrowed part of the bladder called trigone (triangle). The drainage of urine to the outside from the trigone is through a hole that opens

Fig. 10.1 Kidney's, ureters, bladder and urethra. (Courtesy of Wikibooks. Licensed under https://creativecommons. org/licenses/by-sa/4.0/)

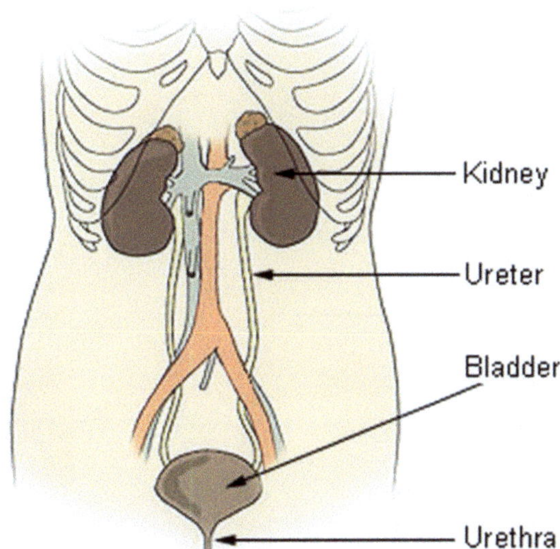

into a single tube called urethra. Urethra is short in women 1.5 cm and longer in men (10 cm) since it goes through the length of penis.

The bladder is an ovoid shape structure, located in the lower part of the pelvis. The wider part of the bladder is located on the top, while the narrower part is at the bottom (Fig. 10.1). Storage and emptying of the urine are managed by three essential muscles:

1. Detrusor muscle (Fig. 10.2): This is the main muscle of the bladder wall which, while relaxed, allows the bladder to expand and store urine; the contraction of this muscle is essential for the drainage of urine.
2. Internal urethral sphincter (Fig. 10.2): This small muscle which is around the neck of the bladder contracts during urine storage and relaxes during micturition letting the urine out of the bladder.
3. External urethral sphincter (Fig. 10.2): This muscle is located further down on the path of urine drainage, and its function is similar to that of the internal sphincter. However, it is under voluntary control.

The detrusor and internal urinary sphincter are special types of muscles called smooth muscles that are innervated by the autonomic nervous system (sympathetic and parasympathetic), and, hence, are not under voluntary control. The external sphincter, has a structure similar to other muscles of the body referred to as striated muscle and is controlled by volition.

During filling of the bladder, the pressure inside the bladder is constantly sensed by the nerve cells located on the surface of the detrusor muscle. When the bladder pressure reaches a certain point, these nerve cells signal filling of the bladder to the nerve cells located in the spinal cord and brain, which in turn command the bladder muscles to relax resulting in release and drainage of urine. The detrusor muscle

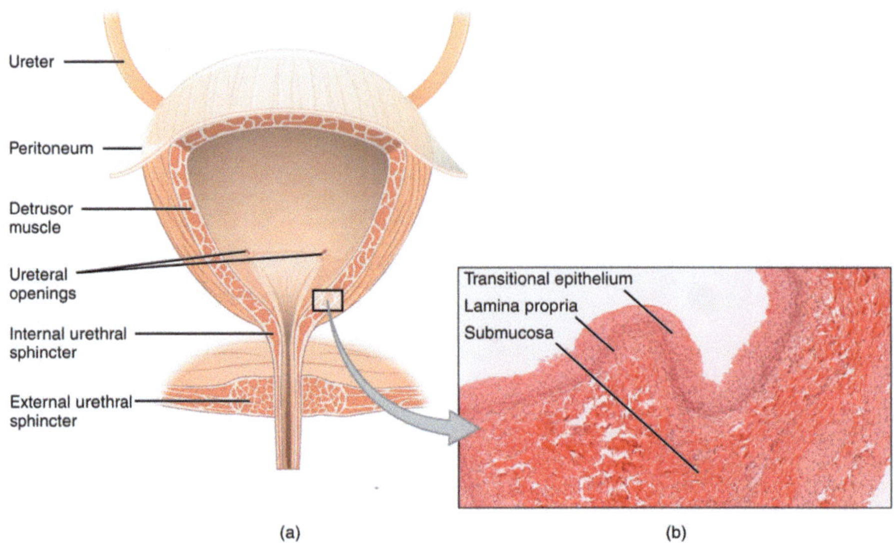

Fig. 10.2 Bladder: Base (at the top), trigone, detrusor muscle, internal and external sphincters. (Courtesy of https://upload.wikimedia.org/wikipedia/commons/d/dc/2605_The_Bladder.jpg)

contracts and pushes the urine towards the trigone, while the internal sphincter relaxes and lets the urine out toward the external sphincter. At this time, the urgent need for micturition is fulfilled by voluntary relaxation of the external sphincter resulting in passage of the urine from bladder to urethra for micturition. The storage and drainage of urine requires proper timing and synergy between detrusor muscle and the two sphincters. In certain neurological conditions, synergy between these muscles does not take place (detrusor -sphincter dyssynergia); this leads to urinary retention. Overactivity or underactivity of detrusor muscles is also the cause of urinary symptoms such as urinary incontinence or retention. Detrusor overactivity is seen in some neurological disorders (neurogenic detrusor overactivity -NDO), but sometimes the cause remains undetermined (overactive bladder—OAB). Detrusor underactivity or paralysis of detrusor muscle, occurs in severe spinal cord injury and is not responsive to botulinum toxin therapy.

Neurogenic Detrusor Overactivity (NDO)

Neurogenic detrusor overactivity (neurogenic bladder- NB) is the most common type of bladder dysfunction in multiple sclerosis (MS) and spinal cord injury (SCI). Research and clinical observation have shown that 50–90% and 70–84% of the patients with MS and SCI develop NB, respectively, sometimes during the course of their illness [6–8]. In both MS and SCI, presence of NB significantly impairs the patient's quality of life due to urinary urgency and incontinence.

Control of bladder function takes place at several levels in the central nervous system that involves the spinal cord, lower part of the brain (brain stem- pons) and cortex of the brain where the large nerve cells are located. Multiple sclerosis and partial spinal cord injury damage the nerve cells and nerve fibers that control bladder function. The result of this damage is increased excitability of the nerve fibers that descend from the brain to the bladder and provide nerve supply to the detrusor muscle of bladder. This is similar to what happens to other muscles of the body in case of central nervous system damage; the affected muscles became overactive. The term reflex bladder is also used sometimes for NB characterizing the overactivity of the bladder's detrusor muscle in NDO/NB.

The symptoms of NDO consist of urinary urgency, urinary frequency and inability to hold urine (incontinence), caused by involuntary and abnormal contractions of a hyperactive detrusor muscle. Urinary urgency (desire to urinate) is the most common symptom and half of the people with urinary urgency have "urge incontinence" wetting themselves during the urge to urinate.

Neurogenic detrusor overactivity often leads to decreased bladder capacity and to retention of some urine with incomplete bladder emptying. Many patients experience discomfort at the time of urination. These symptoms make the patient prone to developing recurrent bladder infections. Furthermore, increased detrusor pressure can cause backing of urine, dilation of ureters (hydronephrosis) resulting to subsequent damage to the kidneys.

Conventional treatments of neurogenic detrusor overactivity include bladder training, pelvic floor exercises and medications. Among general measures, losing weight in overweight patients and avoiding drinking excessive tea or coffee are often recommended. Bladder training is usually a 3–12-week course that includes different behavioral approaches such as trying to delay voiding upon the urge to urinate. Patients start with 5–10 min micturition delay, gradually extends the delay time to several hours. This may not be successful in some patients since it requires the ability to tighten the pelvic floor. Scheduling regular voiding times even in the absence of an urge to void is also a part of bladder training. Pelvic floor exercises aim to strengthen muscles of the pelvic floor which are located in the proximity or are attached to the bladder (Fig. 10.3). The most common exercise is known as Kegel exercise, usually taught to the patient by the physician or a physical therapist. It may take up to 8 weeks before seeing satisfactory results with this exercise.

Medical therapy is focused on "urge incontinence" which is the most disturbing symptom. The drugs that are used for treatment of urge incontinence are usually in the category of anticholinergics since they block the action of acetylcholine- the previously mentioned neurotransmitter that activates muscles after receiving the nerve signal. Several drugs of this category (anticholinergics) are available in the market under different trade names such as Detrol and Ditropan. Dryness of the mouth, dryness of the eyes and constipation are common side effects. Elderly patients may experience impairment of memory and confusion. Mirabegron, a newer drug for preventing urinary incontinence does not cause dryness of the mouth and constipation. Unfortunately, long-term effects of medications in treatment of

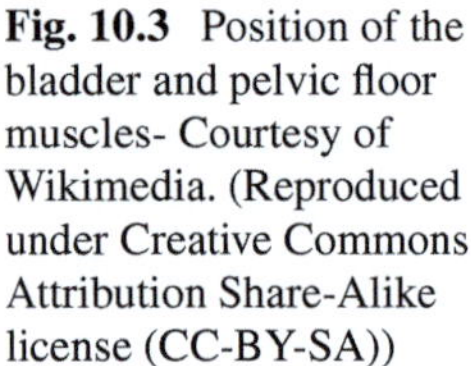

Fig. 10.3 Position of the bladder and pelvic floor muscles- Courtesy of Wikimedia. (Reproduced under Creative Commons Attribution Share-Alike license (CC-BY-SA))

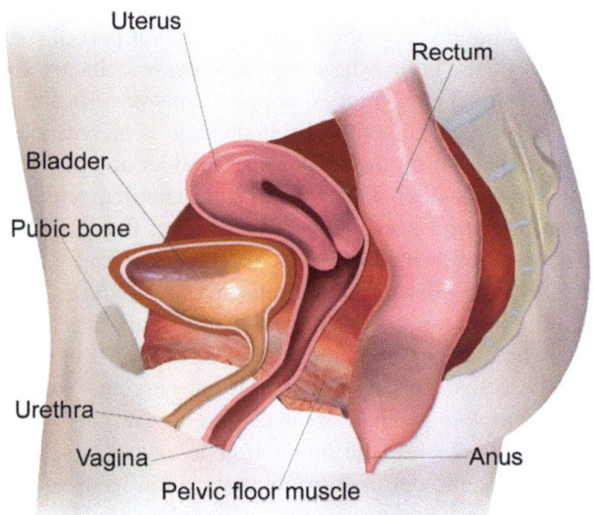

overactive bladder related to nerve damage is disappointing. Research has shown that within 2 years after initiating the treatment, half of the patients stop taking these medications either due to inefficacy or due to undesirable side effects [8].

Botulinum Toxin Treatment of Neurogenic Detrusor Overactivity (NDO)

In 2000, Schurch and his colleagues first demonstrated the effectiveness of Botox injections into the bladder wall in patients with detrusor muscle overactivity. Seventeen of their 19 patients completely regained urinary continence 6 weeks after treatment and, in 11 patients, continence of urine persisted for 36 weeks after a single session of injections. Furthermore, they have shown that patients' maximum bladder capacity increased up to 482 milliliters.

In 2010, FDA approved Botox injections into the bladder wall for management of NDO symptoms based on two large, multicenter and double- blind studies (both doctor and patient being unaware of the type of injection - toxin or placebo) consisting of 217 and 416 patients affected by multiple sclerosis and/or spinal cord injury. These carefully crafted studies that also compared the effect of 200 units of Botox with 300 units, demonstrated significant reduction of incontinence episodes after Botox injections as well as marked improvement of patients' quality of life as measured by standard quality of life rating scales [9–11]. Furthermore, Botox injections were safe and no patient developed any serious side effects. As 200 units was as effective and had less side effects compared to the 300 units, the FDA approval was issued for the 200 unit dose. Subsequently, several follow up studies in both adults and children have demonstrated maintenance of efficacy after repeated injections of Botox over years (3–6 years) with the time interval between injections varying from 6 to 11 months [12–14].

During the past 5 years, high quality studies (double-blind, placebo-controlled) have explored the efficacy of other type A botulinum toxins in treatment of neurogenic bladder. In one study of 47 patients with NB/NDO, investigators found the injections of 750 units of Dysport (each unit of Disport approximates 2.5 units of Botox) improved patients' urinary incontinence significantly [15]. This positive response of NB to Dysport was duplicated later in a larger, high quality study that included nearly 500 patients [16]. In this study, reduction of urinary incontinence correlated with significant improvement of patients' quality of life. In a recent study [15], investigators compared the results of Botox injection into the bladder with bladder injection of Xeomin (another type A toxin with comparable units to Botox) in 57 patients with neurogenic bladder secondary to spinal cord injury or multiple sclerosis. Patients received a total dose of 200 units distributed over 30 sites. Patients were followed for 12 weeks. Both botulinum toxins were equally effective in reducing urinary urgency, incontinence and improvement of patient's quality of life. The side effect profile was also similar for the two toxins. In 2021, FDA approved Botox injections in children over 5 years of age for neurogenic bladder leading to incontinence based on publication of high quality studies [12, 17].

The main side effect of Botox treatment of neurogenic detrusor overactivity/neurogenic bladder is urinary retention. In a study of over 500 patients with NB secondary to MS or SCI,, authors noted urinary retention following Botox injection into the bladder in 29.5% and 7.2% patients with MS and SCI, respectively [18]. When this complication occurs, patients need to do self-catheterization for removing trapped urine from the bladder. For many patients with severe spinal cord injury or advanced multiple sclerosis, this may not be a major issue since they are already doing self-catheterization. The need for self-catheterization after Botox injections, however, decreases with the passage of time. In one study of 227 patients with NDO, researchers have shown that the need for self-catheterization in the third and fourth year after initiation of Botox therapy dropped to 8% and 0% respectively [14]. Increased urinary tract infections (reported in approximately half of the treated patients [18]) and bleeding (usually mild) into the bladder are other complications that require close attention and monitoring.

Injection Technique

Prior to bladder injections, the bladder wall is numbed with an anesthetic via an endoscope. Endoscope is a device that allows to explore and visualize the bladder wall while simultaneously allowing injection into the bladder muscle.

Prior to botulinum toxin injection, injection of an anesthetic, such as lidocaine or alkalinized lidocaine is recommended to numb the bladder wall [19, 20]. For Botox injections, one group of experienced injectors recommends diluting 100 units of Botox in 10 cc of normal saline [21]. Injections are superficial and on the surface of the detrusor muscle at multiple sites almost in a grid-like pattern. The initial FDA approved protocol spares the trigone of the bladder (lower part of bladder, Fig. 10.3) and recommends a total dose of 200 units of Botox. As described earlier, recently published high quality studies indicate that Xeomin and Dysport (two other type A botulinum toxins) may be equally effective as Botox for treatment of urge incontinence in NB.

Currently, there is a debate on the optimum number of injection sites. While some authors advocate 20–30 injection sites, others have found that injecting the toxin into 15 sites may be sufficient.

In recent years, several authors have recommend including the trigone of the bladder in the injected plan since this region of bladder is rich in nerve fibers. Dr. Smith and his colleagues from Baylor College of Medicine in Houston, Texas include the trigone and adjust the dose based on the type and severity of the bladder dysfunction. Their protocol for patients with mild symptoms recommends 9–10 injection sites with a total Botox dose of 100 units (Fig. 10.4). For patients with severe symptoms who are already catheterizing themselves, 30–40 injection sites are recommended with a total Botox dose of 200 units.

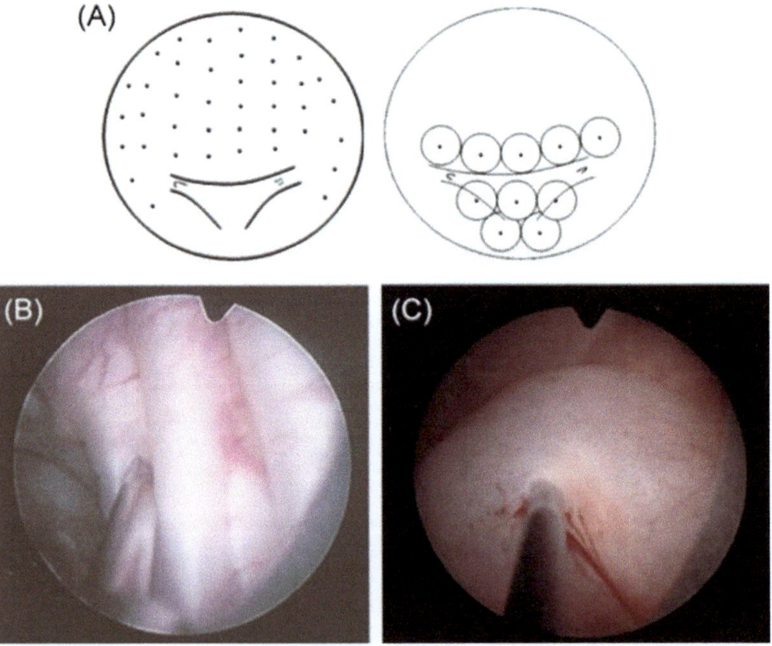

Fig. 10.4 Technique of bladder injection: (**a**) (top left) 30 injections for patients with severe symptoms. (**a**) (top right) 10 injections for patients with mild symptoms. From Dasilva and coworkers. Toxicon 2015. (Reproduced with permission from the publisher Elsevier. (**b** and **c**) site of injection just under the mucosa of bladder surface)

Overactive Bladder of Unknown Cause (OAB)

This category includes patients with undetermined cause of bladder overactivity. Among adults, a prevalence of up to 16.9% has been reported in general population increasing to 30% among those 75 years of age or older [22]. The symptoms of OAB are very similar to those of NDO: mainly urinary urgency, frequency and incontinence. These symptoms are managed similarly with bladder training, pelvic floor exercise, anticholinergic medication, and more recently introduced drugs such as mirabegron and oxybutyrin. As mentioned earlier side effects of these drugs and lack of sustained action is a reason for exploring new modes of treatment.

In 2003, Dykstra and his colleagues were first to show that injection of botulinum toxin B) into the bladder wall can reduce the urinary frequency and incontinence of patients with OAB (for descriptions of different types of botulinum toxins and their units see Chap. 3) [23]. The authors compared the effect of different doses of myobloc starting with 2500, 5000, 10,000 and rarely up to 15,000 units; the first three roughly approximate 50–100 and 200 units of Botox, respectively. They found no difference in efficacy between different doses. Subsequently, several carefully designed, high quality, double blind studies with Botox in large number of patients confirmed the efficacy of Botox for management of OAB symptoms [24–26]. Based on these studies, Botox was approved by FDA for treatment of overactive bladder in 2013. The technique of Botox injection into bladder is similar to what was described earlier for management of urinary incontinence in neurogenic detrusor overactivity (NDO)/ neurogenic bladder (NB).

Cost Effectiveness

Several studies have shown that despite high cost of Botox therapy, this treatment is cost effective for management of NDO and OAB symptoms. It is used infrequently, every 6–9 months, has fewer side effects, and, in many instances, eliminates the need for taking oral medications. Successful Botox therapy of NDO or OAB leads to reduced number of doctor's office and emergency room visits and less hospitalizations [27].

Improper Contraction of External Sphincter of the Bladder at the Time of Expected Relaxation

This condition is medically named sphincter-detrusor dyssynergia (SDD) meaning loss of synergy between these two muscles. As was mentioned earlier, when bladder muscle (detrusor) contracts in response the nerve signal, external sphincter muscle (Fig. 10.2) relaxes and lets urine out of the bladder. In SDD, external sphincter undergoes contraction instead of relaxation in response to detrusor contraction. SDD is caused by medical disorders that damage the nerve fibers that control bladder function; these nerve fibers originate from nerve cells of the brain and spinal cord. Disease conditions such as spinal cord trauma, stroke or multiple sclerosis are common causes of DSD. The result of impaired bladder emptying is urine retention, recurrent infections and potential damage to the kidneys due to back up of the urine.

Technique of Toxin Injection in DSD Injections can be done by a cystoscope which, in men is inserted through the penis. After reaching external sphincter, injections are usually performed at 4 points (3, 6, 9 and 12 o'clock locations). In women, because of the short length of urethra, external sphincter is closer to the surface.

Several studies have shown efficacy of Botox in relieving the symptoms of DSD (lasting 3–9 months) [28–32]. At present time, Botox treatment of DDS is not FDA approved, but it is performed in some centers off label, by experienced physicians. The main side effect of this treatment is urinary incontinence which results from unwanted degree of weakening of the external sphincter muscle.

Botulinum Toxin Indications in Urogenital Pain Syndromes

As mentioned earlier, injection of US marketed botulinum toxins (Botox, Xeomin, Dysport and Myobloc) into the muscle, not only inhibits the release of acetylcholine (a neurotransmitter that activates muscle but also reduces and inhibits the function of a number of pain neurotransmitters. These agents help to convey pain sensation from periphery to the brain. Because of this action, researchers began to explore the effect of botulinum toxin therapy on urogenital pain syndromes. There is now supporting evidence that, at least in three of these conditions, local injection of botulinum toxins alleviates pain; these three conditions consist of male pelvic pain, female pelvic pain and local pain related to chronic bladder infection (interstitial cystitis).

Male Pelvic Pain

Male Pelvic Pain pain is usually the result of chronic inflammation or infection of prostate (chronic prostatitis). This condition is classified by the National Institute of Health (NIH) as chronic prostatitis/chronic pelvic pain syndrome. It is the most common urological disorder among men under the age of 50 with a prevalence of 2.5–16% [33]. The pain is felt in the lower part of the abdomen, pelvis and genitalia and impairs the quality of life due to its severity and persistence.

The efficacy of botulinum toxin therapy for male pelvic pain is supported by publication of two high quality studies. Both studies used Botox but the technique of injection was different. In the smaller study which comprised 13 patients, the injection was directed into one of the muscles of the pelvic floor (bulbospongiosus), whereas in the larger study (60 patients), the site of injections was the lateral lobes of prostate (at 3 locations). Both studies used Botox with comparable doses of 100–200 units. Investigators of both studies reported that patients described a marked reduction in severity and frequency of pain at 1, 3 and 6 months after injection; concurrent with notable improvements of their quality of life [34, 35]. Using the criteria of the Development and Guidelines Subcommittee of the American Academy of Neurology (AAN) (see Chap. 3), botulinum toxin therapy for male pelvic pain would have a level B efficacy (probably effective based on I and one class II). For this indication, however, Botox does not have FDA approval yet. The treatment of male pelvic pain with botulinum toxin is, hence, currently off label based on the supporting literature.

Female Pelvic Pain Chronic pelvic pain in women is most often (71–87%) associates with a medical condition called endometriosis [36]. In endometriosis, a tissue identical to the lining of the uterine cavity (endometrium) is found abnormally in other pelvic organs including the ovaries, the tubes that connect ovaries to uterus and in the peritoneum. This abnormally located and misplaced issue, increases in size and bleeds just as the normal endometrium does during the menstrual cycle.

The pelvic floor contains a dozen small muscles that surround the rectum and vagina and connect the bony structures of front and back of the pelvis (pubis and tailbones). Dr. Abbott and his coworkers from Australia were the first to show that injecting Botox into two of the pelvic floor muscles (one connecting pubis to rectum and one connecting pubis to tailbone) relieves pelvic pain in a group of women, a majority of whom had endometriosis. Their study consisted of 60 women, 30 of whom received 80 units of Botox and 30 received placebo (normal saline) [37]. The patients were followed at 4-week intervals for 26 weeks. In addition to relief from pelvic pain, women who received Botox, reported having less pain during intercourse (dyspareunia) compared to those who received saline. Dr. Abbott and his colleagues, observation, was supported by several other observations, among them a study that reported pain relief and improvement of quality of life following Botox injection in women with pelvic pain [38]. Close to 5% of the patients reported transient urinary and fecal incontinence as side effects of Botox injections. In another study that combined injection of Botox into pelvic floor muscles with pelvic floor physiotherapy, 58% of the affected women reported improvement of their pelvic pain [39]. Dr. Barbara Karp and her colleagues at the National Institutes of Health investigated the effects of botulinum toxin injections in women with pelvic pain and endometriosis in a double-blind, placebo-controlled, carefully crafted protocol. The preliminary results of this protocol are encouraging; the full results will be available, hopefully, in the near future. In a recent review of literature on this subject, Dr. Karp has emphasized the need for more high quality studies in this area [40].

Pain Related to Bladder Infection (Interstitial Cystitis/Bladder Pain Syndrome) Bladder pain syndrome (BPS) or interstitial cystitis (IC) is a debilitating condition that affects millions of people worldwide. It is believed to be due to chronic inflammation of the internal bladder lining (part in contact with urine) that leads to irritation, pain in the area of the bladder, urinary frequency and urinary urgency. Failure of body's immune system is suspected in some patients, but the cause of this bladder problem is currently unknown. No effective treatment is currently available. Instillation of hyaluronic acid into bladder helps some patients and reduces the irritation of the bladder lining, but the results are often temporary and pain recurrence is common. Hydrodistention (distending the bladder with water) also produces some degree of pain relief in some patients. The effects of painkillers in interstitial cystitis (IC) is often not sustained.

In recent years, several studies have shown that injection of bladder wall with botulinum toxins can relieve pain and improve quality of life in patients with interstitial cystitis/bladder pain syndrome [41–45]. This is probably via the dual action of botulinum toxin: 1- relaxing the bladder wall and 2- blocking the effect of chemicals known as pain transmitters (described earlier in this chapter and in detail in Chap. 3). Preference for injection locations varies among different investigators. Some prefer to inject the body of bladder and others have found injecting into bladder trigone which is rich in nerve fibers (usually 10 injection sites) more helpful [45–47].

One comparable study has shown no difference between the two locations (trigone versus body of the bladder) [48]. The recommended dose for Botox is 100 units and for Dysport (another type A toxin) 300 units [48]. In one study, combining Botox injection with hydrodistention was more effective in relieving the symptoms of IC than hydrodistention alone [49]. Repeated injections of Botox for treatment of IC have been found to be generally safe [50] with sustained long-term efficacy (over years) achievable [51].

Botulinum Toxin Therapy for Enlarged Prostate

Among male patients, increased size of the prostate (prostatic hypertrophy) exerts pressure against urethra (the tube draining urine from the bladder), and causes a variety of symptoms including slowness of voiding, weak urine stream, incomplete emptying and, sometimes, incontinence. Researchers have tried to show if injection of botulinum toxin into prostate by decreasing the size of prostate can help the urinary problems. The results of research in this area have ben conflicting. Currently, botulinum toxin therapy (injections) is not recommended for management of urinary symptoms solely related to enlarged prostate.

Conclusion

Many drugs have been tested for treatment of urinary urgency or incontinence resulting from neurogenic bladder [NP] or overactive bladder [OAB], but the results have often been disappointing due to poor sustained efficacy and disturbing side effects [52]. Botulinum toxin injection into bladder wall improves symptoms related to bladder dysfunction and discomfort (urgency, frequency). Botulinum toxin therapy is approved by FDA for treatment of bladder overactivity either related to nerve damage (neurogenic bladder/neurogenic detrusor overactivity-NB/NDO) or bladder overactivity of undetermined cause (overactive bladder-OAB). FDA has not yet approved botulinum toxin therapy for treatment of interstitial cystitis (bladder pain syndrome), but the American Urological Association advocates it as one mode of therapy for this painful condition. Botulinum toxin therapy (injections) is probably effective in relieving male pelvic pain (level B evidence- see Chap. 3). For female pelvic pain the preliminary data are encouraging, but experts encourage waiting for the results of more high quality studies.

References

1. Jankovic J. An update on new and unique uses of botulinum toxin in movement disorders. Toxicon. 2018 Jun 1;147:84–8. https://doi.org/10.1016/j.toxicon.2017.09.003. Epub 2017 Sep 6. PMID: 28888928.
2. Hallett M. Mechanism of action of botulinum neurotoxin: unexpected consequences. Toxicon. 2018 Jun 1;147:73–6. https://doi.org/10.1016/j.toxicon.2017.08.011. Epub 2017 Aug 11. PMID: 28803760. PMCID: PMC5808894.
3. Kaku M, Simpson DM. Spotlight on botulinum toxin and its potential in the treatment of stroke-related spasticity. Drug Des Devel Ther. 2016;10:1085–99.
4. Palazón-García R, Alcobendas-Maestro M, Esclarin-de Ruz A, Benavente-Valdepeñas AM. Treatment of spasticity in spinal cord injury with botulinum toxin. J Spinal Cord Med. 2019 May;42(3):281–7. https://doi.org/10.1080/10790268.2018.1479053. Epub 2018 Jun 5. PMID: 29869974. PMCID: PMC6522928.
5. Ginsberg D. The epidemiology and pathophysiology of neurogenic bladder. Am J Manag Care. 2013;19(10 Suppl):s191–6. PMID: 24495240.
6. Manack A, Motsko SP, Haag-Molkenteller C, Dmochowski RR, Goehring EL Jr, Nguyen-Khoa BA, Jones JK. Epidemiology and healthcare utilization of neurogenic bladder patients in a US claims database. Neurourol Urodyn. 2011 Mar;30(3):395–401. https://doi.org/10.1002/nau.21003. Epub 2010 Sep 29. PMID: 20882676.
7. de Sèze M, Ruffion A, Denys P, Joseph PA, Perrouin-Verbe B, GENULF. The neurogenic bladder in multiple sclerosis: review of the literature and proposal of management guidelines. Mult Scler. 2007 Aug;13(7):915–28. https://doi.org/10.1177/1352458506075651. Epub 2007 Mar 15. PMID: 17881401.
8. Chancellor MB, Yehoshua A, Waweru C. Limitations of anticholinergic cycling in patients with overactive bladder (OAB) with urinary incontinence (UI): results from the CONsequences of treatment refractory overactive bladder (CONTROL) study. Int Urol Nephrol. 2016;48:1029–36.
9. Ginsberg D, et al. Phase 3 efficacy and tolerability study of onabotulinumtoxinA for urinary incontinence from neurogenic detrusor overactivity. J Urol. 2012;187:2131–9.
10. Cruz F, et al. Efficacy and safety of onabotulinumtoxinA in patients with urinary incontinence due to neurogenic detrusor overactivity: a randomised, double-blind, placebo-controlled trial. Eur Urol. 2011;60:742–50.
11. Nitti VW, et al. OnabotulinumtoxinA for the treatment of patients with overactive bladder and urinary incontinence: results of a phase 3, randomized, placebo controlled trial. J Urol. 2013;189:2186–93.
12. Franco I, Hoebeke PB, Dobremez E, Titanji W, Geib T, Jenkins B, Yushmanova I, Austin PF. Long-term safety and tolerability of repeated treatments with OnabotulinumtoxinA in

children with neurogenic detrusor overactivity. J Urol. 2023 Apr;209(4):774–84. https://doi.org/10.1097/JU.0000000000003157. Epub 2023 Jan 19. PMID: 36655470.

13. Honda M, Yokoyama O, Takahashi R, Matsuda T, Nakayama T, Mogi T. Botulinum toxin injections for Japanese patients with urinary incontinence caused by neurogenic detrusor overactivity: clinical evaluation of onabotulinumtoxinA in a randomized, placebo-controlled, double-blind trial with an open-label extension. Int J Urol. 2021 Sep;28(9):906–12. https://doi.org/10.1111/iju.14602. Epub 2021 Jun 1. PMID: 34075630. PMCID: PMC8453759.

14. Kennelly M, Dmochowski R, Schulte-Baukloh H, et al. Efficacy and safety of onabotulinumtoxinA therapy are sustained over 4 years of treatment in patients with neurogenic detrusor overactivity: final results of a long-term extension study. Neurourol Urodyn. 2017;36:368–75.

15. Kennelly M, Cruz F, Herschorn S, Abrams P, Onem K, Solomonov VK, Del Rosario Figueroa Coz E, Manu-Marin A, Giannantoni A, Thompson C, Vilain C, Volteau M, Denys P, Dysport CONTENT Program Group. Efficacy and safety of AbobotulinumtoxinA in patients with neurogenic detrusor overactivity incontinence performing regular clean intermittent catheterization: pooled results from two phase 3 randomized studies (CONTENT1 and CONTENT2). Eur Urol. 2022 Aug;82(2):223–32. https://doi.org/10.1016/j.eururo.2022.03.010. Epub 2022 Apr 7. PMID: 35400537.

16. Denys P, Del Popolo G, Amarenco G, Karsenty G, Le Berre P, Padrazzi B, Picaut P, Dysport Study Group. Efficacy and safety of two administration modes of an intra-detrusor injection of 750 units dysport® (abobotulinumtoxinA) in patients suffering from refractory neurogenic detrusor overactivity (NDO): a randomised placebo-controlled phase IIa study. Neurourol Urodyn. 2017 Feb;36(2):457–62. https://doi.org/10.1002/nau.22954. Epub 2016 Jan 12. PMID: 26756554.

17. Giannantoni A, Gubbiotti M, Rubilotta E, Balzarro M, Antonelli A, Bini V. IncobotulinumtoxinA versus onabotulinumtoxinA intradetrusor injections in patients with neurogenic detrusor overactivity incontinence: a double-blind, randomized, non-inferiority trial. Minerva Urol Nephrol. 2022 Oct;74(5):625–35. https://doi.org/10.23736/S2724-6051.21.04227-2. Epub 2021 Mar 26. PMID: 33769020.

18. Ginsberg D, Cruz F, Herschorn S, Gousse A, Keppenne V, Aliotta P, Sievert KD, Brin MF, Jenkins B, Thompson C, Lam W, Heesakkers J, Haag-Molkenteller C. OnabotulinumtoxinA is effective in patients with urinary incontinence due to neurogenic detrusor overactivity [corrected] regardless of concomitant anticholinergic use or neurologic etiology. Adv Ther. 2013 Sep;30(9):819–33. https://doi.org/10.1007/s12325-013-0054-z. Epub 2013 Sep 27. Erratum in: Adv Ther. 2014 Feb;31(2):242. PMID: 24072665. PMCID: PMC3824824.

19. Austin PF, Franco I, Dobremez E, Kroll P, Titanji W, Geib T, Jenkins B, Hoebeke PB. OnabotulinumtoxinA for the treatment of neurogenic detrusor overactivity in children. Neurourol Urodyn. 2021 Jan;40(1):493–501. https://doi.org/10.1002/nau.24588. Epub 2020 Dec 11. PMID: 33305474. PMCID: PMC7839517.

20. Pereira E Silva R, Ponte C, Lopes F, Palma Dos Reis J. Alkalinized lidocaine solution as a first-line local anesthesia protocol for intradetrusor injection of onabotulinum toxin A: results from a double-blinded randomized controlled trial. Neurourol Urodyn. 2020 Nov;39(8):2471–79. https://doi.org/10.1002/nau.24519. Epub 2020 Sep 21. PMID: 32956506.

21. Smith CP, Chancellor MB. Botulinum toxin to treat neurogenic bladder. Semin Neurol. 2016 Feb;36(1):5–9. https://doi.org/10.1055/s-0035-1571216. Epub 2016 Feb 11. PMID: 26866490.

22. Abrams P. Describing bladder storage function: overactive bladder syndrome and detrusor overactivity. Urology. 2003;62(Supplement 2):26–37.

23. Dykstra D, Enriquez A, Valley M. Treatment of overactive bladder with botulinum toxin type B: a pilot study. Int Urogynecol J Pelvic Floor Dysfunct. 2003 Dec;14(6):424–6. https://doi.org/10.1007/s00192-003-1099-3. Epub 2003 Nov 25. PMID: 14677005.

24. Dmochowski R, Chapple C, Nitti VW, Chancellor M, Everaert K, Thompson C, Daniell G, Zhou J, Haag-Molkenteller C. Efficacy and safety of onabotulinumtoxinA for idiopathic overactive bladder: a double-blind, placebo controlled, randomized, dose ranging trial. J Urol. 2010 Dec;184(6):2416–22. https://doi.org/10.1016/j.juro.2010.08.021. Epub 2010 Oct 16. PMID: 20952013.

25. Yokoyama O, Honda M, Yamanishi T, Sekiguchi Y, Fujii K, Nakayama T, Mogi T. OnabotulinumtoxinA (botulinum toxin type A) for the treatment of Japanese patients with overactive bladder and urinary incontinence: results of single-dose treatment from a phase III, randomized, double-blind, placebo-controlled trial (interim analysis). Int J Urol. 2020 Mar;27(3):227–34. https://doi.org/10.1111/iju.14176. Epub 2020 Jan 20. PMID: 31957922; PMCID: PMC7154639.

26. Flynn MK, Amundsen CL, Perevich M, Liu F, Webster GD. Outcome of a randomized, double-blind, placebo controlled trial of botulinum A toxin for refractory overactive bladder. J Urol. 2009 Jun;181(6):2608–15. https://doi.org/10.1016/j.juro.2009.01.117. Epub 2009 Apr 16. PMID: 19375091. PMCID: PMC2730562.

27. Carlson JJ, Hansen RN, Dmochowski RR, et al. Estimating the cost-effectiveness of onabotulinumtoxinA for neurogenic detrusor overactivity in the United States. Clin Ther. 2013;35:414–24.

28. Dykstra DD, Sidi AA. Treatment of detrusor-sphincter dyssynergia with botulinum A toxin: a double-blind study. Arch Phys Med Rehabil. 1990 Jan;71(1):24–6. PMID: 2297305.

29. Schurch B, Hauri D, Rodic B, Curt A, Meyer M, Rossier AB. Botulinum-a toxin as a treatment of detrusor-sphincter dyssynergia: a prospective study in 24 spinal cord injury patients. J Urol. 1996 Mar;155(3):1023–9. https://doi.org/10.1016/s0022-5347(01)66376-6. PMID: 8583552.

30. Yang WX, Zhu HJ, Chen WG, Zhang DW, Su M, Feng JF, Liu CD, Cai P. Treatment of detrusor external sphincter dyssynergia using ultrasound-guided trocar catheter transurethral botulinum toxin a injection in men with spinal cord injury. Arch Phys Med Rehabil. 2015 Apr;96(4):614–9. https://doi.org/10.1016/j.apmr.2014.10.003. Epub 2014 Oct 24. PMID: 25450132.

31. Huang M, Chen H, Jiang C, Xie K, Tang P, Ou R, Zeng J, Liu Q, Li Q, Huang J, Huang T, Zeng W. Effects of botulinum toxin A injections in spinal cord injury patients with detrusor overactivity and detrusor sphincter dyssynergia. J Rehabil Med. 2016 Oct 5;48(8):683–7. https://doi.org/10.2340/16501977-2132. PMID: 27563834.

32. Goel S, Pierce H, Pain K, Christos P, Dmochowski R, Chughtai B. Use of botulinum toxin A (BoNT-A) in detrusor external sphincter dyssynergia (DESD): a systematic review and meta-analysis. Urology. 2020 Jun;140:7–13. https://doi.org/10.1016/j.urology.2020.03.007. Epub 2020 Mar 19. PMID: 32197987.

33. Pontari MA, Ruggieri MR. Mechanisms in prostatitis/chronic pelvic pain syndrome. J Urol. 2008 May;179(5 Suppl):S61–7. https://doi.org/10.1016/j.juro.2008.03.139. PMID: 18405756.

34. Gottsch HP, Yang CC, Berger RE. A pilot study of botulinum toxin A for male chronic pelvic pain syndrome. Scand J Urol Nephrol. 2011;45:72–6.

35. Falahatkar S, Shahab E, Gholamjani Moghaddam K, Kazemnezhad E. Transurethralintraprostatic injection of botulinum neurotoxin type A for the treatment of chronic prostatitis/chronic pelvic pain syndrome: results of a prospective pilot, double-blind and randomized, placebo-controlled study. BJU Int. 2015;116:641–9.

36. Aredo JV, Heyrana KJ, Karp BI, et al. Relating chronic pelvic pain and endometriosis to signs of sensitization and myofascial pain and dysfunction. Semin Reprod Med. 2017;35:88–9.

37. Abbott JA, Jarvis SK, Lyons SD, Thomson A, Vancaille TG. Botulinum toxin type A for chronic pain and pelvic floor spasm in women: a randomized controlled trial. Obstet Gynecol. 2006;108:915–23.

38. Morrissey D, El-Khawand D, Ginzburg N, et al. Botulinum toxin A injections into pelvic floor muscles under electromyographic guidance for women with refractory high-tone pelvic floor dysfunction: a 6-month prospective pilot study. Female Pelvic Med Reconstr Surg. 2015;21:277–82.

39. Halder GE, Scott L, Wyman A, Mora N, Miladinovic B, Bassaly R, Hoyte L. Botox combined with myofascial release physical therapy as a treatment for myofascial pelvic pain. Investig Clin Urol. 2017 Mar;58(2):134–9. https://doi.org/10.4111/icu.2017.58.2.134. Epub 2017 Feb 1. PMID: 28261683. PMCID: PMC5330376.

40. Karp BI, Stratton P. Applications of botulinum toxin to the female pelvic floor: botulinum toxin for genito-pelvic pain penetration disorder and chronic pelvic pain in women. Toxicon.

2023 Jul;230:107162. https://doi.org/10.1016/j.toxicon.2023.107162. Epub 2023 May 16. PMID: 37201800. PMCID: PMC10330736.

41. Smith CP, Radziszewski P, Borkowski A, Somogyi GT, Boone TB, Chancellor MB. Botulinum toxin a has antinociceptive effects in treating interstitial cystitis. Urology. 2004 Nov;64(5):871–5. https://doi.org/10.1016/j.urology.2004.06.073. discussion 875. PMID: 15533466.

42. Giannantoni A, Cagini R, Del Zingaro M, Proietti S, Quartesan R, Porena M, Piselli M. Botulinum A toxin intravesical injections for painful bladder syndrome: impact upon pain, psychological functioning and quality of life. Curr Drug Deliv. 2010 Dec;7(5):442–6. https://doi.org/10.2174/156720110793566317. PMID: 20950262.

43. Kuo HC, Jiang YH, Tsai YC, Kuo YC. Intravesical botulinum toxin-a injections reduce bladder pain of interstitial cystitis/bladder pain syndrome refractory to conventional treatment—a prospective, multicenter, randomized, double-blind, placebo-controlled clinical trial. Neurourol Urodyn 2016 Jun;35(5):609–14. https://doi.org/10.1002/nau.22760. Epub 2015 Apr 24. PMID: 25914337.

44. Giannantoni A, Costantini E, Di Stasi SM, Tascini MC, Bini V, Porena M. Botulinum A toxin intravesical injections in the treatment of painful bladder syndrome: a pilot study. Eur Urol. 2006 Apr;49(4):704–9. https://doi.org/10.1016/j.eururo.2005.12.002. Epub 2006 Jan 4. PMID: 16417964.

45. Jiang YH, Jhang JF, Lee CL, Kuo HC. Comparative study of efficacy and safety between bladder body and trigonal intravesical onabotulinumtoxina injection in the treatment of interstitial cystitis refractory to conventional treatment-a prospective, randomized, clinical trial. Neurourol Urodyn. 2018 Apr;37(4):1467–73. https://doi.org/10.1002/nau.23475. Epub 2018 Jan 13. PMID: 29331031.

46. Pinto RA, Costa D, Morgado A, Pereira P, Charrua A, Silva J, Cruz F. Intratrigonal OnabotulinumtoxinA improves bladder symptoms and quality of life in patients with bladder pain syndrome/interstitial cystitis: a pilot, single center, randomized, double-blind, placebo controlled trial, J Urol. 2018 Apr;199(4):998–1003. https://doi.org/10.1016/j.juro.2017.10.018. Epub 2017 Oct 13. PMID: 29031769.

47. Pinto R, Lopes T, Frias B, Silva A, Silva JA, Silva CM, Cruz C, Cruz F, Dinis P. Trigonal injection of botulinum toxin A in patients with refractory bladder pain syndrome/interstitial cystitis. Eur Urol. 2010 Sep;58(3):360–365. https://doi.org/10.1016/j.eururo.2010.02.031. Epub 2010 Mar 6. PMID: 20227820.

48. Zargham M, Mahmoodi M, Mazdak H, Tadayon F, Mansori M, Kazemi M, Khorami MH, Saberi N. Evaluation of therapeutic effect of intratrigonal injection of AbobotulinumtoxinA(Dysport) and hydrodistention in refractory interstitial cystitis /bladder pain syndrome. Urol J. 2020 Nov 23;18(2):203–8. https://doi.org/10.22037/uj.v16i7.5879. PMID: 33236337.

49. Kuo HC, Chancellor MB. Comparison of intravesical botulinum toxin type A injections plus hydrodistention with hydrodistention alone for the treatment of refractory interstitial cystitis/painful bladder syndrome. BJU Int. 2009 Sep;104(5):657–61. https://doi.org/10.1111/j.1464-410X.2009.08495.x. Epub 2009 Mar 30. PMID: 19338543.

50. Kuo HC. Repeated intravesical onabotulinumtoxinA injections are effective in treatment of refractory interstitial cystitis/bladder pain syndrome. Int J Clin Pract. 2013 May;67(5):427–34. https://doi.org/10.1111/ijcp.12113. PMID: 23574103.

51. Abreu-Mendes P, Ferrão-Mendes A, Botelho F, Cruz F, Pinto R. Effect of intratrigonal botulinum toxin in patients with bladder pain syndrome/interstitial cystitis: a long-term, single-center study in real-life conditions. Toxins (Basel). 2022 Nov 10;14(11):775. https://doi.org/10.3390/toxins14110775. PMID: 36356025. PMCID: PMC9692970.

52. Michel MC, Cardozo L, Chermansky CJ, Cruz F, Igawa Y, Lee KS, Sahai A, Wein AJ, Andersson KE. Current and emerging pharmacological targets and treatments of urinary incontinence and related disorders. Pharmacol Rev. 2023 Jul;75(4):554–674. https://doi.org/10.1124/pharmrev.121.000523. Epub 2023 Mar 14. PMID: 36918261.

Chapter 11
Botulinum Toxin Therapy for Problems Related to the Gastrointestinal System (Alimentary Tract)

Abstract Injection of Botulinum toxins into the sphincters of the alimentary tract improves symptoms due to contraction and spasm of these circular muscles located in upper and lower esophagus, between stomach and small intestine, opening of bile duct to small intestine and the anal region (anal sphincter). Local injection of botulinum toxin can help healing of anal fissure.

Keywords Botulinum toxin · Botulinum neurotoxin · Achalasia · Upper esophageal sphincter · Lower esophageal sphincter · Pylorus · Sphincter of Oddi · Anal fissure

Introduction

Alimentary tract includes the mouth, throat, esophagus (the tube that connects the throat to the stomach), stomach and the intestines (gut). Food moves through the alimentary tract and is digested in the stomach and further digested and absorbed in the gut. The alimentary tract (AT) has a muscular wall. Two types of muscles are represented in the AT, striated and smooth muscles. Striated muscles, like those of the arm, leg and trunk muscles can be moved at will, whereas smooth muscles' function is not controlled by volition. Most muscles of the stomach, gut or bladder are of the smooth type; the individual is not usually conscious of their movement.

In the alimentary system, from upper part of the esophagus (the tube that connects the mouth to stomach) to its end (anus, the orifice through which solid refuse is excreted), there are five strong circular muscles. These circular muscles are called sphincters. Sphincter is a ring shaped muscle that encircles an opening or a passage in the body. In disease conditions, spasm or unwanted contraction of these sphincters can cause pain and discomfort and interfere with the passage of food.

The first sphincter of AT is located in the upper esophagus (upper esophageal sphincter -UES) just below the lower end of the throat (pharynx) (Fig. 11.1). This sphincter relaxes during swallowing (initiated by contraction of throat muscles) letting food enter into the esophagus. The second sphincter is located at the junction of

B. Jabbari, *Botulinum Toxin Treatment*,
https://doi.org/10.1007/978-3-031-54471-2_11

177

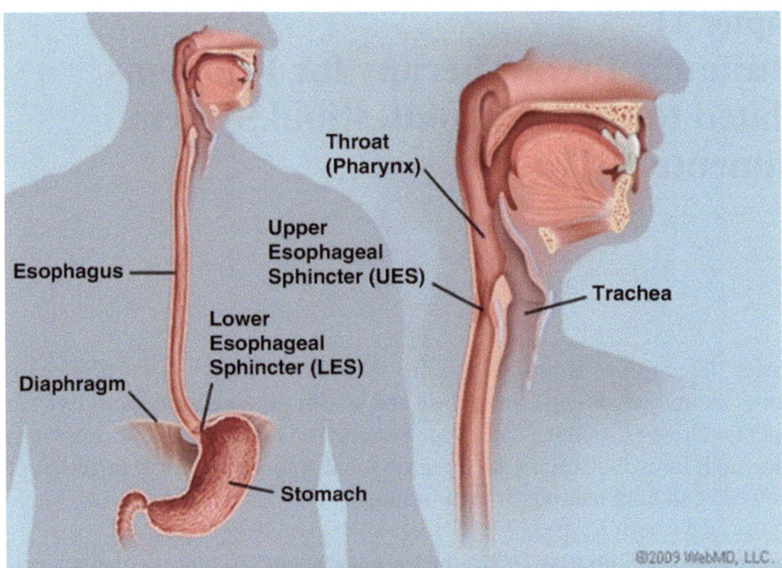

Fig. 11.1 Anatomy of the throat, the esophagus and the two esophageal sphincters (upper and lower). (From Mathew Hoffman M.D. Human Anatomy-Digestive disorders- picture of Esophagus—2009 and 2014 LLC Curtesy of Web Med)

the esophagus and stomach (lower esophageal sphincter- LES). Contraction of this sphincter closes the opening between esophagus and stomach when no food is consumed. During food consumption, and after contraction of the UES, the LES relaxes, opens and lets the food enter into the stomach.

The third sphincter is between the stomach and the small intestine. This sphincter is called pylorus. Pylorus in Greek means gate keeper. From this small circular opening partially digested food passes to the duodenum (first part of small intestine). The fourth sphincter controls the opening and closing of the bile duct. Bile which is important for food digestion and is produced in the gall bladder enters the gut through the bile duct. The sphincter that controls the opening and closing of the bile duct is called sphincter of Oddi, named after an Italian physician who first described it (Fig. 11.2). The fifth sphincter- the anal sphincter -encircles the anus and controls the act of defecation. Relaxation of this sphincter lets the food refuse out of the body.

All these sphincters can be affected and may not function properly if the brain or spinal cord is damaged and the sphincters' nerve supply from central nervous system is interrupted. Common causes of such damages are stroke, trauma, Parkinson's disease and multiple sclerosis. Brain and spinal cord control the function of alimentary sphincters through fine motor fibers.

In normal conditions, the function of every muscle in the body (including alimentary sphincters) is maintained through a balance between excitation and inhibition. Brain excites the muscles through excitatory fibers that induce muscle

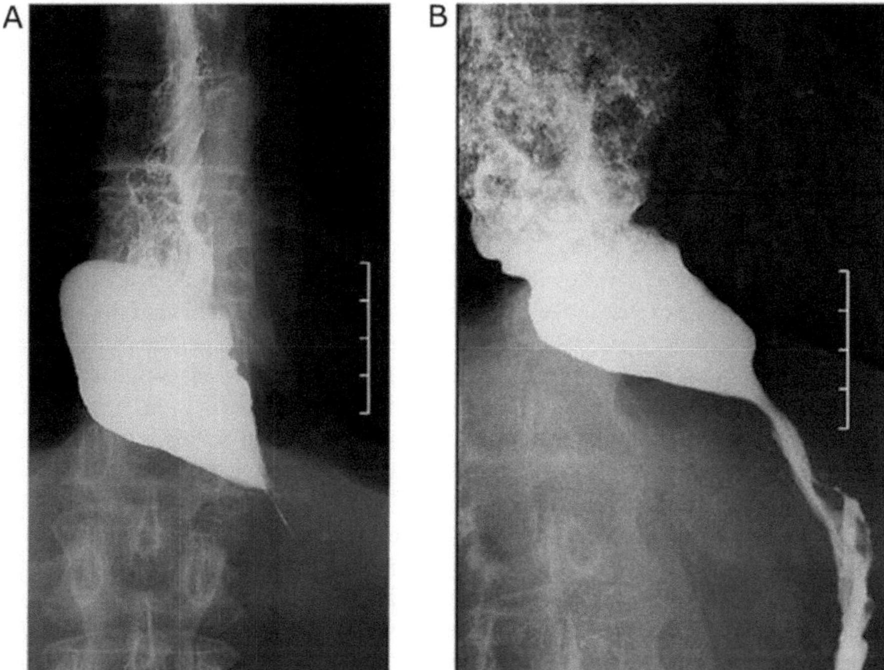

Fig. 11.2 (a) Shows brick-like appearance of esophagus with barium column cut off at the region of LES. (b) After botulinum toxin injection, LES opens and allows passage of barium towards stomach. (From Yamaghughi et al. [13], image reproduced under Creative Commons CC BY 4. Courtesy of PMC publishers)

contraction. These fibers release a chemical at their end that excites the muscle; this chemical (transmitter) is called acetylcholine. The inhibitory fibers also have their own transmitter which is different from acetylcholine. For reasons that are not well understood, conditions that commonly damage the brain or spinal cord, damage the inhibitory fibers more often than the excitatory fibers. This tilts the balance towards excitation that gradually keeps the muscles in a state of continuous tightening and contraction. In the limb muscles, this increased muscle tone is called spasticity. The same tightening that affects the limb muscles can affect the function of all 5 above mentioned sphincters of the alimentary tract. Therefore, tight sphincters can interfere with the function of alimentary system at different levels. Botulinum toxin injection into any muscle (striated or smooth) can block the release of acetylcholine from the nerve endings and results in muscle relaxation. Because of this function, injection of BoNTs into the hyperactive muscles has now become a major (and in many cases the first line of) treatment in conditions that cause involuntary muscle movements [1]. This is the basis of using botulinum toxin therapy for treatment of alimentary symptoms related to hyperactive sphincter disorders.

Upper Esophageal Sphincter (UES)

UES is located in the lower end of the throat (pharynx) and is vertically 1–1.5 inches long (Fig. 11.1). The main muscle of this sphincter is called cricopharyngeal muscle (CP), predominantly making the UES's posterior wall [2]. The main function of UES is to prevent air from the lungs getting into the throat and prevent food from coming back from the esophagus into the throat (reflux) after swallowing. After the initiation of swallowing, UES relaxes and lets the food pass from the throat into the esophagus. The act of swallowing generates a wave of muscle contractions in the esophagus downward that moves the swallowed food or liquid toward the stomach. The medical term for these wave- like contractions of esophageal muscles is peristalsis, a term that also applies to the regular movements of the stomach and gut muscles mixing and moving the food through the alimentary system. A tight UES, caused usually by brain damage (stroke, trauma, multiple sclerosis) is unable to function properly. In some patients the cause is unknown. Patients complain of throat tightness, difficulty swallowing, and food getting stuck in their throat. When the food is forced down, it may inaccurately move into the windpipe causing strong coughs.

Treatment of UES tightness includes swallowing exercises, administration of medications and surgery. A large number of swallowing exercises are prescribed by speech therapists for management of UES tightness. These include forced multidirectional tongue movements, jaw opening and closing exercises, and stimulation of the palate with ice-cold spoons. In Shaker exercise, the patient lays flat on the back without a pillow and lifts the head while looking at the toes for 10–15 s; this exercise is repeated 5–6 times during the day. Other exercises include performing a hard swallow several times a day. In Mendelsohn Maneuver, the individual keeps two fingers against his/her Adam's apple (AA) and then swallows. The Adam's apple (the protruded cartilage in front of the neck) moves up during swallowing and comes down after swallowing is over. Patient is instructed to push gently against it and prevent the AA from coming down after swallowing for a few seconds. This is repeated several times a day.

Medications are not effective in relieving swallowing problems related to the tightness of UES. Balloon dilatation of the constricted sphincter is effective, but the effects are transient. Several surgical procedures have been practiced for improving swallowing problems in this condition. Cutting some of the muscle fibers of this sphincter by surgery offers partial relief, but the procedure has the risk of infection and voice impairment; the latter due to damage to the nerve for the upper part of the windpipe. Endoscopic laser surgery (using a device that visualizes the area), offers a safer approach with fewer side effects.

Botulinum Toxin Treatment of UES Dysfunction

Based on the known effect of botulinum toxins on nerve-muscle junction, i.e. inhibition of the excitatory transmitter acetylcholine, investigators began to look at the effects of injection of BoNT into UES for relief of UES tightness.

The first report on efficacy of Botox in relieving tightness of UES was published in 1994 [3]. The authors injected a total of 20 units of Botox into the cricopharyngeal lower throat muscles and to LES. Five of seven patients had complete relief of symptoms after injection. Dr. Sharzehi and his co-workers review of 2016 included 200 reported patients with LES tightness in whom the success rate with botulinum toxin injection ranged from 43% to 100% [4].

In 2017, Dr. Alfonsi and colleagues published the largest series of patients with UES dysfunction treated with BoNT injections [5]. Sixty seven patients with UES dysfunction were injected with 15–20 units of Xeomin (a botulinum toxin A with units comparable to Botox)) into the cricopharyngeal muscle (located in front of the neck, lower part). The causes of UES in these patients included stroke, trauma and multiple sclerosis. The authors described 52% of the patients as high responders since BoNT injection into the region of LES resulted in >2 levels of improvement in Dysphagia Outcome Severity Scale (DOSS). In 67% of the patients, the positive effect of BoNT injection lasted more than 4 months; some of these patients had relief that lasted up to 1 year. No serious side effects were noted in the responders. However, two patients who did not initially respond and were reinjected developed pneumonia. The authors emphasized risks associated with reinjection of non-responders (exposure to higher dose). More recently, the injection techniques have improved via using ultrasound technique that allows direct visualization of the UES and the tip of the injecting needle [6–8]. In one of these studies [6], over 80% of the 21 injected patients showed significant improvement of swallowing after botulinum toxin therapy of CP muscle. Toxin therapy is now an acceptable alternative to surgery for improving symptoms related to dysfunctional UES. The injector, however, needs to have significant familiarly with the anatomy of throat and esophageal structures.

Tightness of Lower Esophageal Sphincter (LES)– Achalasia

The word achalasia is of Greek origin and means failure to relax (Khalan, Khalasis: relaxing). This entity was first described by the English physician, Thomas Willis, in 1673.

In this condition, LES (Fig. 11.2) fails to relax and allow the passage of food from esophagus to the stomach. Unlike dysfunction of UES which often occurs during the course of well-known neurological problems (stroke, trauma, Parkinson's), in most cases of LES dysfunction (achalasia), the cause is unknown. It is now generally believed that achalasia is a neurological disorder due to the failure of nerve cells located in the lower part of the brain (brain stem) that are responsible for both relaxation of the LES and peristalsis of the esophagus. Peristaltic movements of the esophagus push the swallowed food downward toward LES. Loss of relaxation of LES and peristaltic movements of the esophagus lead to a large, dilated esophagus which contains copious saliva and undigested food. This can be easily visualized by radiography following swallowing a large volume of barium. The test will show stagnant barium column in a dilated esophagus and a very narrow and bird-beak shape LES at the junction of the esophagus and stomach (Fig. 11.3). Fluoroscopy (video) of the esophagus can show the absence of peristalsis, the wave like movements that move the food down the esophagus toward the lower esophageal sphincter.

Achalasia is rare with an incidence of 0. 5–1.63 in 100,000 individuals [9, 10]. The symptoms start slowly with most patients seeking medical attention years after the onset of symptoms (average 4–6 years) [11]. The most frequent symptom is difficulty in swallowing which is more prominent for solid food than liquids. Heart burn and regurgitation of food are the next two common symptoms. A smaller percentage of patients (30–40%) complain of weight loss and chest pain. As the disease progresses difficulty in swallowing becomes a disabling symptom.

The aim of treatment in achalasia is to reduce the tone and tightness of the lower esophageal sphincter. To achieve this goal, two approaches are commonly implemented. The area of narrowing can be dilated via a procedure called pneumatic (balloon insertion) approach. Alternatively, some of the fibers of the lower esophageal sphincter can be cut (myotomy) through a surgical approach. Although initial success rate is high—85% for dilation (pneumatic approach) and 90% for myotomy (cutting some muscle fibers, part of sphincter), a substantial number of patients demonstrate recurrence of symptoms after 4–6 years. Medical treatment of

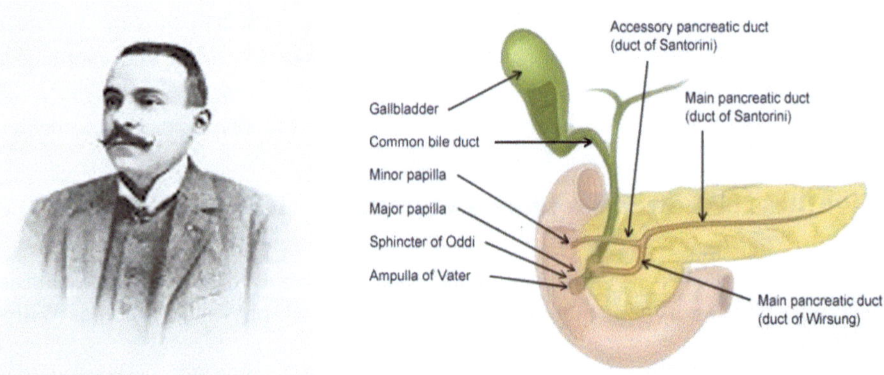

Fig. 11.3 Sphincter of Oddi(SO) (**a**) Ruggio Oddi the Italian anatomist who described location and function of SO Sphincter of Oddi. (Image courtesy of Wikimedia produced under Creative Commons Attribution Share-Alike license (CC-BY-SA); en.wikipedia.org/wiki/sphincter_of_Oddi_dysfunction)

achalasia is not very effective. Calcium channel blockers and nitrates have been prescribed with very modest results. It is due to limitation of the medical and surgical treatment approach in treatment of achalasia that a new mode of treatment that provides efficacy with reasonable safety is sought.

Botulinum Toxin Treatment of Achalasia

The first high quality study investigating the efficacy of BoNT injection into LES in achalasia was published by Dr. Pasricha and co-workers in 1995 [12]. These investigators have shown that injection of Botox into LES markedly reduces the sphincter pressure, relaxes it and improves the patient's symptoms. The findings were statistically highly significant when compared to the placebo (salt water) injections. Six months after BoNT injection, 14 of 21 patients were still in remission. Botox was injected into LES using endoscopy, an approach that uses a device that after insertion into the mouth, is moved through the throat and directed to the lower esophagus to visualize the changes in this area. Four injections, each 20 units, were used covering all four quadrants of the esophagus. No serious side effects were noted. These positive results were duplicated by several investigators over the past 20 years [6, 13–15]. Other investigators have reported a transient over-relaxation of LES after BoNT injection as a side effect resulting in reflux and heart burn. The success rate of Botulinum toxin injections into LES in achalasia has been found to be comparable with balloon dilatation and surgery (over 80%). Botulinum toxin injections are believed to have less side effects compared to surgery. Reinjection after 6–12 months is required.

Recent studies have shown that two types of botulinum toxin A, Botox and Dysport (see Chap. 3 for toxin types), are equally effective in improving the symptoms of achalasia.

In a recent publication, Roland and co-workers described different therapeutic options for treatment of achalasia [16].

Sphincter of Oddi (SO) Dysfunction

As described earlier, this is another sphincter that is important in proper progression of alimentation. Described by Italian anatomist Ruggio Oddi (Fig. 11.2a), this circular muscle controls an opening through which both bile and enzymes from the pancreas enter the gut, both important players in food digestion (Fig. 11.2b). The term sphincter of Oddi dysfunction (SOD) applies to abnormal over contraction of this circular muscle. It occurs in 1.5% of general population and is most common in women between 20 and 50 years of age [16]. Approximately 25% of the patients after complicated cholecystectomy (removal of gallbladder) and over half of the patients with pancreatitis have been found to have SOD.

Clinically, tightness of this sphincter can result in different symptoms. The most benign symptom is isolated chronic pain, felt below the rib cage on the right side, usually after eating. Other common symptoms include nausea and/or vomiting. The diagnosis is made by measurement of the pressure inside the sphincter. A pressure equal or exceeding 40 mm of mercury is consistent with increased pressure and contraction of sphincter of Oddi. More serious clinical conditions related to dysfunction of SO arise from liver and pancreas damage due to backed up bile or pancreatic enzymes into these vital organs. In such cases, patients may develop severe fatigue, poor digestion and/or jaundice (yellow skin) due to liver failure in addition to local abdominal pain and discomfort.

Treatment of SO contraction is difficult. Oral medications are not helpful. Surgery alone (cutting the muscle fibers of the SO) is also often not helpful and is associated with serious risks such as bleeding, perforation or inflammation of the pancreas. Studies in dogs have shown that injection of Botox into sphincter of Oddi decreases the tone of this muscle and relaxes it [17]. Several pilot studies (not placebo controlled) have shown that injection of Botox into the SO relaxes this muscle and reduces the inside pressure of SO substantially [18–20]. Pain relief occurs in 50% of the patients following Botox injection; also, some patients do better after surgery if they have Botox injection prior to surgery. Higher quality studies with long-term follow ups are needed to determine the role of Botox injections in relieving the symptoms of SO dysfunction.

The effects of Botox injection into SO for patients who have had partial removal of their pancreas due to tumor or inflammation have been explored recently. Many of such patients develop a fistula in the pancreas after surgery that complicates their recovery. Two studies reported that injection of Botox into SD before surgery significantly decreased development of fistula in the pancreas after partial resection and improved the patient outcome [21, 22].

Hypertonic Esophagus

This group of esophageal motility disorders includes diffuse esophageal spasm and nutcracker esophagus. The problem seems to be related to hyperexcitability of the esophageal muscle itself related to decreased activity of inhibitory nerve cells in the brain or enhanced effects of previously described nerve-muscle transmitter acetylcholine. Affected patients complain of difficulty in swallowing (dysphagia), nausea, chest pain and regurgitation [23].

Medical treatment includes drugs that are commonly used for treating depression such as tricyclic agents and calcium channel blocking agents. Oral nitrate, sildenafil (50 mg) and isosorbide (10 mg) are the next line of treatment. If these measures fail, some specialists recommend Botox injections. Usually, 100 units of Botox is diluted in 4 ml of saline and injected into multiple sites in the lower esophagus, extending from the region of LES to 5 cm and sometimes even farther upward. In one study, between 70% and 90% of patients respond well to Botox injections with improvements apparent within 30 days [24]. The injections are particularly effective in improving swallowing, but have little effect on other symptoms [25]. A repeat injection is required in 6–24 months to maintain the acceptable level of efficacy. Injection of botulinum toxin into the body of esophagus, however, encompasses a higher risk (rupture of esophagus and infection inside the chest—mediastinitis) than injection into to the upper or lower esophageal sphincters [26].

Partial Paralysis of the Stomach—Gastroparesis

Both sympathetic and parasympathetic nervous systems provide innervation to the stomach. Normal function of these nerves which activate and relax smooth muscles of the stomach controls gastric emptying. Gastroparesis is defined by delayed gastric emptying in the absence of a mechanical obstruction. Gastroparesis is much more common in women than men with a prevalence of 38 and 9.6/100,000, respectively [27].

The symptoms of gastroparesis include nausea, vomiting, bloating, excessive fullness after eating, weight loss, abdominal pain and early satiety. Patients may ignore the mild early symptoms for a longtime before seeking medical care. The diagnosis of gastroparesis is made most efficiently by a 4-h gastric emptying scan.

In approximately half of the patients with gastroparesis, despite modern medical work up, the cause remains elusive. Common diseases associated with delayed gastric emptying are diabetes, Parkinson's disease, multiple sclerosis, surgical or accidental injury to the vagus nerve (a part of the parasympathetic nervous system) that contracts the stomach muscles and controls the function of pyloric sphincter—the circular muscle that controls opening of the stomach into the gut. Movements of the stomach and control of the pylorus are not under conscious control. Excess of certain medications also can cause delayed stomach emptying; most notable among these medications are high doses of narcotics and certain drugs that are used for treatment of Parkinson's disease (Dopamine agonists).

Treatment of delayed gastric emptying starts with dietary counseling and nutritional management. In advanced cases, feeding may have to be done via a tube that delivers food directly to the first part of the gut through a hole opened in the abdomen. The most effective medication for improvement of gastroparesis is a drug called metoclopramide (Reglan) that works on the dopamine system. Surgical treatment focuses on cutting the muscle fibers of the pylorus, electrical stimulation of the stomach or even, in severe cases, removal of the stomach. Many patients remain unsatisfied with the results of these medical and surgical treatments.

The first data on the use of Botox injections in gastroparesis was published in 2002 [28]. In this study, injection of 100 units of Botox into the pylorus (the sphincter between the stomach and the first part of the gut) in patients with gastroparesis secondary to diabetes improved the symptoms of 50% of the patients as well as showing improvement of the gastric emptying tests. Three other open label studies (without placebo arm and no blinding of the patient or physician to the type of injection) have reported similar positive results [29–31]. Some of these studies used a higher dose of 200 units of Botox. Younger patients, women and those patients with unknown cause for their gastroparesis responded better to Botox therapy. The response usually lasted 4–5 months. Unfortunately, these positive results were challenged by the results of two high quality studies that compared the effect of Botox injections with placebo. These studies demonstrated improvement of gastric emptying tests after Botox injection, but failed to show substantial improvement in the patients' symptoms [32, 33]. Furthermore, some investigators claim that stomach lining may harden after Botox injections, the long-term effects of which are not clear. Due to these issues and concerns, currently, Botox injection into the pylorus remains a debatable approach for treatment of gastroparesis.

Botulinum Toxin Therapy for Disorders of Anal Sphincter

Anismus

In this condition, external anal sphincter and the muscle attached to it (puborectalis muscle) that connects pubis to rectum, develop high tone and spasm interfering with defecation. In many cases of anismus, instead of relaxing at the initiation of defecation, anal sphincter and puborectalis (PR) muscle contract and make defecation painful and uncomfortable. Anismus can result from surgery of the ano-rectal area, hysterectomy, trauma to the region and even stress but, in many cases, the cause remains undetermined.

Treatment of anismus is difficult. Soft dietary regimen and improving stress is helpful in some patients. Special biofeedback sessions have been reported to help, but success is limited. In severe cases, surgery is recommended. Cutting some fibers of the sphincter and PR muscles reduces the tightness of these muscles and can provide relief in over 50% of the patients. Surgery, however, carries the risk of fecal incontinence and infection.

Application of botulinum toxin therapy for treatment of anismus was first studied by Dr. Hallan and his associates in 1988; they reported significant improvement of constipation in seven patients with anismus after botulinum toxin injection into anal sphincter [34]. In a review paper published in 2016, Emile and coworkers discussed the published data from seven papers in which authors studied the effect of Botox injection into the anal sphincter for improving anismus [35]. A total of 189 patients were included in these seven studies. The Botox dose varied from 20 to 100 units. Injections were carried out in multiple locations, mostly posterior and lateral into the sphincter. The average rate of success was 77% after the first injection. Approximately 45% of the patients were still satisfied 4 months after treatment. The incidence of side effects was 7.4% and included two patients with fecal incontinence (mild and transient) and one with rectal prolapse.

The side effects with Botox injections are, in general, lower than that of surgery, but treatment needs to be repeated in over half of the patients every 4–6 months. Injections are performed using a thin 27.5 or 30 gauge needle following application of local anaesthesia. The use of electromyography which shows the electrical activity of the muscle, or ultrasound which visualizes the muscle, adds to the procedure's accuracy. For Botox, most clinics use a total of 100 units, often divided between anal sphincter and the PR muscle.

Botulinum Toxin Therapy in Hirschsprung's Disease (HD)

Hirschprung's disease is a congenital condition that results from lack of migration of nerve cells (ganglionic cells) to the rectum (last part of alimentary tract) and to the anal sphincter. As a result, rectum and anal sphincters (internal and external) are devoid from nerve cells and, hence, cannot function normally. It affects approximately 2–2.8 individuals among 10,000 newborns [36]. The disease often presents in babies with inability to defecate leading to enlarged rectum and predisposition to a serious and life-threatening infection entrocollitis [37]. Affected children become febrile, suffer from abdominal pain, nausea and diarrhea, in addition to constipation. Boys are affected five times more than girls by HD.

Medical treatment of HD is difficult. Rectal irrigation and application of laxatives or topical nitric oxide offer some comfort. Some authors recommend to combine these measures with pelvic flood physiotherapy. Posterior myotomy of internal anal sphincter (cutting muscle fibers) improves the condition, but in many patients, obstructive symptoms recur. In 1997, Langer and Birbaum first reported that injection of Botox (15 units) into the anal sphincter of 4 children with HD and persistent symptoms after surgery, improved the symptoms significantly in 3 of 4 children [38]. Since then, several studies have replicated these results in a larger number of patients. The recommended total dose of Botox used for treatment of anal sphincter in HD differs among different injectors varying from 20 to 200 units. In an extensive review of this subject, the authors suggested a total dose of 100 units delivered into the posterior and lateral part of the tight anal sphincter to avoid damage to the urethra (the tube through which urine leaves the bladder) [39]. The total dose is delivered at 3–4 points. Botulinum toxin injections into anal sphincter is also reported to be associated with decreased incidence of entrocolitis in HD [40].

Botulinum toxin injections into anal sphincter has been effective in reducing or eliminating obstructive symptoms after sphincter surgery in HD [41]. In a recent review of 14 studies that reported results on 278 post-surgical patients, 66% of the patients with obstructive symptoms demonstrated significant improvement after botulinum toxin injection. Adverse effects (anal pain and mild incontinence) were seen in 17% of the patients, but were mild with short duration [42].

Anal Fissure

Anal fissure is a tear in the skin of the anal area usually related to increased pressure of the anal sphincter. The torn area leaves a small ulceration and causes significant pain and discomfort during bowel movement. Anal fissures can develop acutely or gradually. Once developed, the healing is difficult due to spasms of the anal sphincter which pulls apart the edges of the fissure exposing the area to inflammation/infection. Passage of hard stool, chronic diarrhea, prolonged vaginal delivery and anal sex are among common causes of anal fissure. Local pain, local bleeding, skin irritation and persistent itch are common complains of the affected patients.

First line of treatment of anal fissure is loosening the stool by using diets high in fiber and drinking lots of water. Taking Sitz baths several times daily helps local discomfort. Application of local analgesic creams such as lidocaine jelly (2%) and local creams that make blood vessels relax (vasodilators), nifedipine and diltiazem (calcium channel blockers) and nitroglycerin ointment are helpful in management of anal fissure. Persistent and unresponsive anal fissures will require surgery which includes cutting the fibers of anal sphincter in order to make it relax. The procedure is helpful but has a high incidence of fecal incontinence specially in elderly patients and women with multiple childbirths.

Botox injection into the anal sphincter, aiming to relax this sphincter and for management of anal fissure was first described by Drs. Jost and Schimrigk in 1993 [43]. Injection of a small amount of Botox (2.5 units) into the external anal sphincter improved the patient's symptoms and helped healing of the anal fissure. Subsequent studies recommended higher doses of 10–20 units. A high quality study (comparing the effect of Botox with placebo) has shown that patients who received Botox injections demonstrated 5 or more times improvement of the symptoms and healing of the anal fissure compared to placebo [44]. Another study of 100 patients with anal fissure demonstrated that patients who received Botox injections into the anal sphincter had significantly less incidence of fecal incontinence compared to surgical sphincterectomy- 7% versus 33% [45]. Botox injections need to be repeated every 4–6 months. A recent study compared the analgesic effect of local lidocaine application, anal dilation and Botox injection in three groups of patients with anal fissure (30 patients in each group). Botox injections were found superior to the other two modes of treatment in relieving local pain. Botox therapy for management of anal fissure (both pain and healing) is, therefore, effective and remains a good alternative for patients who do not want surgery or those who are at high risk for development of fecal incontinence after sphincter surgery [46]. A recent published survey by the Society of American Colon and Rectal Surgeons showed that 90% of 216 Society members who responded used Botox injection for healing and analgesic effect in anal fissure. Two thirds of the injectors injected into the inner rectal sphincter at 4 points, circling the sphincter [47].

Alimentary Problems Related to Tongue Dyskinesia (Involuntary Movements)

Involuntary movements of the tongue are seen most commonly following exposure to certain medications which interfere with the action of an organic chemical called dopamine. Dopamine is present in abundance in brain cells and contributes to the function of the motor system. Drugs that block the action of dopamine are now widely used in psychiatry for treatment of schizophrenia and mood disorders. Unfortunately, chronic exposure to these drugs may damage brain cells and cause involuntary movements (tardive dyskinesia). Sometimes, these movements are short-lived; sometimes, they can persist for a long time, even for life. Involuntary movements of the tongue are often associated with involuntary movements of the face and lips. Tongue movements are often multidirectional, side to side, rolling and sometimes protruding. Involuntary tongue movements are also seen sometimes in certain neurological disorders that involve the brain.

Treatment of tongue movements in tardive dyskinesias (often related to chronic use of neuroleptic drugs) is very difficult. In lucky patients, the movements are self-limiting and disappear within days or months after onset. For those with persistent tongue movements, a drug called tetrabenazine that works on the dopamine system offers partial relief.

Injection of botulinum toxins into the tongue can slow down the tongue movements and improve patients' alimentation as well as speech. Recent studies have shown that injection of the tongue in tardive dyskinesia by diminishing the tongue movement can significantly improve the patients' quality of life [48, 49]. The treatment, however, is risky and over dosing can lead to tongue paralysis for 2–3 months causing significant feeding problems. In experienced hands, however, most patients are happy since reduction of involuntary tongue movements improves alimentation and quality of life. The author of this chapter recommends using ½ inch or ¾ inch long needle (gauge 27.5 mm) through a lateral approach (one injection into each side of the tongue). If using Botox, a starting dose of 5 units on each side of the tongue is usually effective and pleases the patient (although the tongue movements may not totally cease). The dose may be increased to 7.5 units per each side of the tongue in subsequent injections (not in small tongues). The effect of Botox usually lasts 3–4 months. Tongue injection should be done only by experienced injectors after fully explaining to the patients the possible potentially serious side effects.

Conclusion

Hyperactivity of sphincter muscles can cause problems with passage of food through different parts of the alimentary system. Botulinum toxin injections, by reducing sphincter's muscle tone, can help proper passage of food and improve patient's alimentation. Botulinum toxin therapy is effective in management of anal fissure both alleviating pain and enhancing healing. In medical disorders that result in involuntary tongue movements, injection of botulinum toxin into the tongue can reduce movements and improve the patients' quality of life.

References

1. Safarpour Y, Jabbari B. Botulinum toxin treatment of movement disorders. Curr Treat Options Neurol. 2018 Feb 24;20(2):4. https://doi.org/10.1007/s11940-018-0488-3. PMID: 29478149.
2. Sivarao DV, Goyal RK. Functional anatomy and physiology of the upper esophageal sphincter. Am J Med. 2000 Mar 6;108(Suppl 4a):27S–37S. https://doi.org/10.1016/s0002-9343(99)00337-x. PMID: 10718448.
3. Schneider I, Thumfart WF, Pototschnig C, Eckel HE. Treatment of dysfunction of the cricopharyngeal muscle with botulinum A toxin: introduction of a new, noninvasive method. Ann Otol Rhinol Laryngol. 1994;103(1):31–5.
4. Sharzehi K, Schey R. The role of botulinum toxin in gastrointestinal tract. In: Jabbari B, editor. Botulinum toxin treatment in clinical medicine. Springer; 2018. p. 67–80.
5. Alfonsi E, Restivo DA, Cosentino G, De Icco R, Bertino G, Schindler A, Todisco M, Fresia M, Cortese A, Prunetti P, Ramusino MC, Moglia A, Sandrini G, Tassorelli C. Botulinum toxin is effective in the management of neurogenic dysphagia. Clinical-electrophysiological findings and tips on safety in different neurological disorders. Front Pharmacol. 2017 Feb 22;8:80. https://doi.org/10.3389/fphar.2017.00080. PMID: 28275351. PMCID: PMC5319993.
6. Zhu L, Chen J, Shao X, Pu X, Zheng J, Zhang J, Wu X, Wu D. Botulinum toxin A injection using ultrasound combined with balloon guidance for the treatment of cricopharyngeal dysphagia: analysis of 21 cases. Scand J Gastroenterol. 2022 Jul;57(7):884–90. https://doi.org/10.1080/00365521.2022.2041716. Epub 2022 Feb 25. PMID: 35213271.
7. Xie M, Zeng P, Wan G, An D, Tang Z, Li C, Wei X, Shi J, Zhang Y, Dou Z, Wen H. The effect of combined guidance of botulinum toxin injection with ultrasound, catheter balloon, and electromyography on neurogenic cricopharyngeal dysfunction: a prospective study. Dysphagia. 2022 Jun;37(3):601–11. https://doi.org/10.1007/s00455-021-10310-7. Epub 2021 Apr 29. PMID: 33928464.
8. Xie M, Dou Z, Wan G, Zeng P, Wen H. Design and implementation of botulinum toxin on cricopharyngeal dysfunction guided by a combination of catheter balloon, ultrasound, and electromyography (BECURE) in patients with stroke: study protocol for a randomized, double-blinded, placebo-controlled trial. Trials. 2021 Mar 31;22(1):238. https://doi.org/10.1186/s13063-021-05195-8. PMID: 33789722. PMCID: PMC8010959.
9. Farrukh A, DeCaestecker J, Mayberry JF. An epidemiological study of achalasia among the south Asian population of Leicester, 1986-2005. Dysphagia. 2008 Jun;23(2):161–4. https://doi.org/10.1007/s00455-007-9116-1. Epub 2007 Nov 20. PMID: 18027026.
10. Sadowski DC, Ackah F, Jiang B, Svenson LW. Achalasia: incidence, prevalence and survival. A population-based study. Neurogastroenterol Motil. 2010 Sep;22(9):e256–61. https://doi.org/10.1111/j.1365-2982.2010.01511.x. Epub 2010 May 11. PMID: 20465592.
11. Eckardt VF, Köhne U, Junginger T, Westermeier T. Risk factors for diagnostic delay in achalasia. Dig Dis Sci. 1997 Mar;42(3):580–5. https://doi.org/10.1023/a:1018855327960. PMID: 9073142.
12. Pasricha PJ, Ravich WJ, Hendrix TR, Sostre S, Jones B, Kalloo AN. Intrasphincteric botulinum toxin for the treatment of achalasia. N Engl J Med. 1995 Mar 23;332(12):774–8. https://doi.org/10.1056/NEJM199503233321203. Erratum in: N Engl J Med 1995 Jul 6;333(1):75. PMID: 7862180.
13. Yamaguchi D, Tsuruoka N, Sakata Y, Shimoda R, Fujimoto K, Iwakiri R. Safety and efficacy of botulinum toxin injection therapy for esophageal achalasia in Japan. J Clin Biochem

Nutr. 2015 Nov;57(3):239–43. https://doi.org/10.3164/jcbn.15-47. Epub 2015 Oct 17. PMID: 26566311; PMCID: PMC4639589.

14. Ribolsi M, Andrisani G, Di Matteo FM, Cicala M. Achalasia, from diagnosis to treatment. Expert Rev Gastroenterol Hepatol. 2023 Jan;17(1):21–30. https://doi.org/10.1080/1747412 4.2022.2163236. Epub 2023 Jan 1. PMID: 36588469.

15. Huai J, Hou Y, Guan J, Zhang Y, Wang Y, Zhang X, Zhang Y, Yue S. Botulinum toxin A injection using esophageal balloon radiography combined with CT guidance for the treatment of cricopharyngeal dysphagia. Dysphagia. 2020 Aug;35(4):630–5. https://doi.org/10.1007/s00455-019-10070-5. Epub 2019 Oct 16. PMID: 31620859.

16. Rolland S, Paterson W, Bechara R. Achalasia: current therapeutic options. Neurogastroenterol Motil. 2023 Jan;35(1):e14459. https://doi.org/10.1111/nmo.14459. Epub 2022 Sep 25. PMID: 36153803.

17. Brodsky JA, Marks JM, Malm JA, Bower A, Ponsky JL. Sphincter of Oddi injection with botulinum toxin is as effective as endobiliary stent in resolving cystic duct leaks in a canine model. Gastrointest Endosc. 2002 Dec;56(6):849–51. https://doi.org/10.1067/mge.2002.129869. PMID: 12447296.

18. Pasricha PJ, Miskovsky EP, Kalloo AN. Intrasphincteric injection of botulinum toxin for suspected sphincter of Oddi dysfunction. Gut. 1994 Sep;35(9):1319–21. https://doi.org/10.1136/gut.35.9.1319. PMID: 7959245. PMCID: PMC1375716.

19. Murray WR. Botulinum toxin-induced relaxation of the sphincter of Oddi may select patients with acalculous biliary pain who will benefit from cholecystectomy. Surg Endosc. 2011 Mar;25(3):813–6. https://doi.org/10.1007/s00464-010-1260-2. Epub 2010 Jul 28. PMID: 20665051.

20. Wang HJ, Tanaka M, Konomi H, Toma H, Yokohata K, Pasricha PJ, Kalloo AN. Effect of local injection of botulinum toxin on sphincter of Oddi cyclic motility in dogs. Dig Dis Sci. 1998 Apr;43(4):694–701. https://doi.org/10.1023/a:1018841325525. PMID: 9558021.

21. Hackert T, Klaiber U, Hinz U, Kehayova T, Probst P, Knebel P, Diener MK, Schneider L, Strobel O, Michalski CW, Ulrich A, Sauer P, Büchler MW. Sphincter of Oddi botulinum toxin injection to prevent pancreatic fistula after distal pancreatectomy. Surgery. 2017 May;161(5):1444–50. https://doi.org/10.1016/j.surg.2016.09.005. Epub 2016 Nov 16. PMID: 27865590.

22. Volk A, Distler M, Müssle B, Berning M, Hampe J, Brückner S, Weitz J, Welsch T. Reproducibility of preoperative endoscopic injection of botulinum toxin into the sphincter of Oddi to prevent postoperative pancreatic fistula. Innov Surg Sci. 2018 Jan 18;3(1):69–75. https://doi.org/10.1515/iss-2017-0040. PMID: 31579768; PMCID: PMC6754046.

23. Amarasinghe G, Sifrim D. Functional esophageal disorders: pharmacological options. Drugs. 2014 Aug;74(12):1335–44. https://doi.org/10.1007/s40265-014-0272-y. PMID: 25103415.

24. Sharzehi and schey. The role of botulinum toxin in gastrointestinal tract. In: Jabbari B, editor. Botulinum toxin treatment in clinical medicine. Springer; 2018.

25. Vanuytsel T, Bisschops R, Farré R, Pauwels A, Holvoet L, Arts J, Caenepeel P, De Wulf D, Mimidis K, Rommel N, Tack J. Botulinum toxin reduces Dysphagia in patients with nonachalasia primary esophageal motility disorders. Clin Gastroenterol Hepatol. 2013 Sep;11(9):1115–21.e2. https://doi.org/10.1016/j.cgh.2013.03.021. Epub 2013 Apr 13. PMID: 23591282.

26. van Hoeij FB, Tack JF, Pandolfino JE, Sternbach JM, Roman S, Smout AJ, Bredenoord AJ. Complications of botulinum toxin injections for treatment of esophageal motility disorders†. Dis Esophagus. 2017 Feb 1;30(3):1–5. https://doi.org/10.1111/dote.12491. PMID: 27337985.

27. Jung HK, Choung RS, Locke GR, et al. The incidence, prevalence, and outcomes of patients with gastroparesis in Olmsted County, Minnesota, from 1996 to 2006. Gastroenterology. 2009;136(4):1225–33.

28. Ezzeddine D, Jit R, Katz N, Gopalswamy N, Bhutani MS. Pyloric injection of botulinum toxin for treatment of diabetic gastroparesis. Gastrointest Endosc. 2002;55(7):920–3.

29. Bromer MQ, Friedenberg F, Miller LS, Fisher RS, Swartz K, Parkman HP. Endoscopic pyloric injection of botulinum toxin A for the treatment of refractory gastroparesis. Gastrointest Endosc. 2005 Jun;61(7):833–9. https://doi.org/10.1016/s0016-5107(05)00328-7. PMID: 15933684.
30. Lacy BE, Zayat EN, Crowell MD, Schuster MM. Botulinum toxin for the treatment of gastroparesis: a preliminary report. Am J Gastroenterol. 2002 Jun;97(6):1548–52. https://doi.org/10.1111/j.1572-0241.2002.05741.x. PMID: 12094882.
31. Reichenbach ZW, Stanek S, Patel S, Ward SJ, Malik Z, Parkman HP, Schey R. Botulinum toxin A improves symptoms of gastroparesis. Dig Dis Sci. 2020 May;65(5):1396–404. https://doi.org/10.1007/s10620-019-05885-z. Epub 2019 Oct 15. PMID: 31617132.
32. Friedenberg FK, Palit A, Parkman HP, Hanlon A, Nelson DB. Botulinum toxin A for the treatment of delayed gastric emptying. Am J Gastroenterol. 2008 Feb;103(2):416–23. https://doi.org/10.1111/j.1572-0241.2007.01676.x. Epub 2007 Dec 5. PMID: 18070232.
33. Arts J, Holvoet L, Caenepeel P, Bisschops R, Sifrim D, Verbeke K, Janssens J, Tack J. Clinical trial: a randomized-controlled crossover study of intrapyloric injection of botulinum toxin in gastroparesis. Aliment Pharmacol Ther. 2007 Nov 1;26(9):1251–8. https://doi.org/10.1111/j.1365-2036.2007.03467.x. PMID: 17944739.
34. Hallan RI, Williams NS, Melling J, et al. Treatment of anismus in intractable constipation with botulinum a toxin. Lancet. 1988;2(8613):714–7.
35. Emile SH, Elfeki HA, Elbanna HG. Efficacy and safety of botulinum toxin in treatment of anismus: a systematic review. World J Gastrointest Pharmacol Ther. 2016;7(3):453–62. https://doi.org/10.4292/wjgpt.v7.i3.453.
36. Tang CS, Karim A, Zhong Y, Chung PH, Tam PK. Genetics of Hirschsprung's disease. Pediatr Surg Int. 2023 Feb 7;39(1):104. https://doi.org/10.1007/s00383-022-05358-x. PMID: 36749416.
37. Teitelbaum DH, Coran AG. Enterocolitis. Semin Pediatr Surg. 1998 Aug;7(3):162–9. https://doi.org/10.1016/s1055-8586(98)70012-5. PMID: 9718654.
38. Langer JC, Birnbaum E. Preliminary experience with intrasphincteric botulinum toxin for persistent constipation after pull-through for Hirschsprung's disease. J Pediatr Surg. 1997 Jul;32(7):1059–61; discussion 1061–2. https://doi.org/10.1016/s0022-3468(97)90399-7. PMID: 9247234.
39. Bokova E, Svetanoff WJ, Rosen JM, Levitt MA, Rentea RM. State of the art bowel management for pediatric colorectal problems: functional constipation. Children (Basel). 2023 Jun 19;10(6):1078. https://doi.org/10.3390/children10061078. PMID: 37371309. PMCID: PMC10296980.
40. Svetanoff WJ, Briggs K, Fraser JA, Lopez J, Fraser JD, Juang D, Aguayo P, Hendrickson RJ, Snyder CL, Oyetunji TA, St Peter SD, Rentea RM. Outpatient botulinum injections for early obstructive symptoms in patients with hirschsprung disease. J Surg Res 2022. Jan;269:201–6. https://doi.org/10.1016/j.jss.2021.07.017. Epub 2021 Sep 26. PMID: 34587522.
41. Chumpitazi BP, Fishman SJ, Nurko S. Long-term clinical outcome after botulinum toxin injection in children with nonrelaxing internal anal sphincter. Am J Gastroenterol. 2009 Apr;104(4):976–83. https://doi.org/10.1038/ajg.2008.110. Epub 2009 Mar 3. PMID: 19259081.
42. Roorda D, Oosterlaan J, van Heurn E, Derikx J. Intrasphincteric botulinum toxin injections for post-operative obstructive defecation problems in Hirschsprung disease: a retrospective observational study. J Pediatr Surg. 2021 Aug;56(8):1342–8. https://doi.org/10.1016/j.jpedsurg.2020.11.025. Epub 2020 Nov 27. PMID: 33288128.
43. Jost WH, Schimrigk K. Use of botulinum toxin in anal fissure. Dis Colon Rectum. 1993;36(10):974.
44. Maria G, Cassetta E, Gui D, et al. A comparison of botulinum toxin and saline for the treatment of chronic anal fissure. N Engl J Med. 1998;338(4):217–20.
45. Jost WH. One hundred cases of anal fissure treated with botulin toxin: early and long-term results. Dis Colon Rectum. 1997;40(9):1029–32.

46. Andreevski V, Volkanovska A, Deriban G, Josifovic FL, Krstevski G, Nikolova D, Dimitrova MG, Stardelova KG, Serafimovski V. The value of injection therapy with botulinum toxin in pain treatment of primary chronic anal fissures compared to anal dilation, and local nifedipine in combination with lidocaine. Pril (Makedon Akad Nauk Umet Odd Med Nauki). 2023 Jul 15;44(2):89–97. https://doi.org/10.2478/prilozi-2023-0029. PMID: 37453106.

47. Borsuk DJ, Studniarek A, Park JJ, Marecik SJ, Mellgren A, Kochar K. Use of botulinum toxin injections for the treatment of chronic anal fissure: results from an American Society of Colon and Rectal Surgeons Survey. Am Surg. 2023 Mar;89(3):346–54. https://doi.org/10.1177/00031348211023446. Epub 2021 Jun 7. PMID: 34092078.

48. Nastasi L, Mostile G, Nicoletti A, et al. Effect of botulinum toxin treatment on quality of life in patients with isolated lingual dystonia and oromandibular dystonia affecting the tongue. J Neurol. 2016;263:1702–8.

49. Slotema CW, van Harten PN, Bruggeman R, Hoek HW. Botulinum toxin in the treatment of orofacial tardive dyskinesia: a single blind study. Prog Neuro-Psychopharmacol Biol Psychiatry. 2008 Feb 15;32(2):507–9. https://doi.org/10.1016/j.pnpbp.2007.10.004. Epub 2007 Oct 13. PMID: 18022743.

Chapter 12
The Role of Botulinum Toxin Therapy in Joint and Bone Problems

Abstract Animal studies have shown that local injection of botulinum toxins improves pain behavior via blocking the release of pain transmitters and modulators. In human, carefully designed studies comparing the effect of local injection of botulinum toxins with placebo (salt water) have demonstrated efficacy of toxin injection in relieving the pain of chronic osteoarthritis, local pain of tennis elbow, chronic pain after knee surgery and knee pain related to tightness of lateral thigh muscles.

Keywords Botulinum toxin · Botulinum neurotoxin · Tennis elbow · Lateral epicondylitis osteoarthritis · Pain after knee surgery · Patellofemoral syndrome

Introduction

Botulinum neurotoxin (BoNT) is produced by a bacteria present in nature. It causes serious illness when it enters the human body in large amounts through contaminated food. When used as a medicine, the toxin is quantified in units, each unit reflecting certain degree and percentage of mortality among exposed mice. The contaminated food that causes illness in human usually contains hundreds of thousands or even millions of toxin units, whereas the amount used for medical treatment (through injection) is in most cases below 400 units.

The molecular structure of the botulinum toxin, history of its development as a therapeutic agent in medicine, and the different kinds of botulinum toxin are described in detail in the first three chapters of this book. In brief, of the 9 subtypes of the toxin, only types A and B are currently used in medicine due to their long duration of action. Five type A toxin are FDA approved under the trade names of Botox, Xeomin, Dysport, Jeuveau and Dyxxify whereas only one type B toxin—Myobloc—is FDA approved. Jeuveau is currently approved only for cosmetic use. The toxin units for different toxin types are not exactly comparable. However, in research and in medical practice, the following approximations are often used: Each

B. Jabbari, *Botulinum Toxin Treatment*,
https://doi.org/10.1007/978-3-031-54471-2_12

1unit of Botox = 1 unit of Xeomin = 2.5–3 units of Dysport = 40–50 units of Myobloc.

For medical use, botulinum toxin is only used via injection either into the muscle or into/under the skin. Details of different botulinum toxin preparations, their need for refrigeration and their unit differences are discussed in Chap. 3 of this book. After injection, the carefully prepared and titrated toxin reaches the nerve ending and the region of nerve -muscle junction. It is at this junction that after entering the nerve ending the active moiety of the toxin—its light chain (see Chap. 2 for botulinum toxin structure)—prevents release of certain chemicals which are essential for transmission of the nerve signal to the muscle and for muscle activation. In the sensory system, botulinum toxin molecule blocks the function of sensory transmitters that relay the pain sensation to the brain. It is this effect over the pain transmitters that is of great interest in many medical disorders—inclusive of joint and bone disorders—in which the patients are afflicted by pain.

In his chapter, we will discuss the effect of botulinum toxin therapy on pain associated with chronic osteoarthritis, tennis elbow, pain after total knee replacement and joint pain caused by imbalance of attached muscles.

Pain of Chronic Arthritis (Osteoarthritis)

The word arthritis describes inflammation of body joints. Each joint consist of two bones and a fluid filled space (synovia) in between the two; cartilage (hard and slick tissue), over the bone surfaces, along with a joint capsule (synovial membrane). There are also ligaments, narrow bands of fibrous tissue that connect the bones together (Fig. 12.1). Except for the cartilages, all structures of the joint including the

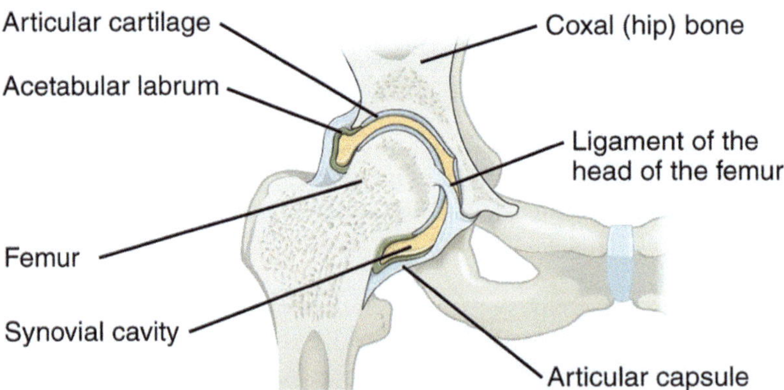

Fig. 12.1 Anatomy of hip joint—A thick synovial fluid is between the head of the long bone of the thigh (femur) and the adjacent pelvic bone, to facilitate movements of the hip joint. (Courtesy of WikiMSK. Permission to reuse is granted under Creative Commons Attribution-ShareAlike (CC-BY-SA-4.0) license)

bones are richly supplied by sensory nerves that sense pain. In addition, in chronic conditions, a cascade of events leads to a phenomenon called sensitization in which many structures that have low pain threshold become sensitive to pain and induce pain. Peripheral sensitization (PS) is a complicated phenomenon, the details of which are beyond the scope of this chapter. In brief, changes in several chemicals known as pain transmitters and modulators enhance the sensitivity of peripheral nerve endings to pain signals. Continued PS leads to central sensitization (CS) of spinal cord nerve cells leading to pain chronicity.

Osteoarthritis (inflammation of bone and joint) is the most common cause of pain among all pains involving the musculoskeletal (muscle and bone) system, affecting approximately 250 million people worldwide [1]. During life, 10–12% of all adults, experience osteoarthritic pain [2]. In the US, the number of patients with osteoarthritic pain is growing due to the aging population and effects of obesity. Osteoarthritis is among the leading causes of disability in elderly individuals [1]. The conditions that can be confused with osteoarthritis include trauma to the joint, pain due to ailment of muscles close to the joint and fibromyalgia, a diffuse painful muscle ailment associated with fatigue and sleep disorder.

Among body joints, the joints that are weight bearing, such as hip and knee joints are most often affected by osteoarthritis. Over time and with age, the bones around the joint grow small bone spurs which irritate the nerves and the soft tissues around them. Gradually, local inflammation develops. Inflammation may affect the synovial membrane (Fig. 12.1) and gradually lead to accumulation of fluid in the joint (effusion). The involved joint becomes swollen and painful with pain getting worse during joint activity. In some patients, genetic predisposition attributes to the development of osteoarthritis.

The second most common form of arthritis is rheumatoid arthritis. Rheumatoid arthritis can be seen in many young individuals. Rheumatoid arthritis is a disease of the body's immune system leading to inflammation of the joint capsule with subsequent destruction of cartilage and bone (Fig. 12.2).

Symptoms and signs of osteoarthritis include focal joint pain, joint stiffness, redness, joint swelling and limitation of joint movements. These symptoms increase with age and often lead to disability. Tests that are used for visualizing the joints are useful in showing the extent of bone and cartilage damage. Among these tests, MRI is most accurate since it provides detailed definition of the bone and soft tissues.

Conventional treatment of arthritis includes multiple strategies. The results of these treatment strategies are usually modest and, in most patients, the level of pain relief is not satisfactory [1]. Medical treatment is often combined with physical therapy that includes exercises designed to improve the range of motion along with strengthening of the joints. Heat pads and ice packs may help to alleviate pain. In obese individuals, loss of weight is recommended. Massage of the affected joint, acupuncture and Yoga can also provide various degrees of pain relief.

Mild cases of osteoarthritis are treated by commonly used pain killers such as aspirin or Tylenol. The drugs that specifically target inflammation but are not in the steroid category such as motrin and advil are also frequently used for treatment of osteoarthritis. More severe cases require steroid therapy [3]. Steroids can be taken

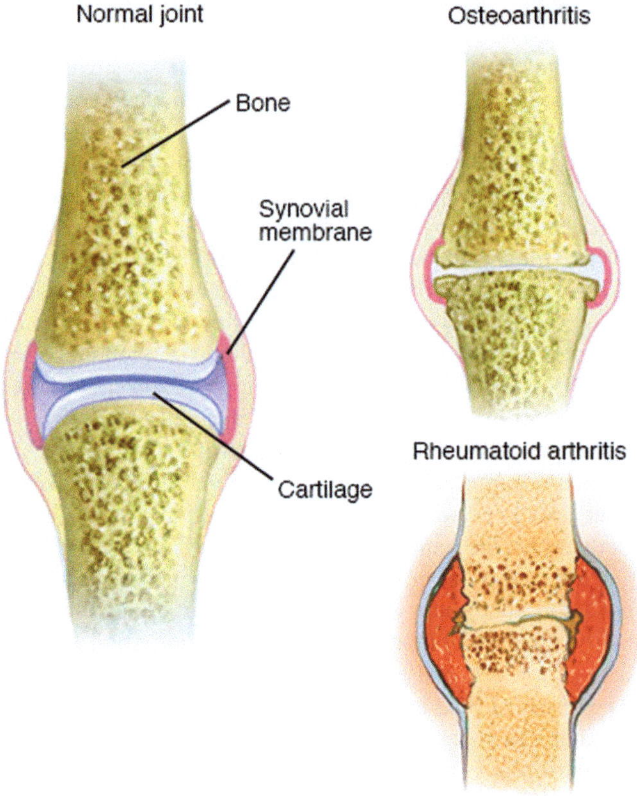

Fig. 12.2 Normal joint and joints affected by osteoarthritis and rheumatoid arthritis. (Courtesy of Mayo foundation)

orally (prednisone) or injected directly into the joint. Their chronic use, however, may damage the cartilage and enhance progression of osteoarthritis. Injection of hyaluronic acid into the joint has been shown to be helpful in some patients. This material which has a viscosity similar to synovia (joint fluid) coats the bone surfaces and may prevent further bone damage.

For the past few years, several new material have been tried for treatment of osteoarthritis including cytokine inhibitors, platelet-enriched plasma, aspirates from bone marrow, insertion of fatty material inside the joint (adipose tissue) or so called expanded mesenchymal stromal cells (MSC); none have been found to have clinically relevant long-term effects [4].

Surgery includes joint fusion, repair and replacement. Joint fusion is used for smaller joints such as those of fingers and wrists. During the procedure, the surgeon cuts across the bone above and below the joint, removes part of the bone and insert new bone in order to shift the weight away from the damaged part of the joint. For worn out joints, joint surfaces are replaced by metal or plastic parts.

Botulinum Toxin Therapy in Osteoarthritis (OA)

The modest effect of medical therapy in osteoarthritis, and reluctance of many patients with OA to have surgery, encouraged investigators to explore the efficacy of botulinum toxin injections for alleviation of pain in OA. As was discussed earlier, animal studies have shown that injection of BoNTs into muscle or skin inhibits release of pain transmitters from nerve endings and alleviates pain [5–7].

Following the observation that Botox injected into dog's arthritic joints relieves joint pain [8], researchers began to study its effect on human joints affected by osteoarthritis. In 2006, Dr. Mahowald and his colleagues first reported that injection of Botox into the shoulder (100 units) or limb joints (25–50 units) can alleviate pain of arthritis in humans [9]. Another study, published in 2010, compared the effect of Botox versus placebo and found Botox to be superior to placebo (saline injection) in 60 patients with knee osteoarthritis [10]. In a recent, high quality, larger study authors compared the effects of Botox with placebo (salt water) injection into the knee joints of 121 patients with OA. The study was blinded meaning neither the injecting doctor nor the patient knew what was injected (Botox or placebo). Half of the patients received Botox. The effect of injections was assessed by another doctor not involved in preparing the Botox or performing the injections. Standard scales for evaluation of joint pain, patients 'quality of life and patients' degree of disability were used to assess the efficacy of the treatment over months of follow up after injections. The researchers found that Botox injection was statistically superior to placebo in regard to pain relief, improvement of quality of life and patient disability [11]. Botox and placebo groups had the same number of side effects which were all minor and self-limiting. The finding of this study are in agreement with the results of a recent review on the safety of BoNT injections in OA. This review [12] found no patient in any of studies on BoNT therapy for OA with any significant side effects after joint injections. Subsequently, several other studies also showed that injection of different type A botulinum toxins, Botox or Dysport into the knee joint of patients with OA can relieve joint pain [13–15].

These positive results were contradicted by a more recent study (blinded and placebo-controlled) of 158 patients that found both botulinum toxin and placebo (salt water-saline) injections into the knee joints of patients with knee arthritis produced the same degree of pain improvement [16]. There are, however, two issues with this study: 1- the pain scale used in this study was not validated for use in knee osteoarthritis, 2- most patients in the placebo arm of the study improved with the injection of salt water. Whenever the placebo has the exact effect as the study's drug, the studied population is suspect to be unusually sensitive to placebo effect invalidating the observation.

Over the past 10 years, several comparative studies have compared the effect of intra-articular (IA) injection of botulinum toxins with other agents that are commonly used for relieving the symptoms (mostly pain) of osteoarthritis. In a study of 30 patients with advanced osteoarthritis of the knee, investigators found that combined injection of Botox with triamcinolone(a potent steroid) was significantly superior in pain relief compared to triamcinolone alone over 6 weeks to 6 month post-injection period [17]. In another study [18], IA injection of botulinum toxin plus exercise was found to be superior to IA injection of hyaluronate, a compound that is frequently used for achieving symptom relief in knee OA. Yet in another study, IA injection of a triamcinolone was compared with IA injection of 100 units of Botox in patients with knee OA [19]. Both injections were equally effective on pain at 12 weeks, but authors found injection of the steroid offered more pain relief at 4 weeks. In this study, the injected dose of Botox however, was 100 units, less than 200–300 units used in most studies of knee arthritis. Moreover, chronic and repeated steroid injections may lead to cartilage degeneration, bone damage or unwanted metabolic changes, not seen with IA injection of botulinum toxins. Most recently, an extensive review of this subject including 7 studies and 548 patients with application of advanced statistical methods (meta-analysis) concluded that IA injection of botulinum toxins is effective in relieving pain of knee osteoarthritis [20]. The authors encouraged the need for conduction of more high quality (double-blind, placebo-controlled) studies.

Much less research has been done on the role of IA injection of botulinum toxin for relieving distressing symptoms of OA in other joints (shoulder, hip, ankle). One study, cited earlier in this chapter, reported improvement of pain and function after IA injection of Botox in 9 shoulder joints [9]. A recent systematic review of IA injections for ankle osteoarthritis concluded that the limited data on the currently studied compounds (botulinum toxin, hyaluronate, plasma-rich protein) do not support evidence for a clinically relevant improvement of symptoms [21]. On hip osteoarthritis, preliminary data from two open label (not placebo- controlled) studies suggest improvement of pain after injection of 400 units of Dysport [22] into the hip joint or into the adductor muscles of the thigh (large muscles that bring the hips together) [23]. Dysport is another botulinum toxin type A; each 2.5–3 units of Dysport approximates 1 unit of Botox. For defining the role of botulinum toxins in hip osteoarthritis, data from blinded and placebo-controlled studies are needed.

Tennis Elbow (Lateral Epicondylitis- LE)

Rungue, in 1873, coined the term "tennis elbow" for a pain disorder which involves the elbow and causes an ailment in tennis players. It is believed that players with a strong back hand repeatedly traumatize the tendon of one of the extensor muscles of the wrist (short extensor/ extensor brevis) which is attached to the lowest part of the long bone of the arm called lateral epicondyle (Fig. 12.3). As a result of repeated trauma, multiple small tears develop in the tendon (where muscle attaches to the bone) causing pain at the elbow region. Pathological evaluation of the involved tendon often shows presence of mild inflammation.

Subsequent observations revealed that this form of muscle and bone injury is not limited to tennis players and a wide range of trauma to this region can cause it such as weight lifting or certain jobs that require repetitive pulling and bending of the

Lateral Epicondylitis (Tennis Elbow)

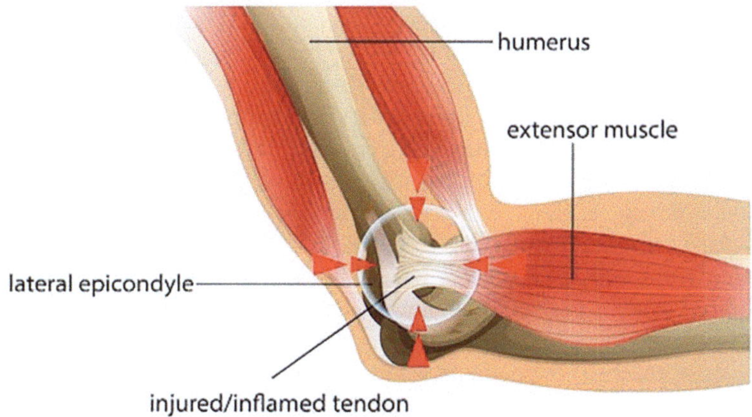

Fig. 12.3 Tennis elbow is caused by tears in the extensor wrist muscles close to lateral epicondyle of the elbow. (Figure designed by Free Pik)

elbow can cause the same problem. It is believed that laborers lifting weights in excess of 20 kg, more than 10 times per day can develop tear (s) in the tendon leading to LE [24]. Currently, the term lateral epicondylitis (LE) which means inflammation of lateral epicondyle (Fig. 12.3) is used more frequently instead of tennis elbow since the damaged muscle close to lateral epicondyle often manifests some degree of inflammation (accumulation of reactive blood cells in the issue). However, this term has also been challenged since inflammatory finding are subtle and may not explain the severity of symptoms (pain and limitation of elbow function). More recently, the term lateral epicondylosis (disease or dysfunction of lateral epicondyle) is preferred by some investigators [24].

Lateral epicondylitis (epicondylosis) affects 1–3% of general population over their life time. Men and women are equally affected with the age of onset being between 35 and 55 years. Most patients gradually recover from this condition over 6–24 months. In 5–10% of the patients, however, the condition continues and becomes the cause of chronic elbow and forearm pain [25]. Affected patients feel the pain in the area of the elbow with radiation to the forearm. In some patients with chronic pain, examination shows some limitation of wrist and finger movements. In chronic cases, X-ray examination of the elbow shows local deposits of calcium in 25% of the patients. The MRI usually shows no significant bone or soft tissue pathology. For most patients, surgery is not necessary unless a serious pathology is suspected (tumor, infection, etc.).

Several medical and non-medical approaches have been tried for management of the pain in chronic LE. These include exercise therapy, physiotherapy, taping the elbow, bracing, laser therapy, applying braces, acupuncture, and ultrasound therapy. Platelet-rich plasma injections is an expensive approach in which the patients' own blood is centrifuged and the buffer zone on the top (rich in platelets- blood cells which help to stop bleeding) is injected in the area of pain. The results of these strategies in chronic LE are at best, modest, and consist of temporary pain relief. Furthermore, the lack of high quality studies makes it hard to discern the utility of these approaches. Local patches of glyceryl trinitrate have helped to relieve pain in patients with LE according to high quality studies (using placebo as control), but the results are temporary [26]. Among non-steroidal analgesics, diclofenac was shown to improve pain of LE better than naproxen [24]. Injection of hyaluronic acid into the joint, in a manner similar to that used in OA, has been reported to reduce the elbow pain in patients affected by LE [27], but the effect is also short lived [28]. In severe cases, injection of steroids (triamcinolone) into the joint for pain relief has been used with temporary success in LE, but it has a high incidence of relapse. Furthermore, repeated injection of steroids can cause unwanted bone degeneration and metabolic abnormalities.

Surgery is reserved for patients who have failed medical treatment and is performed in less than 10% of the patients [29]. Three different surgical approaches are employed to alleviate the symptoms of LE. These include open surgery, percutaneous surgery and arthroscopic surgery. In arthroscopic surgery debridement of the damaged tendon is performed via an instrument (arthroscope) without widely opening the area. Follow up studies of large number of patients have shown comparable results for all three surgical approaches in management of LE [30, 31]. Cohen and co-workers have found, however, that the time to return to work was twice longer in patients that underwent open surgery compared to those who had arthroscopic surgery (mean 66 days versus 35 days) [29].

Botulinum Toxin Treatment of Tennis Elbow (LE)

Recognition of the pain killer potential of local botulinum toxin injection (now approved by FDA for treatment of migraine) encouraged investigators to study this mode of treatment for pain relief in LE. Over the past 20 years, several studies have been published on the efficacy of botulinum toxin injections in alleviating LE symptoms. Among them, five could be classified as high quality since they blindly compared the effect of the botulinum toxin injection with placebo (salt water injection) in LE. One of these studies used Botox [32], whereas the other four used Dysport [33–36]. As indicated earlier, Dysport is a type A botulinum toxin similar to Botox (see Chap. 3 for details). Injections were performed either close to the painful epicondyle or a few centimeters lower into the short wrist extensor muscle that is attached to the lateral epicondyle (Fig. 12.3). The Botox study used a total of 60 units, whereas in the four Dysport studies, the authors used 50–60 units, roughly equivalent to 20–25 units of Botox. Each patient received 2–3 injections either close to the elbow or a down the forearm over the short extensor tendon. Among the five studies that compared the effect of Dysport or Botox with placebo, four have shown that BoNT therapy is clearly superior to placebo in reducing pain and improving the quality of life in patients with LE. The one study that did not show improvement of

LE after botulinum toxin injection [34] assessed the pain only once, 3 months after injection. This may explain the negative result of the study since by 3 months, most of the effect of botulinum toxins is usually vanished (4 and 8 weeks assessment are much more accurate).

The optimum location of the injection (at the area of epicondyle or down the forearm into the short extensor muscle) and the optimum dose of the toxin (low dose versus high dose) have been studied, recently. In one review of the literature [37], researchers have found that toxin's injection into the wrist extensor muscle at a point(s) 1/3 of the length of forearm down from the involved epicondyle was more effective than injection at or close to involved epicondyle. In another study, both low dose (10 units) and high dose (50 units) of Medytoxin (Korean toxin with units close to Botox) were effective, but the higher dose of 50 units better alleviated the patients' symptoms (pain and limitation of arm movement) [38].

Several investigators compared the effect of Botulinum toxin injection in LE with other commonly used injectable substances (steroids, hyaluronic acid, etc.). These studies showed that the two most effective treatments were injection of botulinum toxin type A (Botox or Dysport) or steroids (triamcinolone) [39–41]. Steroid and botulinum toxin therapy had comparable efficacy in alleviating the symptoms of LE, though in one review steroids were found to have better analgesic effect over the initial 4 weeks after injection [41]. Botulinum toxin injection is probably less painful than steroid therapy since it is performed with a thin and short needle. Furthermore, repeated injection of botulinum toxin has less side effects than steroid therapy (see steroid side effects described earlier in this chapter). Weakness of middle finger extension is a common side effect of botulinum toxin therapy in LE (30–40%) which may last for several weeks. Future studies using smaller doses and more refined methods of botulinum toxin injection may overcome this side effect.

Pain After Total Knee Replacement (Arthroplasty)

Advanced osteoarthritis of the knee which is associated with degeneration and destruction of the knee joint limits the patients' activity and may progress to total immobility. Total knee replacement—total knee arthroplasty (TKA)—is a common procedure for retaining the knee function. In 2010, the number of total knee replacements in the US was 719,000 [42]. It is estimated that over half of all patients with chronic knee osteoarthritis will undergo TKA. Modern knee replacement techniques using the latest and most advanced hardware's have been very successful in improving both the range of knee movements and patients' ambulation. Surgery is usually done under general anesthesia; an alternative is spinal anesthesia which numbs the body below the waist. With spinal anesthesia, the patient has the option to remain conscious during the operation.

Unfortunately, 10–34% of the patients develop chronic knee pain after TKA that greatly impairs their quality of life. The pain can be a newly developed pain or an enhancement of the pain that the patient experienced before surgery [43]. A number of factors have been associated with development or exaggeration of knee pain after total knee surgery; these factors include having a high level of pain before surgery, presence of other painful muscle or joint disorders and poor mental condition of the patient [44].

Management of sustained pain after total knee arthroplasty consists of physical therapy, stretch exercises and use of pain killers including opioids. Steroid injection into the soft tissue and around the painful knee joint has been reported to relieve pain in some patients. However, studies of medical therapy for pain after TKA are open label (with no placebo for comparison) and, hence, the results are colored by a moderate to high degree of bias.

Botulinum Toxin Therapy for Pain Following Total Knee Replacement

In 2010, Dr. Singh and his colleagues published the results of a high quality study on 49 patients among whom, 60 knees had total arthroplasty [45]. Thirty legs received 100 units of Botox, diluted in 5 ccs of saline injected into the knee joint, whereas the other 30 legs received 5 cc of saline (salt water, placebo) only. The patients' mean age was 67 years. Patients' response was evaluated by several outcome measures among them scales designed specifically to assess pain. A WOMAC scale (western Ontario and McMaster Universities osteoarthritis index) was also used to assess functionality, joint stiffness and pain. Patients were followed for 6 months after a single set of injections.

At 2 months, the WOMAC osteoarthritis scale showed significant improvement of all three of its subsets (pain, functionality and stiffness) in patients who received Botox injections, but not in the placebo group. There was also a marked difference between the Botox group and the saline group in regard to response to pain in the pain specific scales. A notable pain relief was noted in 71% of the patients who had received Botox injections versus 35% in the placebo group—a finding that was statistically significant. Side effects were minor, consisting of transient local pain after injection and occurred with comparable frequency between the two groups (Botox and placebo).

A sizeable number of patients after TKA surgery gradually develop progressive increased tone in the muscles that flex the knee (hamstring muscle—the large muscle located in the back of the thigh) leading to forced flexion of the knee and difficulty in walking. Progressive stiffness of this muscle can lead to loss of elasticity with replacement of some of the muscle fibers by non-elastic fibrous tissue, referred to as contracture. Injection of botulinum toxin A into the flexor muscles of the knee (hamstrings) decreases the muscle tone and prevents severe and disabling contractures (stiff muscle, lost volume and elasticity) [46, 47]. In a high quality study (double-blind, placebo-controlled), patients who received 50 units of Botox into each hamstring muscle demonstrated significant improvement of flexion contracture along with 18° improvement in knee extension [47].

Chronic Knee Pain Due to Imbalance of Vastus Muscles (Patellofemoral Syndrome-PFS)

A common cause of chronic knee pain is poor balance between the activity of lateral and medial muscles of the thigh (vastus muscles). Vastus muscles along with the rectus muscles (located in front of the thigh) extend the knee.

Overactivity of the lateral vastus muscle (vastus lateralis-VL) or/and delayed activity of medial vastus muscle (VM) leads to misalignment of the patella (knee cap bone) and causes chronic pain in front of the knee. The knee cap gradually shifts laterally and tilts. The pain is felt in the front of the patella and is provoked by ascending or descending stairs, kneeling, squatting and prolonged sitting [48, 49]. Patellofemoral syndrome (PFS) has an incidence of 9.2% [49] and is twice more common among women especially, especially young women and those engaging in sports (running, tennis, etc.).

Imaging of the knee joint by ultrasound or MRI may show displacement of the patella. The goal of treatment is to reduce pain and swelling, improve the balance between vastus medialis and vastus lateralis muscles, restore normal gait, and improve postural control of the lower extremity. Treatment is difficult. Short -term taping/bracing of the patella associated with special exercises to strengthen the thigh muscles provides partial pain relief. Many patients rely on commonly used pain killers with modest degrees of success. Surgery is usually not indicated. High quality studies are not available to compare different methods of treatment in PFS syndrome.

Botulinum Toxin Treatment of Pain Associated with PFS

In 2011, Dr. Singer and his colleagues reported on the results of a study that compared injection of Dysport (a botulinum toxin type, A) with placebo (salt water) in 24 patients with vastus lateralis (VL) imbalance (PFS) [50]. Vastus lateralis is a large muscle located on the lateral part of the thigh that extended lower leg below the knee. The toxin injected group received 500 units of Dysport (roughly equal to 200 units of Botox) at 8 points into the VL muscle (Fig. 12.4). The same injection method was used for the saline (placebo) group. The pain and leg function was evaluated through standard scales, blindly, at 3 months. Patients who received Dysport injections showed significant improvement in walking, stair climbing and squatting, whereas those who received placebo did not. Furthermore, there was a marked reduction of knee pain on the visual analogue scale (VAS), a scale that measures pain at 0–10 levels, reported by the patient. There was no significant side effects after Dysport injections.

This observation was supported by subsequent open label (not blinded) studies [51, 52]. In the most recently published study on this subject [52], Pal and co-workers investigated the effect of botulinum toxin injection in both vastus lateralis

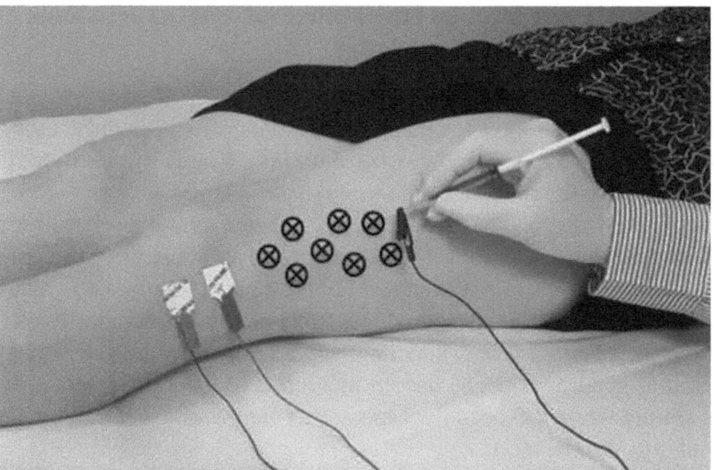

Fig. 12.4 Method of botulinum toxin injection used by Singer and co-workers for treatment of vastus lateralis imbalance. From Singer et al. [50]. The injecting syringe is connected to an EMG needle that identifies the muscle via the sound of its electrical activity. A total dose of 500 units of Dysport is injected into eight sites (marked by Xs) into the vastus lateralis muscle. Courtesy of BMJ Publishing group. Licensed under. (http://creativecommons.org/licenses/by/4.0/)

muscles in 13 patients with PFS. Patients' main complaint was pain in the area of knee cap. Patients' position of the knee cap and degree of their patellar tilt was documented by CT scan. The type of toxin, method of injection and the toxin dose was identical to that used by Singer et al. [50]. Botulinum toxin was injected on both sides and into the most distal part of the lateral rectus muscles (close to the knee). Patients' response to pain and their leg function were measured by standard scales. Botulinum injection was combined with special home exercises designed to strengthen the vastus lateralis muscles. This combination therapy improved patellar tilt and patellar angle; it also markedly reduced the patients' pain at the patellar and lateral thigh region. Patients' pain reduction continued over a follow up period of 2 years.

Conclusion

Botulinum toxin injection into the joint effectively improves pain of chronic knee osteoarthritis as well as chronic knee pain after total knee replacement surgery (arthroplasty). There is limited evidence that this treatment approach may improve pain of hip and shoulder osteoarthritis. High quality studies indicate that botulinum toxin injection close to the elbow can improve persistent pain at the region of the elbow in lateral epicondylitis (Tennis elbow). Botulinum toxin injection into the knee joint improves persistent pain in the knee region experience by some patients after total knee replacement. Injection of Botulinum toxin into the lateral muscle of the thigh (vastus lateralis) corrects the imbalance between lateral and medial thigh muscles in patellofemoral syndrome (PFS) via decreasing the tone of this muscle, consequently relieving the chronic knee pain at the region of the knee cap (patella). Evidence from the literature indicates that with the reported doses applied for these indications, botulinum toxins therapy is safe and well tolerated by the patients.

References

1. Neogi T. Structural correlates of pain in osteoarthritis. Clin Exp Rheumatol. 2017 Sept–Oct; 35(Suppl 107, 5):75–8. Epub 2017 Sep 29.
2. Dunlop DD, Manheim LM, Song J, Chang RW. Arthritis prevalence and activity limitations in older adults. Arthritis Rheum. 2001;44:212–21.
3. Sharma L. Osteoarthritis of the knee. N Engl J Med. 2021 Jan 7;384(1):51–9. https://doi.org/10.1056/NEJMcp1903768. PMID: 33406330.
4. Ossendorff R, Thimm D, Wirtz DC, Schildberg FA. Methods of conservative intra-articular treatment for osteoarthritis of the hip and knee. Dtsch Arztebl Int. 2023 Sep 4;(Forthcoming). https://doi.org/10.3238/arztebl.m2023.0154. Epub ahead of print. PMID: 37427991.
5. Lacković Z. Botulinum toxin and pain. Handb Exp Pharmacol. 2021;263:251–64. https://doi.org/10.1007/164_2019_348. PMID: 32016565.
6. Matak I, Lacković Z. Botulinum toxin A, brain and pain. Prog Neurobiol. 2014 Aug–Sep;119–120:39–59. https://doi.org/10.1016/j.pneurobio.2014.06.001. Epub 2014 Jun 7. PMID: 24915026.
7. Safarpour Y, Jabbari B. Botulinum toxin treatment of pain syndromes -an evidence based review. Toxicon. 2018 Jun 1;147:120–8. https://doi.org/10.1016/j.toxicon.2018.01.017. Epub 2018 Feb 1. PMID: 29409817.
8. Hadley HS, Wheeler JL, Petersen SW. Effects of intra-articular botulinum toxin type A (Botox) in dogs with chronic osteoarthritis. Vet Comp Orthop Traumatol. 2010;23(4):254–8. https://doi.org/10.3415/VCOT-09-07-0076. Epub 2010 Jun 21. PMID: 20585713.
9. Malhowald ML, Singh JA, Dykstra D. Long term effects of intra-articular injection of botulinum toxin A for refractory joint pain. Neurotox Res. 2006;9(2–3):179–88.
10. Boon AJ, Smith J, Dahm DL, Sorenson EJ, Larson DR, Fitz-Gibbon PD, Dykstra DD, Singh JA. Efficacy of intra-articular botulinum toxin type A in painful knee osteoarthritis: a pilot study. PM R. 2010 Apr;2(4):268–76. https://doi.org/10.1016/j.pmrj.2010.02.011. PMID: 20430328.
11. Arendt-Nielsen L, Jiang GL, DeGryse R, et al. Intra-articular Onabotulinum toxin A in osteoarthritis knee pain: effect on human mechanistic pain biomarkers and clinical pain. Scand J Rheumatol. 2017;46:303–16.
12. Nguyen C, Rannou F. The safety of intra-articular injections for the treatment of knee osteoarthritis: a critical narrative review. Expert Opin Drug Saf. 2017;16(8):897–902.
13. Chou CL, Lee SH, Lu SY, Tsai KL, Ho CY, Lai HC. Therapeutic effects of intra-articular botulinum neurotoxin in advanced knee osteoarthritis. J Chin Med Assoc. 2010 Nov;73(11):573–80. https://doi.org/10.1016/S1726-4901(10)70126-X. PMID: 21093825.
14. Hsieh LF, Wu CW, Chou CC, Yang SW, Wu SH, Lin YJ, Hsu WC. Effects of botulinum toxin landmark-guided intra-articular injection in subjects with knee osteoarthritis. PM R. 2016 Dec;8(12):1127–35. https://doi.org/10.1016/j.pmrj.2016.05.009. Epub 2016 May 19. PMID: 27210235.
15. Najafi S, Sanati E, Khademi M, Abdorrazaghi F, Mofrad RK, Rezasoltani Z. Intra-articular botulinum toxin type A for treatment of knee osteoarthritis: clinical trial. Toxicon. 2019 Jul;165:69–77. https://doi.org/10.1016/j.toxicon.2019.04.003. Epub 2019 Apr 14. PMID: 30995453.

16. McAlindon TE, Schmidt U, Bugarin D, Abrams S, Geib T, DeGryse RE, Kim K, Schnitzer TJ. Efficacy and safety of single-dose onabotulinumtoxinA in the treatment of symptoms of osteoarthritis of the knee: results of a placebo-controlled, double-blind study. Osteoarthr Cartil. 2018 Oct;26(10):1291–99. https://doi.org/10.1016/j.joca.2018.05.001. Epub 2018 May 9. PMID: 29753118.

17. Shukla D, Sreedhar SK, Rastogi V. A comparative study of botulinum toxin: A with triamcinolone compared to triamcinolone alone in the treatment of osteoarthritis of knee. Anesth Essays Res. 2018 Jan–Mar;12(1):47–9. https://doi.org/10.4103/aer.AER_210_17. PMID: 29628553. PMCID: PMC5872892.

18. Bao X, Tan JW, Flyzik M, Ma XC, Liu H, Liu HY. Effect of therapeutic exercise on knee osteoarthritis after intra-articular injection of botulinum toxin type A, hyaluronate or saline: a randomized controlled trial. J Rehabil Med. 2018 Jun 15;50(6):534–41. https://doi.org/10.2340/16501977-2340. PMID: 29664106.

19. Mendes JG, Natour J, Nunes-Tamashiro JC, Toffolo SR, Rosenfeld A, Furtado RNV. Comparison between intra-articular botulinum toxin type A, corticosteroid, and saline in knee osteoarthritis: a randomized controlled trial. Clin Rehabil. 2019 Jun;33(6):1015–26. https://doi.org/10.1177/0269215519827996. Epub 2019 Feb 19. PMID: 30782000.

20. Wang C, Zhao J, Gao F, Jia M, Hu L, Gao C. The efficacy and safety of intra-articular botulinum toxin type A injection for knee osteoarthritis: a meta-analysis of randomized controlled trials. Toxicon. 2023 Mar 1;224:107026. https://doi.org/10.1016/j.toxicon.2023.107026. Epub 2023 Jan 11. PMID: 36640812.

21. Paget LDA, Mokkenstorm MJ, Tol JL, Kerkhoffs GMMJ, Reurink G. What is the efficacy of intra-articular injections in the treatment of ankle osteoarthritis? A systematic review. Clin Orthop Relat Res. 2023 Sep 1;481(9):1813–24. https://doi.org/10.1097/CORR.0000000000002624. Epub 2023 Apr 11. PMID: 37039814. PMCID: PMC10427070.

22. Eleopra R, Rinaldo S, Lettieri C, Santamato A, Bortolotti P, Lentino C, Tamborino C, Causero A, Devigili G. AbobotulinumtoxinA: a new therapy for hip osteoarthritis. A prospective randomized double-blind multicenter study. Toxins (Basel). 2018 Oct 31;10(11):448. https://doi.org/10.3390/toxins10110448. PMID: 30384438. PMCID: PMC6266300.

23. Marchini C, Acler M, Bolognari MA, Causero A, Volpe D, Regis D, Rizzo A, Rosa R, Eleopra R, Manganotti P. Efficacy of botulinum toxin type A treatment of functional impairment of degenerative hip joint: preliminary results. J Rehabil Med. 2010 Jul;42(7):691–3. https://doi.org/10.2340/16501977-0546. PMID: 20603701.

24. Ahmad Z, Siddiqui N, Malik SS, Abdus-Samee M, Tytherleigh-Strong G, Rushton N. Lateral epicondylitis: a review of pathology and management. Bone Joint J. 2013 Sep;95B(9):1158–64. https://doi.org/10.1302/0301-620X.95B9.29285. PMID: 23997125.

25. Luk JKH, Tsang RCC, Leung HB. Lateral Epicondylalgia: midlife crisis of a tendon. Honk Kong Med J. 2014;20:145–51.

26. McCulloch C, Hunter MM, Lipp C, Lang E, Ganshorn H, Singh P. Management of lateral epicondylitis using transdermal nitroglycerin: a systematic review. Cureus. 2022 Dec 15;14(12):e32560. https://doi.org/10.7759/cureus.32560. PMID: 36654592. PMCID: PMC9840472.

27. Zinger G, Bregman A, Safran O, Beyth S, Peyser A. Hyaluronic acid injections for chronic tennis elbow. BMC Sports Sci Med Rehabil. 2022 Jan 12;14(1):8. https://doi.org/10.1186/s13102-022-00399-0. PMID: 35022075. PMCID: PMC8753848.

28. Yalcin A, Kayaalp ME. Comparison of hyaluronate & steroid injection in the treatment of chronic lateral epicondylitis and evaluation of treatment efficacy with MRI: a single-blind, prospective, randomized controlled clinical study. Cureus. 2022 Sep 10;14(9):e29011. https://doi.org/10.7759/cureus.29011. PMID: 36249613. PMCID: PMC9550185.

29. Cohen MS, Romeo AA. Open and arthroscopic management of lateral epicondylitis in the athlete. Hand Clin. 2009; 25(3):331–8. https://doi.org/10.1016/j.hcl.2009.05.003. PMID:19643333.

30. Moran J, Gillinov SM, Jimenez AE, et al. No difference in complication or reoperation rates between arthroscopic and open debridement for lateral epicondylitis: a national database study. Arthroscopy. 2023;39(2):245–52.
31. Choudhury AK, Niraula BB, Bansal S, Gupta T, Das L, Goyal T. Arthroscopic release and decortication provide earlier return to work with similar patient satisfaction compared to continued intensive conservative therapy for recalcitrant tennis elbow: a retrospective observational study. Eur J Orthop Surg Traumatol. 2024 Jan;34(1):175–80. https://doi.org/10.1007/s00590-023-03628-5. Epub 2023 Jun 30. PMID: 37389708.
32. Creuzé A, Petit H, de Sèze M. Short-term effect of low-dose, electromyography-guided botulinum toxin a injection in the treatment of chronic lateral epicondylar tendinopathy: a randomized, double-blinded study. J Bone Joint Surg Am. 2018 May 16;100(10):818–26. https://doi.org/10.2106/JBJS.17.00777. PMID: 29762276.
33. Wong SM, Hui AC, Tong PY, Poon DW, Yu E, Wong LK. Treatment of lateral epicondylitis with botulinum toxin: a randomized, double-blind, placebo-controlled trial. Ann Intern Med. 2005 Dec 6;143(11):793–7. https://doi.org/10.7326/0003-4819-143-11-200512060-00007. PMID: 16330790.
34. Hayton MJ, Santini AJ, Hughes PJ, Frostick SP, Trail IA, Stanley JK. Botulinum toxin injection in the treatment of tennis elbow. A double-blind, randomized, controlled, pilot study. J Bone Joint Surg Am. 2005 Mar;87(3):503–7. https://doi.org/10.2106/JBJS.D.01896. PMID: 15741614.
35. Placzek R, Drescher W, Deuretzbacher G, Hempfing A, Meiss AL. Treatment of chronic radial epicondylitis with botulinum toxin A. A double-blind, placebo-controlled, randomized multicenter study. J Bone Joint Surg Am. 2007 Feb;89(2):255–60. https://doi.org/10.2106/JBJS.F.00401. PMID: 17272437.
36. Espandar R, Heidari P, Rasouli MR, Saadat S, Farzan M, Rostami M, Yazdanian S, Mortazavi SM. Use of anatomic measurement to guide injection of botulinum toxin for the management of chronic lateral epicondylitis: a randomized controlled trial. CMAJ. 2010 May 18;182(8):768–73. https://doi.org/10.1503/cmaj.090906. Epub 2010 Apr 26. PMID: 20421357. PMCID: PMC2871199.
37. Song B, Day D, Jayaram P. Efficacy of botulinum toxin in treating lateral epicondylitis-does injection location matter?: A systematic review. Am J Phys Med Rehabil. 2020 Dec;99(12):1157–63. https://doi.org/10.1097/PHM.0000000000001511. PMID: 33214499.
38. Lee SH, Choi HH, Chang MC. The effect of botulinum toxin injection into the common extensor tendon in patients with chronic lateral epicondylitis: a randomized trial. Pain Med. 2020 Sep 1;21(9):1971–76. https://doi.org/10.1093/pm/pnz323. PMID: 31804698.
39. Lin YC, Tu YK, Chen SS, Lin IL, Chen SC, Guo HR. Comparison between botulinum toxin and corticosteroid injection in the treatment of acute and subacute tennis elbow: a prospective, randomized, double-blind, active drug-controlled pilot study. Am J Phys Med Rehabil. 2010 Aug;89(8):653–9. https://doi.org/10.1097/PHM.0b013e3181cf564d. PMID: 20134306.
40. Guo YH, Kuan TS, Chen KL, Lien WC, Hsieh PC, Hsieh IC, Chiu SH, Lin YC. Comparison between steroid and 2 different sites of botulinum toxin injection in the treatment of lateral epicondylalgia: a randomized, double-blind, active drug-controlled pilot study. Arch Phys Med Rehabil. 2017 Jan;98(1):36–42. https://doi.org/10.1016/j.apmr.2016.08.475. Epub 2016 Sep 22. PMID: 27666156.
41. Tavassoli M, Jokar R, Zamani M, Khafri S, Esmaeilnejad-Ganji SM. Clinical efficacy of local injection therapies for lateral epicondylitis: a systematic review and network meta-analysis. Caspian J Intern Med. 2022 Spring;13(2):311–25. https://doi.org/10.22088/cjim.13.2.1. PMID: 35919654. PMCID: PMC9301214.
42. Centers for Disease Control and Prevention. Number of all-listed procedures for discharges from short-stay hospitals, by procedure category and age: United States, 2010. Atlanta: Centers for Disease Control and Prevention; 2010.

43. Beswick AD, Wylde V, Gooberman-Hill R, et al. What proportion of patients report long-term pain after total hip or knee replacement for osteoarthritis? A systematic review of prospective studies in unselected patients. BMJ Open. 2012;2:e000435.
44. Beswick AD, Wylde V, Gooberman-Hill R. Interventions for the prediction and management of chronic postsurgical pain after total knee replacement: systematic review of randomised controlled trials. BMJ Open. 2015 May 12;5(5):e007387. https://doi.org/10.1136/bmjopen-2014-007387.
45. Singh JA, Mahowald ML, Noorbaloochi S. Intraarticular botulinum toxin A for refractory painful total knee arthroplasty: a randomized controlled trial. J Rheumatol. 2010;37(11):2377–86.
46. Seyler TM, Jinnah RH, Koman LA, Marker DR, Mont MA, Ulrich SD, Bhave A. Botulinum toxin type A injections for the management of flexion contractures following total knee arthroplasty. J Surg Orthop Adv. 2008 Winter;17(4):231–8. PMID: 19138496.
47. Smith EB, Shafi KA, Greis AC, Maltenfort MG, Chen AF. Decreased flexion contracture after total knee arthroplasty using botulinum toxin A: a randomized controlled trial. Knee Surg Sports Traumatol Arthrosc. 2016 Oct;24(10):3229–34. https://doi.org/10.1007/s00167-016-4277-9. Epub 2016 Aug 11. PMID: 27515301.
48. Pal S, Besier TF, Draper CE, Fredericson M. Patellar tilt correlates with vastus ateralis: vastus medialis activation ratio in maltracking patellofemoral pain patients. J Orthop Res 2012;30(6):927–33. https://doi.org/10.1002/jor.22008. Epub 2011 Nov 15.
49. Crossley KM, Stefanik JJ, Selfe J, Collins NJ, Davis IS, Powers CM, McConnell J, Vicenzino B, Bazett-Jones DM, Esculier JF, Morrissey D, Callaghan MJ. 2016 Patellofemoral pain consensus statement from the 4th international patellofemoral pain research retreat, Manchester. Part 1: terminology, definitions, clinical examination, natural history, patellofemoral osteoarthritis and patient-reported outcome measures. Br J Sports Med. 2016 Jul;50(14):839–43. https://doi.org/10.1136/bjsports-2016-096384. Epub 2016 Jun 24. PMID: 27343241. PMCID: PMC4975817.
50. Singer BJ, Silbert PL, Song S, et al. Treatment of refractory anterior knee pain using botulinum toxin type A (Dysport) injection to the distal vastus lateralis muscle: a randomised placebo controlled crossover trial. J Sports Med. 2011;45(8):640–5.
51. Chen JT, Tang AC, Lin SC, Tang SF. Anterior knee pain caused by patellofemoral pain syndrome can be relieved by botulinum toxin type A injection. Clin Neurol Neurosurg. 2015 Feb;129(Suppl 1):S27–9. https://doi.org/10.1016/S0303-8467(15)30008-1. PMID: 25683309.
52. Pal S, Choi JH, Delp SL, Fredericson M. Botulinum neurotoxin type A improves vasti muscle balance, patellar tracking, and pain in patients with chronic patellofemoral pain. J Orthop Res. 2023 May;41(5):962–72. https://doi.org/10.1002/jor.25435. Epub 2022 Sep 5. PMID: 36031589.

Chapter 13
Botulinum Toxin Treatment in Aesthetic Medicine

Marie Noland and Marissa Dennis

Abstract This chapter describes the spectrum of botulinum toxin applications in the field of aesthetic medicine including treatment of wrinkles at different locations and facial sculpturing for correction of eyebrow lift, lateral lip lift, gummy smile, eye widening, chin and masseter muscles aesthetic improvement as well as correction of platysma bands (skin of the neck) and reduction of the size of the enlarged glands secreting saliva (parotid and submaxillary). The Microtox and Microdroplet techniques for improving skin and glands are discussed.

Keywords Botulinum toxin · Botulinum neurotoxin · Rhytids · Wrinkles · Facial sculpturing · Crow feet's · Gummy smile · Lateral eyebrow lift · Glabellar line · Microtox · Microdroplet

Injectable botulinum toxin type A is currently the leading non-surgical procedure in aesthetic medicine, and its popularity continues to rise every year [1]. Its use for cosmetic indications was first discovered by ophthalmologist Dr. Jean Carruthers and her husband Dr. Alastair Carruthers, a dermatologist, both based in Vancouver, Canada. Patients being treated for blepharospasm (eyelid twitching) were returning and requesting further treatment as they noticed their frown lines softening. The Carruthers' recognized the benefit of this novel treatment and published the first clinical study of Botox (onabotulinumtoxinA) for the treatment of glabellar lines in 1992 [2]. A decade later, it was approved by the Food and Drug Administration (FDA) for this limited indication. Since then, Health Canada and the FDA have expanded onabotulinumtoxinA's cosmetic indications to include multiple treatment

---

The original version of the chapter has been revised. A correction to this chapter can be found at https://doi.org/10.1007/978-3-031-54471-2_20

M. No1land (✉)
Plastic Surgery, McGill University, Gatineau, QC, Canada
e-mail: noland.marie@gmail.com

M. Dennis
Onyx Beauty Lab, Kelowna, British Columbia, Canada

MAIA Medical Aesthetics & Injectables Academy, Kelowna, British Columbia, Canada

areas of the upper face. Additional botulinum toxin A medications have also been approved in North America for cosmetic indications, including Dysport (abobotulinumtoxinA), Xeomin (incobotulinumtoxinA), Nuceiva/Jeuveau (prabotulinumtoxinA), Letybo (letibotulinumtoxinA), and Daxxify (daxibotulinumtoxinA).

These neuromodulator products generally function the same and can be used relatively interchangeably depending on the practitioner's preference. While Botox, Xeomin, Letybo, and Nuceiva are considered to be clinically interchangeable, Dysport dosing is generally accepted as 2-2.5:1 unit of Botox. Daxxify recommends glabellar dosing that is twice that of Botox and reports increased longevity of the results by 6–9 months [3]. Furthermore, each medication has its own nuances that clinicians should be aware of. Recommendations made in this chapter for Botox dosing can be applied to all current approved medications adjusted as above.

Understanding the mechanism of action of botulinum toxin gives the practitioner the ability to use the product beyond the official indications and optimize results based on patient presentation and specific concerns. Botulinum neurotoxin works by stopping the transmission of the neurotransmitter acetylcholine from the nerve cell to the muscle cell, resulting in local paralysis of the muscle in the treated area. It has been shown to have a dose-dependent effect influenced by injection technique and the size of the muscle [4]. Accurate injections of small volumes of properly concentrated solution is preferred to target specific muscles [5]. Larger volumes and less concentrated solutions favor drug dispersion and are often preferred for use in larger muscles, or muscles with more surface area, for a more aesthetically pleasing result. The effects of botulinum neurotoxin are typically seen within 3–10 days after initial injection and can last from 3 to 6 months.

Techniques and dose recommendations for injections continue to evolve as new formulations are introduced to the market and clinical research continues to expand. As such, treatment plans should be tailored to the individual based on muscle patterns, strength, and intended outcomes. Unless otherwise specified, the recommended needle size is 31–32-gauge and 12–13 mm length [6]. The injection needle should be changed regularly to minimize the risk of infection and decrease patient discomfort.

Prior to injections, the skin should be assessed for any dermatologic pathology as injections through inflamed or irritated skin should be avoided [7]. Complications can be minimized by developing a deep understanding of the structure and function of the underlying facial anatomy.

Botulinum toxin's use within the field of aesthetic medicine will be summarized below. Guidelines for its use on targeting specific rhytides of the face, modification of facial form, improvement of skin quality, scar management, and salivary gland hypertrophy will be outlined. Because aesthetic enhancement is not an exact science, the following should be used as a starting point and allow for flexibility.

Rhytides (Wrinkles)

As demonstrated by Carruthers in 1987, botulinum toxin injections into muscles result in temporary improvement in wrinkles by preventing the contraction of targeted facial muscles. Thus, dynamic lines respond well to neuromodulators, while static lines related to old age, sun damage, and redundant skin are less responsive.

Rhytides (wrinkles) form perpendicular to the underlying muscle. Overactive muscles can be partially or entirely relaxed to achieve the desired aesthetic outcome. It is important to note that muscles contract towards their points of origin, this is helpful in determining the muscle function and whether it elevates or depresses facial features. Although clinical trials emphasize the efficacy of botulinum toxin injections at maximum doses, the frozen look is no longer desired by most patients (2), so doses can be reduced to suit a patient's desires.

Dynamic rhytides are more easily appreciated in the upper third of the face, as influenced by the function of the frontalis, procerus, corrugator supercilii, and orbicularis oculi. These areas account for the majority of treatments with botulinum toxin type A [5, 8]. Major muscles in the midface include the nasalis, levator labii superioris alaeque nasi, and levator labii superioris. The lower third of the face includes the orbicularis oris, depressor anguli oris, masseters, and mentalis muscle. Static rhytides are common in this region and treatment with botulinum toxin is aimed more at prevention. The platysma covers the neck and inserts into the lower face. Treatment of the lower face and neck can result in functional deficits (muscle paralysis) and should be approached with caution (5). More recently, the industry is trending towards full-face treatments, so these areas must still be assessed and considered. Dosage recommendations are illustrated in Table 13.1.

Injection patterns and dosing are often tailored to suit the individual's aesthetic goals, muscular strength, wrinkle pattern, and asymmetries. As such, it is the treating clinician's responsibility to evaluate the patient at rest and in full movement prior to determining a treatment plan.

Forehead Lines

The frontalis muscle is the only elevator muscle in the upper face [8], in other words, it is the only muscle with an upward pull on the eyebrows. It is responsible for the development of horizontal lines in the forehead. The frontalis is the "frontal belly" of the occipitofrontalis muscle. It originates from the galea aponeurotica (essentially at the hairline of the forehead) and inserts into the skin of the eyebrow, intertwining with the fibers of the procerus, corrugator supercilli, and orbicularis oculi [9]. It has bidirectional movement. The upper aspect of the muscle draws the scalp forward and down (approximately the upper third of the visible forehead), and the lower portion lifts the eyebrows up.

To assess the degree of muscle activity, the patient is asked to forcefully raise their eyebrows. During this contraction, the clinician can assess where the upward

Table 13.1 Recommended OnabotulinumtoxinA injections for rhytides

Indications	Dose range[a]	No. of injections
Forehead	2–20	4–12
Glabella	20–30	3–7
Crow's feet	6–15	3–4 per side
Lip lines	4–8	2–4 upper lip, 2 lower lip

[a]All doses are in units

pull of the inferior frontalis meets the downward pull of the superior aspect; this is referred to as the line of Convergence [10] and is often found around the second visible wrinkle down from the hairline. Injections above this line can be deep and higher doses may be used (2–4 Botox units per site). Injections below this line may be dosed lower and/or injected more superficially [10], depending on medication selection and clinician preference. Any discrepancies between the positioning of the brows should also be noted both at rest and during maximal contraction, as this can affect the outcome after treatment and dosing adjustments may be beneficial.

The dosage, placement, depth, and dilution for botulinum toxin use in this area depend on the desired aesthetic outcome. It is important to note that treatment of the frontalis will affect the positioning of the eyebrows. As the lower portion of the frontalis muscle is inactivated, the brows will naturally rest in a lower position. This effect can be either desirable or not [2]. Injectors should be conservative in this region as the goal typically is to soften the forehead lines without causing brow ptosis (droop) and loss of expressiveness [2]. Exercise extreme caution in patients with hooded eyelids or if active forehead contraction is noted at rest.

The needle should be introduced perpendicular to the skin for deeper injections and on a 30–45-degree angle for more superficial injections. The injector can follow the creases of the forehead in 4–12 sites (Fig. 13.1) for a total of 2–20 onabotulinumtoxinA units [2]. If desired, small dose adjustments can be made between sides to adjust for asymmetries.

The glabella should generally be treated in conjunction with the frontalis to avoid central eyebrow depression. Furthermore, overtreatment of the central forehead can result in a "Spock" appearance of the brows which is an unnatural elevation of the arches of the eyebrows. This can be corrected or prevented with a low dose injection of botulinum toxin into the lowest aspect of the frontalis muscle in line with the outside margin of the iris [7]. Have the patient lift their eyebrows while immobilizing the medial aspects of the corrugators (at the head of the eyebrows) and look for the most inferior contraction of the frontalis that appears to be "spocking". Keep injections 2 cm above the orbital rim to avoid inadvertent diffusion into the levator palpebrae superioris, a muscle which if paralysed would result in an eyelid droop (ptosis).

Fig. 13.1 Recommended injection points for the targeted treatment of forehead lines. A total of 4–20 onabotulinumtoxinA units are delivered depending on the severity of the wrinkles and degree of paralysis desired

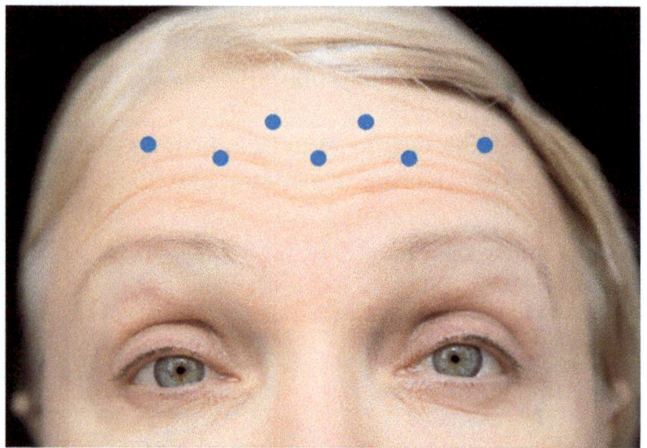

If eyelid ptosis does occur, this can be treated by activating a muscle called the Muller's muscle with 0.5% apraclonidine eye drops into the affected eye three times daily until the effects of the botulinum toxin wear off [7]. Upneeq (oxymetazoline hydrochloride ophthalmic solution) is a more recently FDA-approved option that can be used once daily until the ptosis self-resolves [11]. Lastly, in severe cases, pre-tarsal (just above the eyelashes) injections of botulinum toxin A may be an appropriate intervention [12] by weakening the strength of contraction of the orbicularis oculi muscle-favoring eyelid opening [13].

Glabellar Lines

The glabella refers to the region between the eyebrows. It was the first cosmetic treatment site for botulinum toxin [2]. The glabellar complex includes the corrugator supercilii, depressor supercilii, and procerus. It is responsible for depression of the medial eyebrows when frowning. The procerus originates midline at the nasal cartilage and inserts into the skin of the lower to mid forehead, blending with fibers of the frontalis [6]. The paired corrugator supercilli originate at the medial superior brow bones and insert into the forehead skin along or just above the eyebrow. The depressor supercilli originate at the lateral portion of the nasal bridge and flare across the inner corners of the eyes, inserting into the frontalis and the skin at the level of the eyebrows. They are the medial aspect of the orbicularis oculi [9]. Repeated contraction of the corrugator muscles is what causes the two vertical creases, commonly referred to as the "11 s". Contraction of the procerus muscles pulls the brows downward, resulting in a horizontal crease across the nasal bridge [4, 14]. This region was once treated as an independent indication but is now considered an important component of brow harmonization. The total dosage can be adjusted to allow for movement and expression as desired [2].

The glabella is assessed for the location, orientation, and severity of rhytides. The degree of muscle activity is determined by asking the patient to forcefully furrow their brows. Once again, the positioning and shape of the eyebrows is noted and any asymmetries are recorded.

Treatment of the glabella typically involves five injection sites for a total of 20–30 units of onabotulinumtoxinA. The sites include one point into the base of the procerus muscle, and two sites into each medial and lateral corrugator muscle [7] (Fig. 13.2). To guide the injection placement, the patient is asked to frown as the skin and muscle are gently pinched by the injector's fingers. The patient is then asked to relax and the injection is made deep into the muscle (for the three medial sites) while the clinician continues to gently pinch the muscle with their non-dominant hand. The two lateral injection points can be made by inserting the needle just below the skin, while angling upward due to the lateral corrugator's more superficial location [7]. The superficial injections should produce a bleb or a "wheel". More recently, an injection pattern of 3 sites with 10 units per site has been suggested for more simplicity and a decreased risk of eyelid droop [15]. This pattern

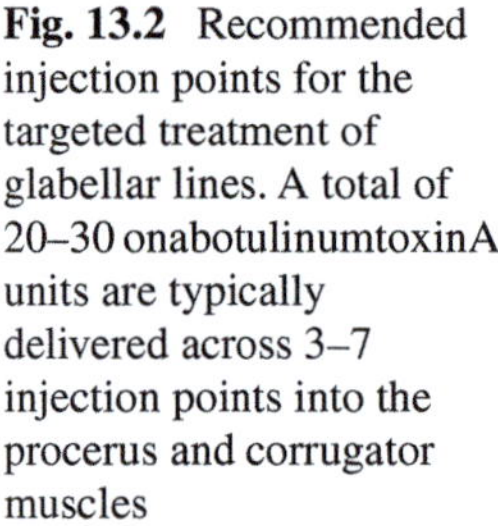

Fig. 13.2 Recommended injection points for the targeted treatment of glabellar lines. A total of 20–30 onabotulinumtoxinA units are typically delivered across 3–7 injection points into the procerus and corrugator muscles

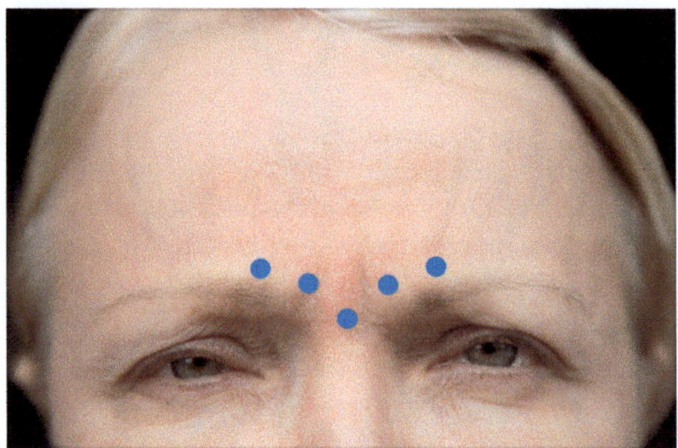

includes the base of the procerus and the medial head of each corrugator. However, some clinicians inject up to 7 sites which may include an injection midway between the head and the tail of longer corrugator muscles.

If the glabellar region is treated without the frontalis, there may be unwanted medial elevation of the eyebrows from the unopposed pull of the forehead elevator muscle. Other complications can include inadvertent diffusion of botulinum toxin that may result in eyelid ptosis if the lateral corrugator injection sites are placed too deeply [7].

Crow's Feet

Lateral canthal lines, also referred to as crow's feet, are one of the earliest signs of aging. As the skin changes with age and becomes more photodamaged, these dynamic lines can become static. They are caused by repeated contraction of the muscles involved in squinting, and smiling. The muscle that has the most effect on these lines is the orbicularis oculi. Its' function is to close the eyelid [9]. Consequently, it also has a downward pull on the eyebrow. This area becomes less responsive to botulinum toxin in older patients with static wrinkling.

The patient's lateral canthal lines should be assessed both at rest and with active contraction. They should be asked to squint while smiling to determine the degree and extent of muscle activity. Note any asymmetries of the eyebrows.

The orbicularis oculi originates from the medial aspect of the orbit, the palpebral part inserts into the skin of the upper and lower eyelids, and the orbital part fans out attaching to the skin of the orbit, forehead and cheeks [6]. The orbicularis is more superficial than most facial muscles. Injections of botulinum toxin should, therefore, be very superficial, just below the skin, producing a visible bleb [7]. These lines are typically treated with 3–4 injection sites of 2–5 onabotulinumtoxinA units into each horizontal rhytid (Fig. 13.3). Keep the injection sites 1 cm lateral to the orbital rim to avoid inadvertent diffusion into the eyelid portion of the orbicularis

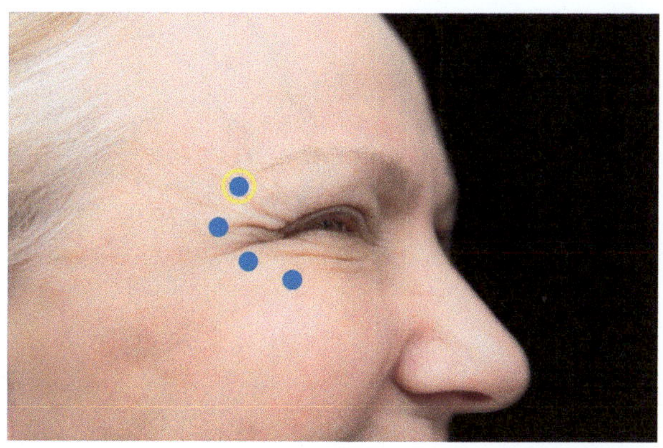

Fig. 13.3 Recommended injection points for the targeted treatment of lateral canthal lines. A total of 5–15 onabotulinumtoxinA units are delivered intradermally across 3–7 injection points. Additionally, the superior-most injection point may be used to achieve a slight brow lift with 3–5 extra units

oculi or the lateral rectus muscle (responsible for movement of the eye to the side) which may lead to eyelid ptosis or diplopia [16]. If no lifting of the lateral eyebrow is desired, then avoid injecting the superior-most lateral canthal line.

This area is prone to bruising due to its high vascularity. Keep pressure on the skin after injection and avoid injecting into visible superficial veins. Furthermore, inadvertent injection into the zygomatic muscle can weaken a patient's smile and result in asymmetries. Avoid injecting deeply for more inferior injections and use caution when at or below the level of the zygoma [2].

Lip Lines or "Lip Flip"

The main muscle found in the lips is the orbicularis oris [17]. It is a circular muscle surrounding the opening of the mouth and it acts as a sphincter to close the lips and keep food inside. It originates from the mandible and maxilla and inserts into the upper and lower lip [6]. The orbicularis oris is also involved in puckering the lips, as would be important in speech production and sucking [18]. With age and photo-damage, the white lip tends to thin and elongate, leading to loss of the Cupid's bow and flatness of the vermillion border (transition from the red to white lip). Vertical wrinkles become evident with repeated contraction of the perioral musculature, as well as soft-tissue volume loss and bony resorption of the mandible and max-illa [19].

Assessment of the lips should be made at rest and during animation. The patient should be asked to smile and pucker, as well as being assessed with normal speech and expression. Assess the presence of dynamic and static vertical perioral rhytids. Make note of any loss of lip and perioral volume, as well as the projection (protrusion) of the lips on profile view.

Perioral lip lines can be treated at one to two sites per side along the upper lip, and at one site per side along the lower lip [17]. The injection is made at the vermillion border and should be placed superficially. Injections may also be made more

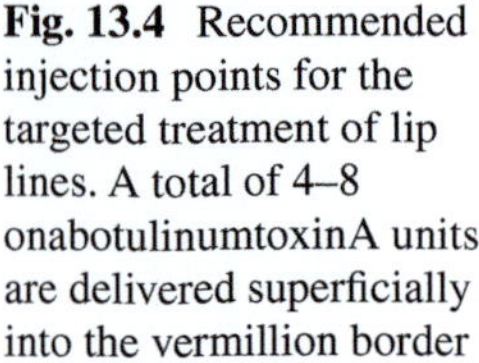

Fig. 13.4 Recommended injection points for the targeted treatment of lip lines. A total of 4–8 onabotulinumtoxinA units are delivered superficially into the vermillion border

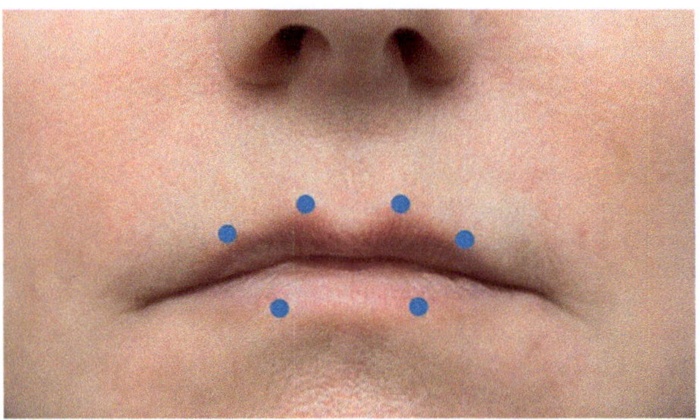

superiorly along the white lip if rhytides extend superiorly. A total of 4–8 units of onabotulinumtoxinA is recommended [20] (Fig. 13.4). Additionally, botulinum toxin injections in this area can have a secondary benefit of everting the lips (commonly referred to as the "lip flip").

Administering high doses can result in difficulty drinking out of straws and lip pursing. This can also affect speech and pronunciation and may cause drooling [17]. This can be avoided by keeping the injection dosages conservative and injection sites further away from where the lips come together.

Facial Sculpting

Beyond the immediate benefit of injectable neuromodulators on wrinkle reduction, they can also be used to improve the shape and position of various facial landmarks. Facial expression is achieved by activation of muscles that either elevate or depress the features of the face. This balance of muscles can be modified strategically by weakening the muscles that alter the face undesirably. For instance, relaxing a depressor muscle leaves unopposed action of the elevator muscles resulting in a lifted appearance of a given facial structure. Furthermore, muscles that are inactive undergo atrophy over time resulting in a slimming effect. This can be desirable when the targeted muscle is hypertrophic or contributing to unaesthetic appearance. Dosage recommendations are illustrated in Table 13.2.

Eyebrow Lift

Botulinum toxin can be used to achieve a more desirable eyebrow shape by manipulating the vectors of pull relating to the muscles of the upper face. The frontalis muscle is the only elevator muscle in the upper face and it is responsible for lifting both the medial and lateral eyebrows [8]. The glabellar muscle complex is

Table 13.2 Recommended OnabotulinumtoxinA injections for facial sculpting

Indications	Total dose[a] range	No. of injections	Injection sites
Eyebrow lift	6–10	1 per side	Superior-most lateral canthal line
Eye widening	2–4	1 per side	Lower eyelid mid-pupil
Gummy smile	6–10	3 if moderate, 5 if severe	Inferior to columella; lateral to ala
Lateral lip lift	4–8	1–2 per side	1 cm lateral to oral commissure along mandibular border
Mentalis muscle	4–10	2–3	1 cm from mandibular border, at least 1.5–2 cm inferior to vermillion, and as close to midline as possible
Masseter hypertrophy	24–48	3–4 per side	Inverted triangle or square centered on masseter body
Platysmal bands	25–30	3–4 per band	Vertically along each band
Parotid hypertrophy	60–80	2–9 per side	Posterior to masseter, midway between tragus and mandibular angle
Submandibular gland hypertrophy	24–30	2 per side	Ultrasound guided or 1 finger breadth medial to the midpoint of a line from mandibular angle to chin

[a]The doses are in units

responsible for depressing the medial eyebrows, while the lateral orbicularis oculi is responsible for depressing the lateral eyebrows. A lateral eyebrow lift can be achieved by either deactivating the lateral orbicularis oculi or the medial frontalis muscle. The ideal eyebrow shape has varied over the years with various trends; however, a classic youthful aesthetic shape always remains. An aesthetically desirable female eyebrow should rest medially in line with the inner corner of the eye at the top of the bony orbit. The lateral tail should rest on the same horizontal plane as the medial brow and extend just beyond the outer corner of the eye [7]. The peak of the ideal female brow should be positioned somewhere between the outside edge of the iris and the outside corner of the eye and sit above the bony orbital rim. This may differ based on patient gender, age, or ethnicity [21]. The male eyebrow follows a similar shape but is lower and flatter than that of a female [7].

Assessment of the eyebrows should be made with the patient looking forward with their eyes open. Many patients will compensate for a natural eyelid droop or excess eyelid skin by over activating their forehead muscle. This can result in a surprised appearance and/or asymmetry of the eyebrows. Ask the patient to close their eyes gently and note the positioning of the eyebrows. Determine the positioning of the medial and lateral eyebrows relative to the supraorbital rim and note the vertical positioning of the tail of the brow relative to the medial head. The patient should be asked to squint, and the superior-most crow's foot should be marked.

A single injection point of botulinum toxin is made into the orbicularis oculi muscle at the superior-most lateral canthal line (Fig. 13.3). This point should be 1 cm lateral to the orbital rim to avoid inadvertent diffusion into the palpebral portion of the orbicularis oculi or into the levator palpebrae muscle. Injections should be made intradermally forming a visible bleb due to the superficial location of the orbicularis oculi muscle. A total of 3–5 onabotulinumtoxinA units can be injected per side. To avoid a "Spock" appearance, it is recommended to also place 1–2 units of onabotulinumtoxinA into the frontalis muscle 2 cm above the superior orbital rim in line with the lateral iris [7]. This keeps the lift isolated to the lateral aspect of the brow only and produces a more aesthetically pleasing result. Injection of several units of botulinum toxin can also be made into the medial wrinkles of the forehead and this can result in a compensatory hyperactivation of the lateral frontalis leading to a lateral eyebrow lift.

Keep in mind that if the medial eyebrow is lowered to prevent hyperactivation of the frontalis, the patient may complain of "heaviness" of the forehead or eyelids. If an underlying ptosis is a significant issue, it should be surgically corrected. The injector should also be mindful that paralyzing the glabellar complex will result in separation and elevation of the medial eyebrows. This may not be a desirable aesthetic effect and can be mitigated by deactivating the frontalis muscle medially.

Eye Widening and "Jelly Rolls"

The orbicularis oculi muscle is a sphincter muscle that functions to close the eyelids. It can be separated into orbital and palpebral sections. The palpebral section can be further subdivided into the preseptal (the mobile eyelids) and pretarsal portions (just above the eyelashes) [22]. The orbital section of the orbicularis oculi is more involved in voluntary squeezing and winking of the eyelid while the palpebral section has a greater role in involuntary blink closure as well as keeping the eyelids closed during sleep [22]. With age, strong preseptal fibers are responsible for narrowing of the eye opening (palpebral aperture) [7]. Furthermore, some patients may present with a bulge below their eyelids whereby the orbicularis muscle contracts with smiling, this is often referred to as a "jelly roll". Botulinum toxin injections into the preseptal orbicularis oculi can improve the appearance of a narrowed palpebral aperture as well as correct congenital and senile entropion (inversion of the eyelids) [23].

With the patient looking straight, assess the patient's palpebral aperture bilaterally noting any asymmetries. Perform a snap test before injection to verify lower lid elasticity. A snap test is performed by gently pinching the skin under the eye and observing the speed of recoil, elasticity and turgor response. Identify the presence of any ectropion (eversion of the eyelids), entropion, and lower lid show. Assess the patient upon smiling for any bulging of the lower lid.

A single injection site in the lower eyelid 3–4 mm below the eyelash margin in line with the mid pupil can treat a narrowing palpebral aperture. Have the patient close their eyes and inject superficially into the dermis 1–2 onabotulinumtoxinA units per side [7] (Fig. 13.5). Keep the needle parallel to the skin to avoid injury to

Fig. 13.5 Recommended injection points to achieve widening of the eye aperture. A single injection of 1–2 onabotulinumtoxinA units per side is made into the lower eyelid, 3–4 mm below the eyelash margin

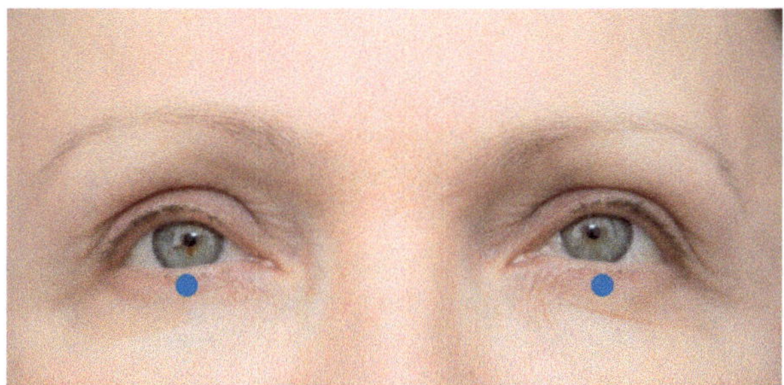

the eye. If the patient presents with bulging of the lower eyelid, this area can be treated directly with 1–3 injection directly into the "jelly roll".

This area should not be treated if the patient has prominent infraorbital fat pads, scleral show, ectropion, or a poor snap test as botulinum toxin injections can worsen these conditions [7].

Nasal Lines ("Bunny Lines")

Nasal lines are caused primarily by the nasalis and levator labii superioris alaeque nasi muscles (LLSAN). The procerus and orbicularis oculi are also contributors [24]. The nasalis originates at the top of the incisor and canine tooth roots and inserts into the wing and bridge of the nose and the lateral nasal cartilage [9]. The LLSAN originates from the frontal process of the maxilla and the orbicularis oculi and inserts into the wings of the nose, upper lip, and the lateral and dorsal circumference of the nostril [9]. Hyperactivity of these muscles can result in radial lines to the upper third of the nose. These lines can also occur following treatment of the glabella or lateral canthal region [6].

Assess by having the patient squint or scrunch up their nose "like a bunny" and observe muscle strength and depth of lines at rest and on animation. Identify any asymmetries.

Injections can be made by inserting the needle almost parallel to the skin up to 45° and utilizing an intradermal technique, creating a wheel or a bleb [6]. The superior portion of the nasalis/LLSAN is targeted with one injection point per side, approximately at the level of the rhinion (where the bony top of the nose meets the middle cartilage of the nose), just medial to a vertical line drawn down from the inner eye corner [24]. Two to five units per site may be used for a total dose of 4–10 units. Doses should be conservative to start, as over injection may lead to upper lip elongation or a dropped upper lip upon smiling.

Gummy Smile

A gummy smile refers to the showing of excess gingiva while smiling [19]. In certain individuals, hyperactivity of the muscles responsible for smiling can result in this problem, specifically the LLSAN muscle which elevates and everts the upper lip and the depressor septi nasi muscle which draws the nasal tip downwards while smiling. In severe cases, the levator labii superioris and zygomaticus minor muscles are also hyperactive [14].

Assess the lips and the amount of teeth and gum visible both at rest and with smiling. Make note of any depression of the nasal tip with smiling, as well as the length of the upper lip. Identify any asymmetries.

Injection of botulinum toxin can be made at three sites if the gummy smile is moderate and at five sites if it is severe [19]. Botulinum toxin is injected deep into the muscles at full depth. One injection site per side, lateral to the ala (lower corner of the nose where it meets the face), targets the inferior portion of the LLSAN, while one central injection, inferior to the nasal columella, targets the depressor septi nasi muscle. A second injection site in line with the ala and the pupil can be made to target the levator labii superioris and zygomaticus minor muscles. Two onabotulinumtoxinA units per injection site can be used for a total of 6–10 units.

Over-injection with botulinum toxin in the LLSAN may lead to elongation of the upper lip. Patients with long upper lips may not be ideal candidates for this procedure [19].

Lateral Lip Lift

The depressor anguli oris (DAO) muscle is involved in frowning and functions to draw the corners of the mouth downwards. It is triangular shaped and originates on the mandible and inserts at the angle of the mouth onto the modiolus (structure at the corner of the mouth where fibers from multiple facial muscles converge) [17]. Excessive contraction of this muscle and soft tissue depletion leads to a sullen appearance and contributes to the creation of marionette lines, forming downwards from the lateral oral commissure (mouth corner) [25].

The patient's mouth should be assessed at rest and with activity. Note the direction of the oral commissure (corner of the mouth) at rest. They should be asked to frown to determine the strength and location of the depressor anguli oris muscle. As always, note any asymmetries between each side. There are two generally accepted injection points used to achieve a subtle lift of the oral commissures (Fig. 13.6).

A total dose of 2–5 onabotulinumtoxinA units (per side) is typically injected. More commonly, the injection points used are 1 cm lateral to the oral commissure along the base of the muscle at the mandibular border [25]. Injections here should be deep and remain lateral to the marionette fold. Alternatively, the clinician can have the patient pull the corners of their mouth down and inject the muscle where

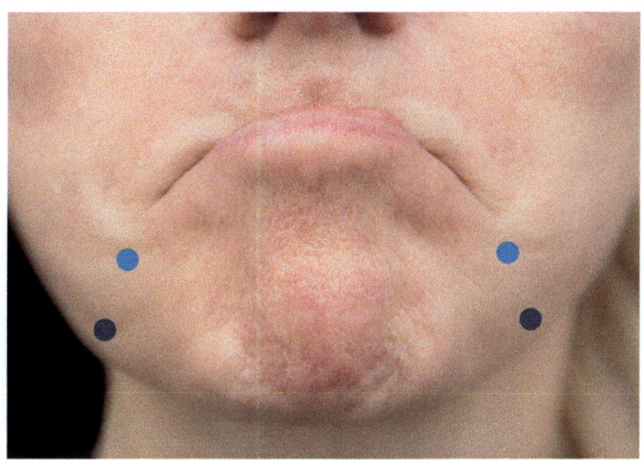

Fig. 13.6 Recommended injection points to achieve a lateral lip lift. A total dose of 4–10 onabotulinumtoxinA units is injected deep into the depressor anguli oris muscle, 1 cm lateral to the oral commissure at the mandibular border. Alternatively, a mid-depth injection more superiorly where visible contraction of the skin is noticed can be made instead

there is a visible contraction. Injection points should remain at least 1 cm inferior to the mouth corner, lateral to the marionette line, with the needle being inserted at a 45 degree angle for a mid-depth injection [24].

Diffusion of the medication medially can result in inadvertent paralysis of the depressor labii inferioris (DLI) muscle leading to an asymmetrical smile. This unwanted effect can be minimized by using a more concentrated reconstitution, avoiding excessive dosing and keeping injections lateral to the marionette lines, as the DLI lies deep and medial to the DAO [19].

Mentalis Muscle

The mentalis muscle is a paired muscle located at the centre of the mandible. It is the only elevator muscle of the lower lip [26]. It originates on the mandible and its fibers insert into the skin of the chin. This muscle functions to maintain oral competence (ensuring that the mouth stays closed during chewing) and supports the lower lip [6]. It also serves to elevate the overlying skin via its thick fibrous septa [27]. A hyperdynamic mentalis muscle can accentuate the mentolabial crease, as well as create unwanted dimpling of the chin area upon animation [17].

Assess the chin by having the patient pull the lower lip up over their upper lip to determine the outline of the mentalis muscle and identify areas of contour irregularities [27].

Injection sites should be at least 1.5–2 cm inferior to the border of the lower lip and approximately 5–10 mm above the lower border of the mandible [24]. The total dosage is 4–8 onabotulinumtoxinA units [19]. The injection sites can be spread out over 2–3 points, with the two inferior points being deep and/or superficial injections, and the superior point, if used, being a deep injection (Fig. 13.7). Keeping the superior injection deep limits any unwanted spread to the orbicular oris muscle, while adding a superficial injection inferiorly can help improve textural issues

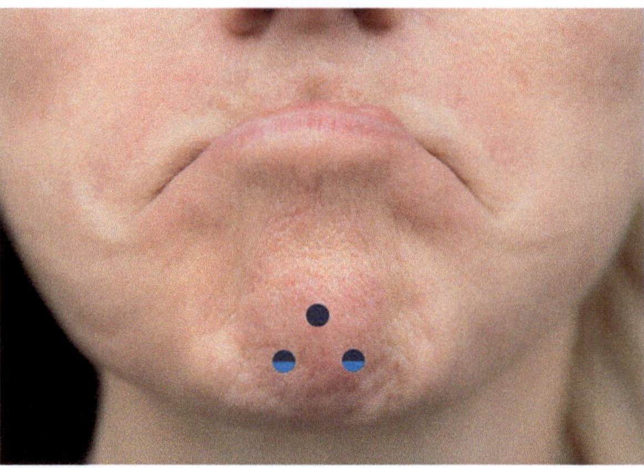

Fig. 13.7 Recommended injection points to treat chin dimpling. Injection sites should be at least 1.5 cm inferior to the border of the lower lip and approximately 5–10 mm above the lower border of the mandible. A total dose of 4–10 onabotulinumtoxinA units are delivered over 2–3 injection sites. The inferior injection points can be made either superficially or deep, while the superior-most injection point should remain deep

related to where the mentalis inserts into the skin. Care must be taken not to inject too laterally as this can result in unwanted spread to the DLI, resulting in an asymmetrical smile [17]. Keep injection points as close to midline as possible.

The mentalis can be a challenging muscle to inject. Over-injection can have significantly undesirable consequences ranging from lower tooth exposure to oral incompetence and drooling [26]. If the lower lip rests too low after treatment, it may be of benefit to also inject the depressor anguli oris muscles to balance the lip position [27].

Masseter Hypertrophy

The masseter muscle is a thick quadrangular muscle that rests superficial to the angle of the mandible. It is divided into deep and superficial portions by the deep inferior tendon [21]. The deep portion of the masseter originates from the surface of the zygomatic arch and inserts into the upper half of the mandible [24]. When treating masseters therapeutically (for clenching or grinding), the deep portion must be targeted. The superficial portion originates from the inferior aspect of the anterior cheekbone and inserts into the mandibular angle and the posterior aspect of the jaw [24]. If treating masseters strictly for cosmetic purposes, it is acceptable to target the superficial aspect of the muscle. The masseter functions to elevate the jaw and assist with chewing [17]. It can become enlarged with repeated clenching or grinding of the jaw resulting in a widened or squaring of the lower face [28].

The patient should be assessed from the front view to determine the width of the lower face. Assess the strength, size, and location of the masseter muscle by asking the patient to clench their jaw. Mark out the anterior border of the muscle. Patients should also be assessed for parotid hypertrophy as this can also contribute to the impression of enlarged mandibular angles [29]. Parotid enlargement can be identified by the presence of diffuse swelling that extends beyond the posterior border of the mandible. Luckily, this too can be treated with botulinum toxin.

For treatment of masseter hypertrophy, injection is made at three or four sites on each side of the face [24]. Four to eight onabotulinumtoxinA units should be administered at each injection site deep to the muscle with the needle injected to its full depth. Palpate the point of maximum muscle contraction as well as the anterior margin of the muscle by asking the patient to clench their jaw. The injection sites should be approximately 1 cm apart from one another and form an inverted triangle or a square centered on the masseter body [17] (Fig. 13.8).

Ensure that the most anterior injection points are at least 1 cm posterior to the anterior border of the muscle. The average initial total dose of onabotulinumtoxinA is 12–24 units into each muscle. This can be repeated at 1 month intervals until no palpable movement of the muscle is felt with clenching. This can take up to three or four treatments. Maintenance dosing is typically a total of 20–30 units every 3–6 months.

Possible complications of injections to this area include asymmetries, hematomas [19], crooked smile, and jowling due to volume reduction and sagging of the skin [29]. Avoid unwanted diffusion into the surrounding muscles by keeping the volume of injection less than 1.5 ml at a time [29] and remaining inferior and lateral along the muscle [17]. Patients may experience weakness with chewing or wide

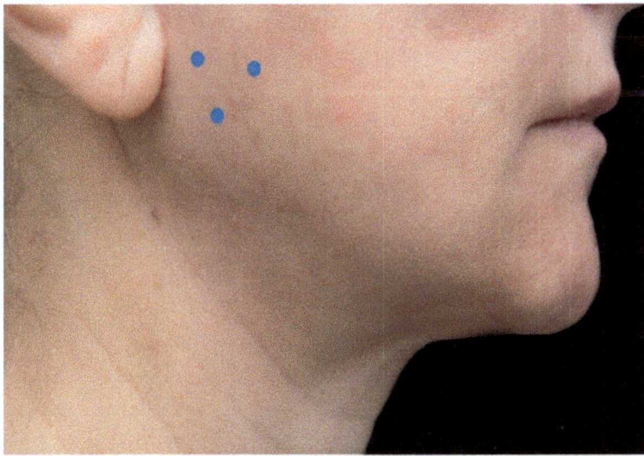

Fig. 13.8 Treatment of masseter hypertrophy is made at three sites on each side of the face. Four to eight onabotulinumtoxinA units should be administered at each injection site deep to the masseter muscle with the needle injected to its full depth. The three to four injection sites should be 1 cm apart from one another and form an inverted triangle or a square centered on the masseter body

mouth opening due to diffusion of the medication into the pterygoid muscles [29]. Temporary fasciculations or paradoxical masseteric bulging may also occur [29] and are typically self-resolving. This is thought to be due to either the deep or superficial portions being treated and the other portion compensating [28].

Platysmal Bands

The platysma muscle acts as a major depressor of the lower face, drawing down the mandible and corners of the mouth [25]. It appears as two superficial thin sheets of muscle that run down the lateral neck below the thin fat layer below the skin [25]. The platysma originates on the pectoralis and deltoid fascia and inserts partially onto the mandible and partially extending up to the muscles of the lower lip and the superficial musculoaponeurotic system (SMAS) [30]. These superior extensions allow the platysma to have a downward pulling effect on the cheek and the corners of the mouth.

One of the first signs of aging is prominent vertical platysmal bands in the neck [31]. This is generally believed to be the result of hyperactivity of the platysma as well as generalized skin laxity [32]. Patients with less skin laxity are better candidates for botulinum treatment, as relaxation of the bands may worsen the appearance of saggy skin [19].

Assess the patient's neck at rest and with maximum contraction. Mark out the trajectory of medial and lateral bands, there may be up to 8 bands observed. Note any skin excess.

Have the patient contract their anterior neck and pinch the band to help guide the injection [25]. Once the band is secured, have the patient release the contraction as this muscle fatigues easily. Inject 2 onabotulinumtoxinA units at 2 cm intervals along the bands, starting at the superior most aspect, between 4–6 injection points per band [24]. Injections should be into the belly of the muscle, but not too deep as to bury the needle.

Additional injections can be added to the supra-mandibular segment of the platysma, resulting in a lifting effect to the midface [33]. Mark 4 points, 1 cm cranial to the superior margin of the bony mandible (1 cm above the jawbone); these points should be at equal distances between the oral commissures and the mandibular angle. Injections should be performed sub-dermally with 2–2.5 units of onabotulinumtoxin A per site for a total of 8–10 units per side.

Dysphagia and dysphonia have been reported as potential complications of botulinum toxin injection in the neck [19]. To mitigate this, avoid injecting more than 50 onabotulinumtoxinA units at one time, keep the doses along the medial bands to a minimum, and avoid injecting too deep [34]. This area is also prone to bruising.

Microtox or Microdroplet

The microbotox technique was first described by Wu in 2015 as a means of improving the overall appearance of the skin in the face and neck. With this technique, multiple microdroplets of diluted botulinum toxin are injected superficially into the dermis to target the sebaceous glands, sweat glands, and superficial fibers of the facial muscles [35]. Patients report an overall improvement in their skin texture, jawline and neck appearance [35], as well as an overall more rested appearance [36]. It remains a simple nonsurgical solution for those patients seeking improvement in mild neck laxity, jowling, horizontal necklines, and rough crepey skin and is a useful adjunct to earlier mentioned techniques.

By affecting the muscles that guard lymphatic drainage, the microdroplet technique affects the osmolality of the skin, leaving patients with a luminous glow [36]. To the relaxation of superficial musculodermal attachments, rhytides are softened and the face appears more relaxed [36, 37]. Inhibition of sweat and sebaceous glands does not only improve skin texture and sheen, it can also reduce the appearance of pores [36]. Muscle function is mostly preserved by sparing their deeper surfaces, resulting in a more natural dynamic appearance.

Microdroplet technique is currently being used for multiple off-label indications including: jawline definition (lower face & neck "lift"), forehead expression lines, midface lift, open pores, rosacea, scarring, and acne [36].

To prepare the solution, 100 units of onabotulinumtoxinA is diluted in four to five milliliters of saline to obtain a concentration of 20–25 U/mL [37]. This concentration can be applied to all areas of the face and neck as described below. An application of a topical anesthetic agent prior to injections is recommended for patient comfort.

Forehead expression lines can be treated with approximately 20–24 units of botulinum toxin type A recommended to be injected into the superficial dermis using a microdroplet technique. Using a 31- or 32-gauge needle, the bevel should be down and the needle inserted just under the skin. Slight resistance should be felt with extrusion and a visible blanched bleb or wheal should appear [36]. Eight to twelve units is recommended for periorbital treatment including canthal lines and the under-eye area [36]. Extra care should be taken in this area as too small of a dose will yield no visible results and too high of a dose may lead to unwanted side effects [36]. Midface can be treated with 20 units across the nose & cheeks in a uniform pattern [36]. For lower face and neck, a total of 24–48 units can be used throughout the entire anterior neck [36]. About 100–150 units place into equally spaced injections should span the width of the platysma muscle defined by a line parallel to the mandibular border 3 fingerbreadths above, a vertical line 1 fingerbreadth posterior to the depressor anguli oris medially, the clavicle inferiorly, and the sternocleidomastoid posteriorly [37] (Fig. 13.9).

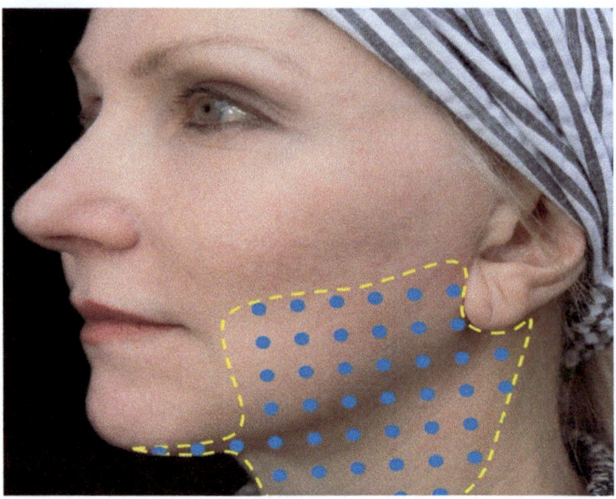

Fig. 13.9 Microbotox injections delivered intradermally at each point indicated. The margins of the area to be injected correspond to the extent of the platysma. The anatomical landmarks are defined by a line parallel to the mandibular border 3 fingerbreadths above, a vertical line 1 finger-breadth posterior to the depressor anguli oris medially, the clavicle inferiorly, and the sternocleido-mastoid posteriorly

Scar Management

Botulinum toxin has been introduced as an effective modality in the prevention and treatment of scars including hypertrophic and keloid scars. It can be a helpful adjunct to other treatment modalities including microneedling and corticosteroid injection [38]. This treatment cannot only improve the appearance of scars (redness, pigmentation, pliability, and height), but it also improves negative symptoms such as pruritis and pain [39]. Injections of botulinum toxin directly into scar tissue improve collagen production and organization, leading to faster wound healing [40].

The exact mechanism is not completely understood, however, there is emerging evidence that botulinum toxin inhibits fibroblast activity in hypertrophic scars and minimises tension around the scar by relaxing local muscles around the wound [41]. Less tension minimizes inflammation and overproduction of collagen [41]. Additionally, the effects of botulinum toxin A on a variety of healing and scarring mechanisms is thought to account for the improved effect on scar tenderness and itch [41, 42]. Of note, these effects of botulinum toxin were not observed in fibro-blasts isolated from normal skin [43].

The exact protocol, timing, and technique for botulinum toxin injections in scar management varies greatly in the literature, however, starting injections upon initial surgery is a common practice [44]. Some studies agree that an intradermal technique within five millimeters of the scar along its length at a dose of 1.5–10 ona-botulinumtoxinA u/cm is quite effective [45, 46]. Concentrations of botulinum toxin should not exceed 20 onabotulinumtoxinA u/ml, as they have been shown to inhibit the development of new blood vessels, and thus affect wound healing [47].

In general, botulinum toxin injections are a safe and effective method for the management and prevention of scarring, however, further large-scale research to determine protocols and assess any long-term effects is warranted.

Conclusion

Botulinum neurotoxins have become a staple product in the medical aesthetic providers' toolbox. Although they are best known for their role in wrinkle reduction, further applications continue to be introduced and explored. Facial balance and form can be improved through strategic applications of botulinum toxin. This versatile medication also plays a role in improving skin tone and texture, luminosity, and scar quality in addition to its effect on salivary gland hypertrophy. This remains a rapidly evolving area for research as new applications for this powerful drug are identified and more specific injection protocols are developed.

References

1. ASPS. Plastic Surgery Statistics Report.; 2018.
2. Monheit G. Neurotoxins: current concepts in cosmetic use on the face and neck-upper face (glabella, forehead, and crow's feet). Plast Reconstr Surg. 2015;136(5):72S–5S. https://doi.org/10.1097/PRS.0000000000001771.
3. Revance Therapeutics Inc, ed. Daxxify Drug Monograph. 2023. https://www.accessdata.fda.gov/drugsatfda_docs/label/2023/761127s002lbl.pdf. Accessed 17 Nov 2023
4. Hui JI, Lee WW. Efficacy of fresh versus refrigerated botulinum toxin in the treatment of lateral periorbital rhytids. Ophthalmic Plast Reconstr Surg. 2007;23(6):433–8. https://doi.org/10.1097/IOP.0b013e31815793b7.
5. Noland ME, Lalonde DH, Yee GJ, Rohrich RJ. Current uses of botulinum neurotoxins in plastic surgery. Plast Reconstr Surg. 2016;138(3):519e–30e.
6. Sattler G, Gout U. Illustrated guide to injectable fillers: basics, indications, uses. Quintessence Publishing; 2016.
7. de Maio M, Swift A, Signorini M, Fagien S. Facial assessment and injection guide for botulinum toxin and injectable hyaluronic acid fillers: focus on the upper face. Plast Reconstr Surg. 2017;140(2):265e–76e.
8. Jaspers G, Pijpe J, Jansma J. The use of botulinum toxin type A in cosmetic facial procedures. Int J Oral Maxillofac Surg. 2011;40:127–33.
9. Zarins U. Anatomy of facial expression. Anatomy Next; 2019.
10. Cotofana S, Freytag DL, Frank K, et al. The bidirectional movement of the frontalis muscle: introducing the line of convergence and its potential clinical relevance. Plast Reconstr Surg. 2020;145(5):1155–62. https://doi.org/10.1097/prs.0000000000006756.
11. Wirta DL, Korenfeld MS, Foster S, et al. Safety of once-daily oxymetazoline hcl ophthalmic solution, 0.1% in patients with acquired blepharoptosis: results from four randomized, double-masked clinical trials. Clin Ophthalmol. 2021;15:4035–48. https://doi.org/10.2147/opth.s322326.

12. Mustak H, Rafaelof M, Goldberg RA, Rootman D. Use of botulinum toxin for the correction of mild ptosis. J Clin Aesthet Dermatol. 2018;11(4):49–51.
13. Turkmani MG. Botulinum toxin treatment for botulinum toxin–induced blepharoptosis. Am. J. Cosmet. Surg. Published Online 2022:074880682211418. https://doi.org/10.1177/07488068221141813
14. de Maio M, Rzany B. Botulinum toxin in aesthetic medicine. Berlin/Heidelberg: Springer; 2009.
15. Cotofana S, Pedraza AP, Kaufman J, et al. Respecting upper facial anatomy for treating the glabella with neuromodulators to avoid medial brow ptosis—a refined 3-point injection technique. J Cosmet Dermatol. 2021;20(6):1625–33. https://doi.org/10.1111/jocd.14133.
16. Khan S, Pathak G, Milgraum D, Tamhankar M, Milgraum S. Double vision due to lateral rectus injury after cosmetic botulinum toxin injections. Australas J Dermatol. 2023;64(3) https://doi.org/10.1111/ajd.14120.
17. Wu DC, Fabi SG, Goldman MP. Neurotoxins: current concepts in cosmetic use on the face and neck-lower face. Plast Reconstr Surg. 2015;136(5):76S–9S.
18. Jain P, Rathee M. Anatomy, head and neck, orbicularis Oris muscle. StatPearls; 2019.
19. de Maio M, Wu WTL, Goodman GJ, Monheit G. Facial assessment and injection guide for botulinum toxin and injectable hyaluronic acid fillers: focus on the lower face. Plast Reconstr Surg. 2017;140(3):393e–404e.
20. Cohen J, Dayan S, Cox S. OnabotulinumtoxinA dose-ranging study for hyperdynamic perioral lines. Dermatologic Surg. 2012;38:1497–505.
21. Packirisamy V, Sadacharan CM. Preference of eyebrow apex positions on different facial shapes in Malaysian population: an inter-ethnic study. J Cosmet Dermatol. 2021;20(12):3991–4000. https://doi.org/10.1111/jocd.14062.
22. Tong J, Bhupendra CP. Anatomy, head and neck, eye orbicularis oculi muscle. StatPearls; 2019.
23. Deka A, Saikia SP. Botulinum toxin for lower lid Entropion correction. Orbit. 2011;30(1):40–2.
24. Yi K-H, Lee J-H, Hu H-W, Kim H-J. Novel anatomical guidelines on botulinum neurotoxin injection for wrinkles in the nose region. Toxins. 2022;14(5):342. https://doi.org/10.3390/toxins14050342.
25. Carruthers JD, Glogau RG, Blitzer A. Facial aesthetics consensus group faculty. Advances in facial rejuvenation: botulinum toxin type a, hyaluronic acid dermal fillers, and combination therapies. Consensus recommendations. Plast Reconstr Surg. 2008;121(5):5S–30S.
26. Hur MS, Kim HJ, Choi BY, Hu KS, Kim HJ, Lee KS. Morphology of the mentalis muscle and its relationship with the orbicularis oris and incisivus labii inferioris muscles. J Craniofac Surg. 2013;24(2):602–4.
27. Kane MAC. The functional anatomy of the lower face as it applies to rejuvenation via Chemodenervation. Facial Plast Surg. 2005;21(1):55–64.
28. Rice SM, Nassim JS, Hersey EM, Kourosh AS. Prevention and correction of paradoxical masseteric bulging following botulinum toxin injection for masseter hypertrophy. Int J Women's Dermatol. 2021;7(5):815–6. https://doi.org/10.1016/j.ijwd.2021.03.002.
29. Wu WT. Botox facial slimming/facial sculpting: the role of botulinum toxin-a in the treatment of Hypertophic masseteric muscle and parotid enlargement to narrow the lower facial width. Facial Plast Surg Clin N Am. 2010;18:133–40.
30. Levy PM. Neurotoxins: current concepts in cosmetic use on the face and neck-jawline contouring/platysma bands/necklace lines. Plast Reconstr Surg. 2015;136(5):80S–3S.
31. Sandulescu T, Stoltenberg F, Buechner H, et al. Platysma and the cervical superficial musculoaponeurotic system—comparative analysis of facial crease and platysmal band development. Ann Anat. 2019;
32. Trévidic P, Criollo-Lamilla G. Platysma bands: is a change needed in the surgical paradigm? Plast Reconstr Surg. 2017;139(1):41–7.
33. Hernandez CA, Davidovic K, Avelar LE, et al. Facial soft tissue repositioning with neuromodulators: lessons learned from facial biomechanics. Aesthet Surg J. 2022;42(10):1163–71. https://doi.org/10.1093/asj/sjac090.

34. Carruthers J, Carruthers A. Aesthetic botulinum A toxin in the mid and lower face and neck. Dermatologic Surg. 2003;29:468–76.
35. Awaida CJ, Jabbour SF, Rayess YA, El Khoury JS, Kechichian EG, Nasr MW. Evaluation of the microbotox technique: an algorithmic approach for lower face and neck rejuvenation and a crossover clinical trial. Plast Reconstr Surg. 2018;142(3):640–9.
36. Kaur I, Kandhari R, Gupta J, Al-Niaimi F. Microdroplet botulinum toxin: a review. J Cutan Aesthet Surg. 2022;15(2):101. https://doi.org/10.4103/jcas.jcas_162_21.
37. Wu W. Microbotox of the lower face and neck: evolution of a personal technique and its clinical effects. Plast Reconstr Surg. 2015;136(5 Suppl):92S–100S.
38. Morsy EE, Hussien TM, Maksoud OMA. Needling combined with Intralesional corticosteroid injections compared to Intralesional botulinum toxin A injections in the treatment of hypertrophic scars and. J Dermatol Plast Surg. 2019;3(1):1–6.
39. Scala J, Vojvodic A, Vojvodic P, et al. Botulinum toxin use in scars/keloids treatment botulinum toxin use in scars/keloids treatment. Maced J Med Sci. 2019, August;
40. Xiao Z, Zhang F, Lin W, Zhang M, Liu Y. Effect of botulinum toxin type A on transforming growth factor beta1 in fibroblasts derived from hypertrophic scar: a preliminary report. Aesth Plast Surg. 2010;34(4):424–7.
41. Zhang S, Li K, Yu Z, et al. Dramatic effect of botulinum toxin type A on hypertrophic scar: a promising therapeutic drug and its mechanism through the SP-NK1R pathway in cutaneous neurogenic inflammation. Front Med. 2022:9. https://doi.org/10.3389/fmed.2022.820817.
42. Sohrabi C, Goutos I. The use of botulinum toxin in keloid scar management: a literature review. Scars Burns Healing. 2020;6:205951312092662. https://doi.org/10.1177/2059513120926628.
43. Huang C, Akaishi S, Hyakusoku H, Ogawa R. Are keloid and hypertrophic scar different forms of the same disorder? A fibroproliferative skin disorder hypothesis based on keloid findings. Int Wound J. 2014;11(5):517–22.
44. Yang W, Li G. The safety and efficacy of botulinum toxin type A injection for postoperative scar prevention: a systematic review and meta-analysis. J Cosmet Dermatol. 2019;June:1–10.
45. Li Y, Yang J, Liu J, et al. A randomized, placebo-controlled, double-blind, prospective clinical trial of botulinum toxin type A in prevention of hypertrophic scar development in median sternotomy wound. Aesth Plast Surg. 2018;42:1364–9.
46. Chen Z, Chen Z, Pang R, et al. The effect of botulinum toxin injection dose on the appearance of surgical scar. Sci Rep. 2021;11(1) https://doi.org/10.1038/s41598-021-93203-x.
47. Gugerell A, Kober J, Schmid M. Botulinum toxin A: dose- dependent effect on reepithelialization and angiogenesis. Plast Reconstr Surg Glob Open. 2016;4:e837.

Chapter 14
Botulinum Toxin Therapy for Autonomic Dysfunction (Excessive Drooling/Sialorrhea and Excessive Sweating (Hyperhidrosis) and for Certain Skin Disorders

Abstract Injection of botulinum toxins to the glands reduces the secretion of saliva or sweat by blocking the release of nerve signal transmitter acetylcholine. This action can help patients who suffer from local excessive sweating or those who are affected by persistent drooling. Salivary and sweat glands are located under the skin and are readily accessible to surface injections. The emerging data suggests that intense, recalcitrant local itch and some forms of psoriasis also respond to local botulinum toxin injections.

Keywords Botulinum toxin · Botulinum neurotoxin · Drooling · Sialorrhea · Perspiration · Excessive sweating · Psoriasis · Itch

Introduction

Salivary glands that secret saliva and sweat glands receive their innervation from the sympathetic and parasympathetic nervous systems. Sympathetic and parasympathetic nervous systems are part of the autonomic nervous system. Autonomic nervous system is a part of nervous system that, unlike the motor system, is not under voluntary control and contains very thin nerve fibers. Saliva and sweat are secreted in response to peripheral stimuli independent of the individuals' wish and/or will. The sympathetic nervous system excites the salivary and sweat glands. Sympathetic nerves also innervate important muscles in the body such as heart and intestine. Stimulation of the sympathetic nerves increases the number of heart beats while slowing down movements of the gut, neither of the two are under voluntary control. Parasympathetic nervous system is another major part of autonomic nervous system that opposes the function of the sympathetic nervous system (for example it slows heartbeat or increases movements of the gut). Sympathetic and parasympathetic nerves are much thinner than motor and sensory nerves and are devoid of the fatty myelin sheet (myelin) that covers motor and sensory nerves and enhances their conduction. Like motor nerves, sympathetic nerves also use a chemical agent at their endings that activates their targets (salivary or sweat glands). This chemical neurotransmitter that excites the seat glands, like that of the motor nerves (exiting muscle), is acetylcholine.

Botulinum neurotoxins (BoNT) which are produced by a bacteria called clostridium botulinum, were purified and prepared for medical use between 1940 and 1970 (see Chaps. 1 and 3 of this book for details). The toxin molecule travels to the nerve endings after injection into the muscle or into the skin; then, through a cascade of complicated mechanisms (see Chap. 2 of this book), it blocks the release of acetylcholine from the nerve endings. This function of botulinum toxin has made it a useful commodity for treatment of a variety movement disorders, characterized by involuntary movements. Blocking acetylcholine release also decreases the muscle tone, and hence, helps spastic muscles to relax, After receiving FDA approval, botulinum toxins are now widely used for reducing stiffness and spasticity of muscles in stroke, multiple sclerosis and cerebral palsy . Since sympathetic nerve endings also use acetylcholine as the chemical neurotransmitter to activate salivary and sweat glands, injection of BoNT into these glands can reduce secretion of saliva and sweat when excessive salivation and sweating become problematic.

Anatomy and Physiology of Salivary Glands

Three glands (parotid, submandibular, and sublingual) are the major producers of saliva (Fig. 14.1). Saliva plays an important role in lubrication, digestion, immunity and maintenance of homeostasis in the human body. The parotid gland is located under the skin in front of lower part of the ear and extends to the angle of the jaw. It is divided by the facial nerve into a superficial lobe and a deep lobe. The submandibular gland, the second largest salivary gland after the parotid, is located in the submandibular (under the jawbone) triangle. The sublingual (under the tongue)

Fig. 14.1 Location of the three major salivary glands: parotid, Submandibular (under the jaw) and sublingual (under the tongue) glands. (Printed with permission from Mayo Foundation)

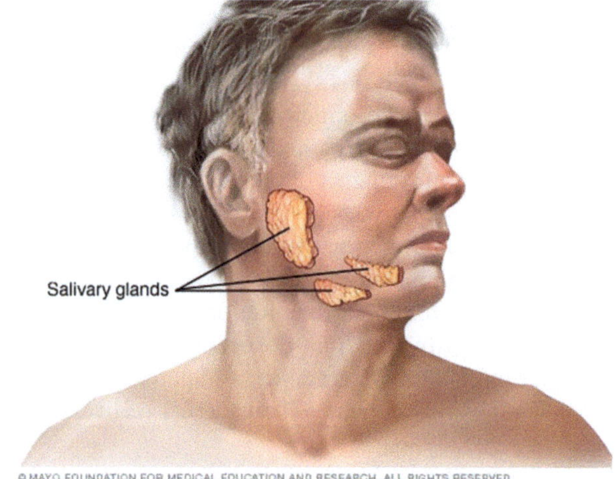

gland is the smallest of the three and lies in the anterior floor of the mouth below the tongue (Fig. 14.1). Each gland produces high volumes of saliva relative to its mass. Since parotid gland is the largest (14–28 g), most saliva is produced by this gland. Production of saliva is not controlled by an individual's will, but rather, it is controlled by the autonomic nervous system, sympathetic and parasympathetic nerve fibers. In stimulated state, i.e. chewing, parotid glands provide most of the saliva. In the unstimulated state, however, 70% of saliva is secreted by the submandibular (weighs 10–15 g) and sublingual glands. The flow of saliva is five times greater in the stimulated state than in the resting state.

Sialorrhea or drooling is a debilitating condition which implies presence of excess saliva in the mouth beyond the lip margin. Drooling is common in babies but subsides between the ages 15 and 36 months with establishment of salivary continence. Drooling is considered abnormal if it persists beyond 4 years of age.

Pathologic drooling can be due to increased production of saliva (usually due to certain drugs) or related to disease conditions that disrupt mechanisms that clear and remove saliva from the mouth. These diseases cause retention of saliva in the mouth and drooling through weakening the tongue or through impairing the swallowing reflexes. Drooling frequently occurs in neurological diseases such as Parkinson's disease (PD), amyotrophic lateral sclerosis (Lou Gehrig's disease -ALS) and with degenerative disease of the nervous system as well as different type of dementias. In a large study of 691 patients with Parkinson, the prevalence of drooling was 40.1% versus 2.4% of controls [1]. In children, the most common cause of drooling is cerebral palsy with an incidence of 10–58% [2]. Among medications used to treat schizophrenia, clozapine has been reported to cause daytime drooling in 40% of the patients; 31.6 awaken from sleep because of drooling [3]. Regardless of the cause, excessive drooling can lead to social embarrassment, aspiration, skin breakout, bad odor, and sometimes local infection, impairing the patients' quality of life.

Sialorrhea is difficult to treat. Management can be conservative or invasive. Conservative treatments include changes in diet or habits of eating, oral-motor exercises, intra-oral devices such as palatal training devices, and oral medications. Behavioral modification has been advocated by some, but results have been inconsistent. Severe cases of drooling non-responsive to medications may require removal of salivary glands by surgery or local radiation of the salivary glands. Surgical approach offers more permanent results, but it is an invasive process that is not without side effects. Local radiation of the glands is now hardly practiced.

The main category of drugs used for reduction of drooling is anticholinergic medications. These medications block the effect of acetylcholine that activates the glands resulting in secretion of saliva. Several anticholinergic drugs are available in the market under the trade names of glycopyrrolate, benztropine, scopalamine and tropicamide. Glycopyrrolate oral solution is the first drug approved in the United States for treatment of drooling in children who have neurologic conditions. Elderly patients tolerate oral anticholinergic agents poorly due to side effects such as confusion and blurring of vision. Glycopyrrolate is a favorite of many physicians since presence of a quaternary ammonium in its molecule prevents its passage through blood-brain barrier in large amounts, ultimately decreasing the occurrence of central side effects such as confusion and memory impairment. Medications that are used for relieving heartburn and reflux have also been suggested for treatment of drooling; however, their effectiveness in managing drooling has not been confirmed by any high quality studies (comparing the drug with placebo).

Botulinum Neurotoxin (BoNT) Therapy for Excessive Drooling (Sialorrhea)

Among different serotypes of botulinum toxins, only type A and B are currently used in medical practice, due to their safety profile and long duration action. Among type A toxins, Botox,Xeomin and Dsyport have been studied in excessive drooling and excessive sweating as well as type B toxin Myobloc. The structural and functional details of these toxins as well as their unit comparability has be described earlier in Chaps. 2 and 3 of this book as well as the preceding chapters. In brief, each 1 unit of Botox = 1 unit of Xeomin = 2.5–3 units of Dysport = 40–50 units of Myobloc.

As described in earlier chapters, both types of botulinum toxins (A and B) can block the effect of acetylcholine, a neurotransmitter at nerve-muscle or nerve-gland junction that activates the muscle and certain glands. Glands that secrete saliva and sweat are activated by acetylcholine. Based on this premise, in 1999, Dr. Bhatia and his colleagues from London first showed that injection of 10–20 units of Dysport (a type A toxin commonly used in England) into the parotid glands (Fig. 14.1) can significantly reduce patients' drooling [4]. The four patients in their study had different disorders involving the central nervous system; one of the four had Parkinson disease. There were no side effects. Since then, the efficacy and safety of BoNTs in management of sialorrhea has been assessed by several larger and high quality studies (comparing toxin injection with placebo). A majority of these studies were conducted using the type B toxin (Myobloc). These studies have found objective evidence (measured by reduction in the saliva volume) for efficacy of BoNT injection into salivary glands for reducing chronic drooling [5–8]. Most studied patients expressed satisfaction with treatment and indicated improvement of their quality of life. In adults, side effects were infrequent and minor consisting of slight local pain at the time of injection, minor local bleeding and subtle, transient swallowing difficulty (very uncommon). Patients with drooling in Parkinson's disease responded better than other patients. The effect of toxin therapy lasted 3–6 months. Based on high quality and large multicenter studies, FDA approved the use of Myobloc for sialorrhea in 2010 and the use of Xeomin (a type A toxin similar to Botox) in 2018.

Comparative studies conducted to define similarity or differences of various toxins' efficacy in reduction of chronic drooling are scarcely reported in the literature. In one study, botulinum toxin B (Myobloc) was shown to have comparable efficacy with botulinum toxinA (Dysport), but it demonstrated a faster onset of action for reduction of drooling [9]. The authors found that Myobloc was also less costly for patients than Dysport. In another study, Myobloc and Dysport had comparable efficacy in treatment of chronic drooling [10]. One review has reported comparable duration of effectiveness between Myobloc (type B toxin) and Xeomin (type A toxin) (the two toxins approved by FDA) in treatment of chronic drooling [11].

Technique of Injection

A small narrow syringe (1 cc) with 10 divisions of 0.1 cc and a short, thin needle (½ to ¾ inch, gauge 30) is used for injection of the toxin into the glands. Although many physicians inject only the parotid gland, injection of both parotid and submaxillary glands probably renders better results. Many physicians perform injections based merely on the anatomical knowledge of the parotid and submaxillary gland locations without the use of ancillary techniques such as ultrasound (Fig. 14.1). Both glands, especially the parotid glands, are readily accessible to a small needle approaching from the surface of skin as they are only a few millimeters under the skin. In adults, numbing of the skin is not necessary since the needles are very small and injections are very quick and superficial.

The author of this chapter had excellent results in many patients with chronic drooling by injecting only parotid glands in chronic drooling. If the parotid injection did not work, even after increasing the dose for the second injection (usually performed 3–4 months later), then a combined injection of parotid and submaxillary gland was carried out; in great majority of the patients the combined injection significantly improved the sialorrhea (Fig. 14.2).

A more precise way to perform parotid and submaxillary injections for drooling is via the use of ultrasound. Under ultrasound guidance, it is possible to visualize the gland, see the tip of the needle as it is approaching and entering into the gland as well as visualization of the injected material into the gland. In adults, usually, no local anaesthesia is necessary before injections. The number of injections per gland varies among different physicians. Most physicians recommend injecting into 2 or more sites for the parotid gland.

One of common causes of drooling in children is cerebral palsy. The term cerebral palsy is applied to an unfortunate medical ailment of children in which, during birth or infancy, brain is damaged causing significant motor deficit and /or disorder such as paralysis or involuntary movements. Most affected children have degrees of mental retardation. The cause of CP, in most cases, is poor oxygenation of the brain during birth or genetic/ metabolic disorders that damage the brain during pregnancy or shortly after birth. In a study of 113 children with cerebral palsy, aged 6–17, 48.7% had chronic drooling that was defined as severe in 27.7% of them [12].

Over the past 15 years, several researchers have explored the role of botulinum toxin therapy in chronic drooling of children, specifically in children with cerebral palsy. Based on the positive results of a large multi-center study including 255 children aged 2–17 years, FDA approved the use of Xeomin, a type A botulinum toxin with units comparable to Botox, for treatment of sialorrhea in children [13].

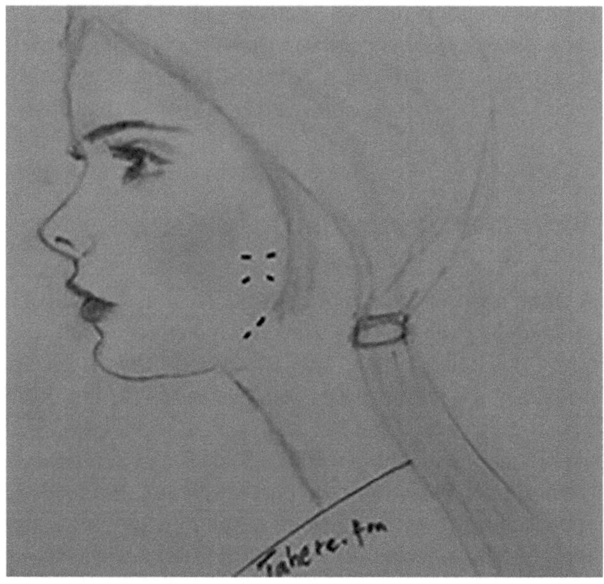

Fig. 14.2 Author's injection technique using 4 injection sites for the parotid gland and 2 injection sites for the submaxillary gland (located below the jawbone close to angle of the jaw). (Drawing courtesy of Dr. Tahereh Mousavi)

Although other type A toxins and the type B toxin are not yet approved by FDA use in children in US, there are several studies strongly suggesting that Botox is also effective for this indication in children [14].

Recently, Fan and coworkers conducted a study in 41 children, 3 years of age and younger, with chronic sialorrhea who had neurologic and congenital disorders. Following botulinum toxin injections into both the parotid and submaxillary glands, the authors noted significant reduction of salivation and decreased number of hospital admissions for pneumonia. Also the treated children no longer needed to use anticholinergic drugs (drugs working against acetylcholine) for treatment of sialorrhea [15].

Technical Issues and Toxin Dose

The technique of injection of botulinum toxins for sialorrea in children is similar to that described earlier for adults. Due to sensitivity of children to injection induced pain, it is advisable to numb the skin with an anesthetic cream (for instance, Emla cream) an hour before injection into the glands. Further application of a numbing skin spray seconds before each injection is also helpful in children.

Side effects of botulinum toxin therapy in children is similar to those experienced adults. In some studies, transient, mild difficulty with swallowing has been mentioned. This could be avoided in most cases by starting with a smaller dose and performing injections under ultrasound that shows the exact location of the glands. This side effect is more common after submandibular gland injection that is closer to the neck.

Excessive Sweating (Hyperhidrosis)

Hyperhidrosis (excessive sweating) is a debilitating condition that can lead to emotional and social embarrassment. In severe cases, it can cause occupational, physical and psychological disability [16].

Hyperhidrosis can be classified into primary and secondary hyperhidrosis. Primary hyperhidrosis has an incidence of 0.6–1% in general population [17]. Many cases of childhood hyperhidrosis are hereditary with more than one family member affected. A genetically dominant form of excessive sweating with onset in childhood is now recognized with a defined abnormality of chromosome 14.

The diagnostic criteria for primary hyperhidrosis include excessive sweating for at least 6 months, no obvious cause and at least two of the following features: sweating occurs at least once per week, sweating is impairs daily activities, a bilateral and relatively symmetric pattern of sweating, an age of onset younger than 25 years, positive family history and cessation of focal sweating during sleep.

Secondary hyperhidrosis can be caused by certain drugs (for example sertraline), induced by toxins (acrylamide)], or caused by a systemic illness (endocrine and metabolic disorders, tumors, spinal cord lesions). Certain congenital disorders that involve the autonomic nervous system such as familial dysautonomia (Riley-Day syndrome) are also often associated with excessive sweating. Among the other causes of secondary hyperhidrosis is compensatory hyperhidrosis. In this condition, there is increased sweating in parts of the body below the level of a surgery called sympathectomy. Gustatory hyperhidrosis is a familial disorder in which, the face sweats during eating. Gustatory hyperhidrosis can be the result of trauma to the face or neck or happen after parotid gland surgery.

The glands that secret sweat are called eccrine and apocrine glands. There are about 4 million sweat glands in the body. Eccrine glands (the most frequent sweat glands) have the highest concentration in the region of the armpit (axilla), palms and sole of the feet; hence, these are the primary areas involved in excessive sweating. Excessive sweating of the face and scalp is less common. Sympathetic nervous system, a division of autonomic nervous system, stimulates the sweat glands. As mentioned earlier in this chapter, the nerves of the autonomic nervous system (sympathetic or parasympathetic) are very thin fibers with slow conduction (compared to motor nerves) and function independent of individual's will. Sympathetic nerves use acetylcholine the chemical transmitter that excites the sweat glands.

Anatomy and Physiology of Sweating

The pathway for control of sweating (sudomotor pathway) starts from the nerve cells located at thin (few millimeters) covering (cortex) of brain. Cortex contains millions of nerve cells. From cortex, the fibers travel down to lower centers of the nervous system which exert autonomic control such as hypothalamus (a region deep in the brain where growth hormone is secreted) and the medulla (elongated lower part of the brain before spinal cord). The sweat fibers cross in medulla and travel on to the other side of the spinal cord. Emerging from the lateral part of the spinal cord, sympathetic nerves involved in secretion of sweat enter sympathetic ganglia. Sympathetic ganglia are a bunch of sympathetic nerve cells that receive the message from the cortex and send their fibers to the sweat glands. These fibers as describes above are very thin with acetylcholine at their end as chemical activator of the sweat gland. A lesion anywhere in this pathway can interrupt the secretion of sweat.

Sweat glands in the palms and soles are mostly activated by emotional stimuli. Primary hyperhidrosis which is usually familial and absent during sleep, most likely results from abnormal function of the areas of the brain responsible for emotional sweating such as hypothalamus. Sweating also happens during exposure to external heat. It is believed this form sweating which has a more diffuse distribution (including face and scalp) has a different anatomic pathway in the brain.

Treatment of Excessive Sweating (Hyperhidrosis)

Treatment strategies to control excessive sweating include application of topical agents on the skin, administration of oral medications, a procedure called iontophoresis and local injection of botulinum toxins into the sweated areas.

Aluminum salts are the main topical agents used for treatment of hyperhidrosis. Their mechanism of action is not clear but is attributed to either an interaction between aluminum chloride and keratin in the sweat ducts leading to sweat duct closure or a direct action on the excretory eccrine gland epithelium (lining cells of the sweat gland). Aluminum salts are only effective for mild cases of hyperhidrosis; the duration of their effect is often limited to 48 h. Skin irritation, probably related to high salt concentration is the main side effect of aluminum salt treatment.

Glycopyrrolate (1–2 mg twice a day), oxybutynin (5–7.5 mg twice a day), and methantheline bromide (50 mg twice a day) are commonly used anticholinergic agents for pharmacological management of hyperhidrosis. Side effects, especially in elderly, can be disabling and include dry mouth, blurring of vision, urinary hesitancy, dizziness, tachycardia, and confusion. Clonidine, given as 0.1 mg twice a day, is also partially effective by inhibiting the sympathetic output; side effects include dry mouth, dizziness, constipation, sedation and a fall in blood pressure.

Iontophoresis is a procedure that introduces an ionized substance through application of a direct electrical current on intact skin. Tap water and anticholinergic agents (glycopyrrolate) are usually used for iontophoresis. Tap water iontophoresis must be performed initially every 2 to 3 days until therapeutic effect is achieved. Once the therapeutic effect is achieved for 2 weeks, treatment can be done once every 2–3 weeks. Duration of the effect for both tap water and anticholinergic iontophoresis is only a few days which makes iontophoresis an undesirable mode of treatment for hyperhidrosis.

Botulinum Toxin Treatment of Hyperhidrosis

Injection of botulinum toxin into the skin is now an established mode of treatment for excessive sweating. Its advantage over other modes of treatment include less frequent side effects and long duration of action (3–6 months) after a single injection session, eliminating the need for taking daily oral medications or daily application of topical creams.

Over the past 20 years, several high quality studies (comparing toxin injections with placebo injections) have demonstrated that injections of BoNTs into or under the skin, reduces the volume of the local sweating way out of proportion to placebo injections. Although the injection are painful, (despite topical application of numbing cream before injections), 90% of the adults tolerate the injections and prefer 15–20 min of discomfort to debilitating excessive sweating. At the present time Botox and Xeomin are FDA approved for management of hyperhidrosis in adults and children older than 9 years,; the medical literature, however, indicates that Dysport (another type A toxin) and the type B toxin (Myobloc) are also effective for this indication. Long-term follow-ups exceeding 10 years are now available and have shown continued efficacy of BoNT injections in hyperhidrosis with no reduction of efficacy after prolonged use.

Technique of Injections

Injections are performed with a thin (gauge 30) and short needle (½ inch) into the skin, using a grid like scheme (Fig. 14.3). Since the skin is sensitive and many injections are needed, it is advisable to numb the skin before injections. Emla cream can be applied to the intended areas (armpit, palm, sole of the foot) an hour before the injections. The author also uses a numbing spray intermittently during the injections that provides additional numbing of the skin for a few seconds. The injected dose of toxin per site should be very small in order to avoid weakening of the muscles underneath the skin. This is particularly important in the palm area to avoid weakness of the fingers. For Botox and Xeomin, the advocated dose per injection site is 2–2.5 units. For Dysport (another type A toxin) and Myobloc (type B toxin) the units used are higher, 2.5–3 times and 40–50 times compared to Botox units, respectively. Most authors inject at 20 sites in each armpit and inject more sites for the

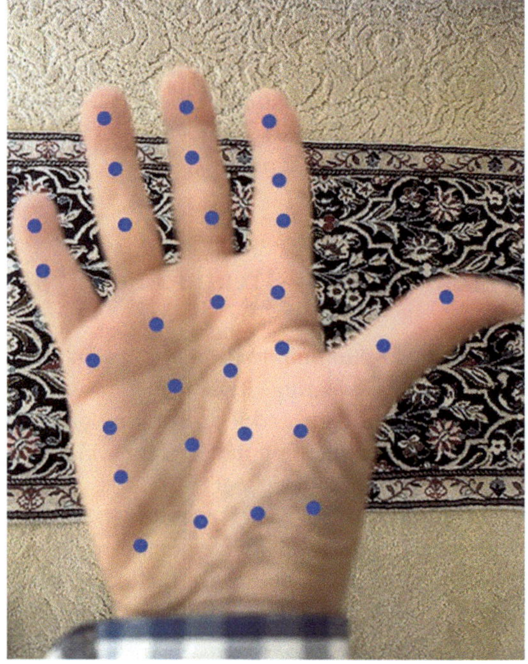

Fig. 14.3 The author has recommended sites of toxin injections for excessive sweating of the palm. From author's collection. The seating hand usually dies up within a week

palm and foot injections. Usually fingers and toes are also covered in the plan of injections (Fig. 14.3). Excessive sweating in a great majority of cases is bilateral; hence injections should cover both sides. In experienced hands, Botox (or other toxins) injections can be performed quickly over 10-15 min for each side. Side effects are uncommon and usually are limited to local pain and minor bleeding.

Case Report

A 42-year-old woman was referred to Yale Botulinum Toxin Clinic for excessive sweating of the sole of the feet since childhood. Her mother and younger brother had the same problem since their early teens. She had no other health problems. She stated that excessive seating was the source of major social embarrassment for her. She has tried different anticholinergic medications for management of her foot hyperhidrosis, but the effect was modest and oral drugs caused disturbing dry mouth and blurring of vision. After numbing the sole of the feet with Emla cream, she was injected with Botox on both feet. The total dose of Botox per foot was between 70 and 75 units; 2.5 units injected per site. She tolerated the procedure and had no side effects. Over the next 6 years of follow up, patient visited the clinic every 4–6 months and received similar injections. She continued to do well; each time expressing satisfaction with the treatment.

Current strategies for management of drooling (sialorrhea) and excessive sweating (hyperhidrosis) are discussed in detail in several publications [18–22].

Potential Indications of BoNT Therapy in some Skin Disorders: Intractable Itch and Psoriasis

Recalcitrant Itch (Pruritus)

Itch is an irritating sensation involving a part of skin often provoking a scratch response to relieve it. In many cases, acute itch is part of a body defense mechanism against an external noxious stimulus. Chronic itch can be seen in a variety of disease conditions such as skin disorders (i.e. psoriasis), systemic disorders (kidney or liver dysfunction), diabetes, infectious conditions and nerve damage from an external cause. It is believed that itching sensation is conveyed to the brain by very thin nerve fibers similar to those that carry pain sensation. Chronic itch is defined as an itch that lasts more than 6 weeks. The prevalence of chronic itch (CP) in general population is 13.5% [23].

Treatment of persistent itch includes non-pharmacological approaches, pharmacological approaches and neurostimulation. Non-pharmacological approaches include wearing protective garments, avoiding warm temperature and ultraviolet exposure. Pharmacological therapy includes application of cooling lotions, emollient creams, capsaicin, lidocaine 5%, cortisone creams and tacrolimus [24]. Anecdotal reports suggest efficacy of antiepileptic drugs pregabalin, carbamazepine and lamotrigine in management of chronic itch disorder [25]. Transient stimulation of peripheral nerves (neural stimulation) has been reported to provide temporary relief from recalcitrant itch in a limited number of patients.

Botulinum Toxin Treatment of Chronic Itch

After injection into the muscle or skin, botulinum toxins block the release and action of several specific proteins which are important in transmission of pain sensation to the brain. Some of these proteins such as histamine and substance P are believed to be important in the pathophysiology of itch as well. One of the earliest reports on the efficacy of Botox in alleviating recalcitrant itch was published by the author of this chapter and his co-workers at Yale University in 2008 [26], and is described below.

Case Report

A 55-year-old woman presented to the clinic evaluation of intense right facial itch for the past 6 years. The affected area extended from the medial part of the right eyebrow up across the forehead ending at the hairline. She had had a right frontal sinus injury 14 years ago. The skin at the region of forehead surgery had a tingling sensation for several years before the intense itch developed in the same area. Treatment with oral medications and local novocaine injections provided minimal relief. With the patient's consent, Botox was injected into the right side of the forehead into the area of intense itch (Fig. 14.4). Similar areas were injected on the left side of the forehead in order to maintain forehead symmetry. The dose per site was 5 units.

After a week, the patient reported marked reduction of the itch intensity which lasted for months. The patient moved out of the area and was lost to follow up for 6 months. She returned to the clinic a year later for a second injection. The injection again relieved her itch. In her words, "Botox injection was the only thing that helped her itch problem."

In 2017, another group of investigators have shown similar results with Botox injection into the skin following intense itch induced by skin injection of cowhage (an itch producing plant) in 35 normal human volunteers [27]. In 2022, Dr. Gazerani published a review on the issue of positive botulinum toxin effects in animal models of itch as well as itch in human subjects including the information from his own

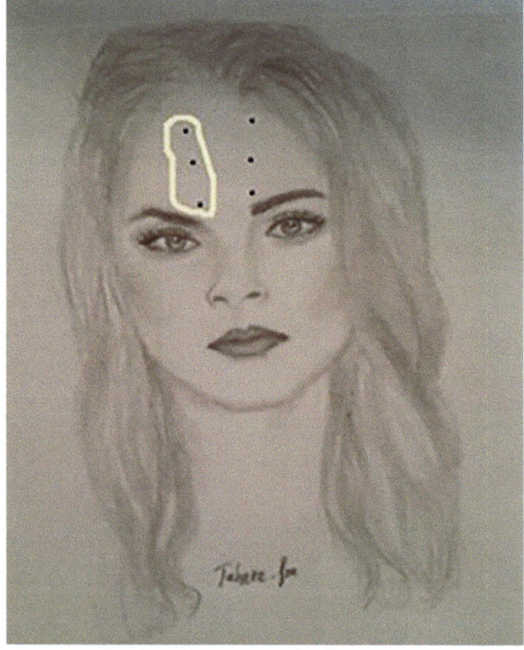

Fig. 14.4 Botox injection for recalcitrant itch of the right forehead (area of itch is marked in yellow). Injection dose is 5 units of Botox per site- Drawing courtesy of Dr. Tahere Mousavi

earlier blinded study that had shown showed injection of botox into the skin reduced intensity of itch in 14 normal volunteers afcted by itch after histamine injection [28].

Psoriasis

Psoriasis is a common skin lesion characterized by proliferation of skin cells causing raised and discolored skin areas. The affected skin areas often itch and cause local pain and are cosmetically unpleasant. In plaque psoriasis, lesions can affect any part of the body, whereas in inverse psoriasis, psoriatic lesions involve the area of skin folds (armpit, groin, etc.). Psoriasis is considered an autoimmune disease in that the immune system of the patient mistakenly attacks the patient's own tissue- skin.

In 1998, Dr. Zanchi and his colleagues published results of their study on 15 patients with inverse psoriasis who were given Botox injections (50–100 units) into the psoriatic skin lesions [29]. The lesions were located in the armpit, groin and, in several women below the breast in the inframammary (under the breast) fold. Injections were performed in a grid-like pattern, 2.8 centimeters apart, with each site receiving 2.4 units of Botox. Patients were followed for 2, 4 and 12 days. All patients reported improvement of itch and local pain. Photographs of the lesions demonstrated notable improvement of redness and healing of the lesions in 13 of 15 patients. In the following years, other investigators have published reports indicating improvement of skin lesion in both plaque and inverse psoriasis after botulinum toxin injections [30–33] (Fig. 14.5).

Contrary to these reports, Todberg and co-workers in a double-blind and placebo controlled investigation of botulinum toxin effect on psoriasis (8 subjects) were unable to achieve positive results [34]. After 8 weeks, none of the patients reported clinical improvement and the injected lesions with botulinum toxin did not change and looked the same as psoriatic lesions injected with saline (salt water). However, in this study the investigators used Dysport (a different type A botulinum toxin). As 2.5-3 units of Dysport approximates 1 unit of Botox. Hence, 36 units of Dysport used in this study is equivalent to 10.2–15 units of Botox, much less than 50–100 units used in the study of Zanchi and coworkers [29]. Since success in Botulinum toxin treatment is highly dose dependent, the failure of this study could be due to the use of inadequate (too low) amount of the toxin.

Conclusion

Local injections of botulinum toxins (A or B) have been shown to be effective in reducing saliva and sweat in patients affected by chronic drooling or excessive sweating. Limited data from uncontrolled studies (no comparison with placebo)

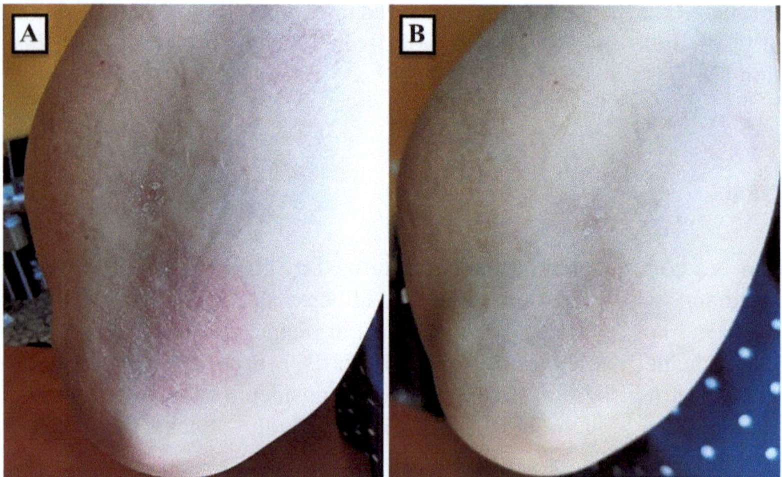

Fig. 14.5 (**a**) Psoriasis of the elbow and extensor surface of the forearm a month before Botulinum toxin injection (**b**) Significant improvement of psoriatic lesion following injection of 1000 units of Dysport (approximately 300–350 units of Botox) for treatment of elbow spasticity (see Chaps. 6 and 7 for spasticity treatment in stroke and multiple sclerosis with botulinum toxins). (Courtesy of Dr. Popescu and colleagues 2022 and publisher-Medicina. Reproduced under Creative Commons Attribution (CC BY) license (https://creativecommons.org/licenses/by/4.0/)

suggest that injection of Botox into the skin can alleviate local recalcitrant itch. Recent observations on psoriatic skin lesions also strongly suggest that injections of Botox into psoriatic skin plaques can heal the lesions and improve patients' symptoms as well as their quality of life. Side effects of botulinum toxin treatment for excessive drooling and sweating as well as botulinum toxin for recalcitrant itch and psoriasis have been infrequent, minor and transient (transient local pain from injection and, in some cases, minor bleeding).

References

1. Santos-García D, de Deus Fonticoba T et al. Prevalence and factors associated with drooling in Parkinson's disease: results from a longitudinal prospective cohort and comparison with a control group. Parkinsons Dis. 2023 Apr 6;2023:3104425. https://doi.org/10.1155/2023/3104425. PMID: 37065970. PMCID: PMC10101739.
2. Dias BL, Fernandes AR, Maia Filho HS. Sialorrhea in children with cerebral palsy. J Pediatr. 2016 Nov–Dec;92(6):549–58. https://doi.org/10.1016/j.jped.2016.03.006. Epub 2016 Jun 6. PMID: 27281791.
3. Maher S, Cunningham A, O'Callaghan N, Byrne F, Mc Donald C, McInerney S, Hallahan B. Clozapine-induced hypersalivation: an estimate of prevalence, severity and impact on quality of life. Ther Adv Psychopharmacol. 2016 Jun;6(3):178–84. https://doi.org/10.1177/2045125316641019. Epub 2016 Mar 30. PMID: 27354906. PMCID: PMC4910403.

4. Bhatia KP, Münchau A, Brown P. Botulinum toxin is a useful treatment in excessive drooling in saliva. J Neurol Neurosurg Psychiatry. 1999 Nov;67(5):697. https://doi.org/10.1136/jnnp.67.5.697. PMID: 10577041. PMCID: PMC1736626.

5. Hosp C, Naumann MK, Henning H. Botulinum toxin treatment of autonomic disorders. Focal hyperhidrosis and sialorrhea. Semin Neurol. 2016;36:20–8.

6. Dressler D. Botulinum toxin therapy. Its use for the neurological disorders of autonomic nervous system. J Neurol. 2013;260:701–13.

7. Naumann M, Dressler D, Hallet M, et al. Evidence–based review and assessment of botulinum toxins for the treatment of secretory disorders. Toxicon. 2013;67:141–53.

8. Lakraj AA, Moghimi N, Jabbari B. Sialorrhea: anatomy, pathophysiology and treatment with emphasis on the role of botulinum toxins. Toxins (Basel). 2013;5:1010–31.

9. Guidubaldi A, Fasano A, Ialongo T, Piano C, Pompili M, Mascianà R, Siciliani L, Sabatelli M, Bentivoglio AR. Botulinum toxin A versus B in sialorrhea: a prospective, randomized, double-blind, crossover pilot study in patients with amyotrophic lateral sclerosis or Parkinson's disease. Mov Disord. 2011 Feb 1;26(2):313–9. https://doi.org/10.1002/mds.23473. Epub 2011 Jan 21. PMID: 21259343.

10. Petracca M, Guidubaldi A, Ricciardi L, Ialongo T, Del Grande A, Mulas D, Di Stasio E, Bentivoglio AR. Botulinum toxin A and B in sialorrhea: long-term data and literature overview. Toxicon. 2015 Dec 1;107(Pt A):129–40. https://doi.org/10.1016/j.toxicon.2015.08.014. Epub 2015 Aug 30. PMID: 26327120.

11. Tamadonfar ET, Lew MF. BoNT clinical trial update: Sialorrhea. Toxicon. 2023 Apr;226:107087. https://doi.org/10.1016/j.toxicon.2023.107087. Epub 2023 Mar 16. PMID: 36931440.

12. Hegde AM, Pani SC. Drooling of saliva in children with cerebral palsy-etiology, prevalence, and relationship to salivary flow rate in an Indian population. Spec Care Dentist. 2009 Jul–Aug;29(4):163–8. https://doi.org/10.1111/j.1754-4505.2009.00085.x. PMID: 19573043.

13. Berweck S, Bonikowski M, Kim H, Althaus M, Flatau-Baqué B, Mueller D, Banach MD. Placebo-controlled clinical trial of IncobotulinumtoxinA for Sialorrhea in children: SIPEXI. Neurology. 2021 Aug 2;97(14):e1425–36. https://doi.org/10.1212/WNL.0000000000012573. Epub ahead of print. PMID: 34341153. PMCID: PMC8520391.

14. Heikel T, Patel S, Ziai K, Shah SJ, Lighthall JG. Botulinum toxin A in the management of pediatric sialorrhea: a systematic review. Ann Otol Rhinol Laryngol. 2023 Feb;132(2):200–6. https://doi.org/10.1177/00034894221078365. Epub 2022 Feb 18. PMID: 35176902. PMCID: PMC9834812.

15. Fan T, Frederick R, Abualsoud A, Sheyn A, McLevy-Bazzanella J, Thompson J, Akkus C, Wood J. Treatment of sialorrhea with botulinum toxin injections in pediatric patients less than three years of age. Int J Pediatr Otorhinolaryngol. 2022 Jul;158:111185. https://doi.org/10.1016/j.ijporl.2022.111185. Epub 2022 May 14. PMID: 35594794.

16. Lakraj AA, Moghimi N, Jabbari B. Hyperhidrosis: anatomy, pathophysiology and treatment with emphasis on the role of botulinum toxins. Toxins (Basel). 2013;5:821–40.

17. Adar R, Kurchin A, Zweig A, Mozes M. Palmar hyperhidrosis and its surgical treatment: a report of 100 cases. Ann Surg. 1977 Jul;186(1):34–41. https://doi.org/10.1097/00000658-197707000-00006. PMID: 879872. PMCID: PMC1396202.

18. Restivo DA, Panebianco M, Casabona A, Lanza S, Marchese-Ragona R, Patti F, Masiero S, Biondi A, Quartarone A. Botulinum toxin A for Sialorrhoea associated with neurological disorders: evaluation of the relationship between effect of treatment and the number of glands treated. Toxins (Basel). 2018 Jan 27;10(2). pii: E55.

19. Rosen R, Stewart T. Results of a 10-year follow-up study of botulinum toxin A therapy for primary axillary hyperhidrosis in Australia. Intern Med J. 2018;48:343–7.

20. Sridharan K, Sivaramakrishnan G. Pharmacological interventions for treating Sialorrhea associated with neurological disorders: a mixed treatment network meta-analysis of randomized controlled trials. Clin Neurosci. 2018;51:12–7.

21. Nawrocki S, Cha J. Botulinum toxin: pharmacology and injectable administration for the treatment of primary hyperhidrosis. J Am Acad Dermatol. 2020 Apr;82(4):969–79. https://doi.org/10.1016/j.jaad.2019.11.042. Epub 2019 Dec 4. PMID: 31811879.
22. Campanati A, Diotallevi F, Radi G, Martina E, Marconi B, Bobyr I, Offidani A. Efficacy and safety of botulinum toxin B in focal hyperhidrosis: a narrative review. Toxins (Basel). 2023 Feb 11;15(2):147. https://doi.org/10.3390/toxins15020147. PMID: 36828461. PMCID: PMC9966525.
23. Rajagopalan M, Saraswat A, Godse K, Shankar DS, Kandhari S, Shenoi SD, et al. Diagnosis and management of chronic pruritus: AN expert consensus review. Indian J Dermatol. 2017;62(1):7–17. https://doi.org/10.4103/0019-5154.198036.
24. Andrade A, Kuah CY, Martin-Lopez JE, Chua S, Shpadaruk V, Sanclemente G, Franco JV. Interventions for chronic pruritus of unknown origin. Cochrane Database Syst Rev. 2020 Jan 25;1(1):CD013128. https://doi.org/10.1002/14651858.CD013128.pub2. PMID: 31981369. PMCID: PMC6984650.
25. Dhand A, Aminoff MJ. The neurology of itch. Brain. 2014 Feb;137(Pt 2):313–22. https://doi.org/10.1093/brain/awt158. Epub 2013 Jun 22. PMID: 23794605.
26. Salardini A, Richardson D, Jabbari B. Relief of intractable pruritus after administration of botulinum toxin A (botox): a case report. Clin Pharmacol. 2008 Sep–Oct;31:303–6. https://doi.org/10.1097/WNF.0b013e3181672225. PMID: 18836352.
27. Papoiu AD, Tey HL, Coghill RC, Wang H, Yosipovitch G. Cowhage-induced itch as an experimental model for pruritus. A comparative study with histamine-induced itch. PLoS One. 2011 Mar 14;6(3):e17786. https://doi.org/10.1371/journal.pone.0017786. PMID: 21423808. PMCID: PMC3056722.
28. Gazerani P, Pedersen NS, Drewes AM, Arendt-Nielsen L. Botulinum toxin type A reduces histamine-induced itch and vasomotor responses in human skin. Br J Dermatol. 2009 Oct;161(4):737–45. https://doi.org/10.1111/j.1365-2133.2009.09305.x. Epub 2009 May 11. PMID: 19624547.
29. Zanci M, Favot F, Bizarrini M, et al. Botulinum toxin type- a for treatment of inverse psoriasis. J Eur Acad Venerol. 2008;31:303–6.
30. Gilbert E, Ward NL. Efficacy of botulinum neurotoxin type A for treating recalcitrant plaque psoriasis. J Drugs Dermatol. 2014 Nov;13(11):1407–8. PMID: 25607710.
31. Khattab FM, Samir MA. Botulinum toxin type-a versus 5-fluorouracil in the treatment of plaque psoriasis: comparative study. J Cosmet Dermatol. 2021 Oct;20(10):3128–32. https://doi.org/10.1111/jocd.14306. Epub 2021 Jul 14. PMID: 34146460.
32. Popescu MN, Beiu C, Iliescu MG, Mihai MM, Popa LG, Stănescu AMA, Berteanu M. Botulinum toxin use for modulating neuroimmune cutaneous activity in psoriasis. Medicina (Kaunas). 2022 Jun 16;58(6):813. https://doi.org/10.3390/medicina58060813. PMID: 35744076. PMCID: PMC9228985.
33. Saber M, Brassard D, Benohanian A. Inverse psoriasis and hyperhidrosis of the axillae responding to botulinum toxin type A. Arch Dermatol. 2011 May;147(5):629–30. https://doi.org/10.1001/archdermatol.2011.111. PMID: 21576592.
34. Todberg T, Zachariae C, Bregnhøj A, Hedelund L, Bonefeld KK, Nielsen K, Iversen L, Skov L. The effect of botulinum neurotoxin A in patients with plaque psoriasis—an exploratory trial. J Eur Acad Dermatol Venereol. 2018 Feb;32(2):e81–2. https://doi.org/10.1111/jdv.14536. Epub 2017 Oct 5. PMID: 28833574.

Chapter 15
Botulinum Toxin Treatment in Dentistry

Abstract Over the past 20 years, researchers and clinicians have found different potential indications for the use of botulinum toxin therapy in dentistry. The areas of interest are management of pain in temporomandibular disorder, pain after fracture of jawbone, local persistent pain at the site of tooth extraction, teeth grinding, angular cheilitis and burning mouth syndrome as well as improvement of gummy smile and management of protruded tongue.

Keywords Temporomandibular disorder · Fracture of jawbone · Pain at the site of dental extraction · Teeth grinding · Angular cheilitis · Gummy smile · Burning mouth syndrome · Protruded tongue

Introduction

Dentistry is an active medical field in the US with the number of dentists increasing yearly. In 2020, California, Texas and New York had the highest number of dentists: 31,059; 15,872, and 14,479, respectively [1]. The average income of dentists in US was $203,000 in 2020. The dental service expenditure in US rose from 62.1 billion in year 2000 to 143.2 billion in the year 2019 (Statistica 2023). Women visited dentists more often than men in 2019 (69.3% versus 61.5%) [1].

Over the past 20 years clinicians have found several new potential indications for botulinum toxin therapy in the field of dentistry. These include alleviating Jaw pain in temporomandibular disorder (TMD), pain after jaw bone fracture, persistent pain at the site of jaw bone extraction, teeth grinding, and burning mouth syndrome as well as improvement of the gummy smile and management of involuntary protruded tongue.

Botulinum Toxin Indications for Pain Issues in Dentistry

Botulinum toxin injection can reduce focal pain through several mechanisms. These mechanisms have been described in detail in Chaps. 4 and 5 of this book. In brief, it has been shown that local injection (into the muscle and skin) of Botox and similar toxins reduces the activity of certain chemicals known as pain transmitters. These chemicals that are present at the end of sensory nerves help to convey specific signals from periphery to spinal cord and brain where they are perceived as pain. Several of these pain transmitters that are influenced by botulinum toxin injection are now recognized such as glutamate, substance P and calcitonin gene-related peptide (CGRP). The injected toxin has the ability to diminish the function of pain transmitters either peripherally (at nerve endings) or it may travel(toxin molecule) from the periphery (skin or muscle) centrally to the spinal cord and lower part of the brain (brain stem) where they influence pain pathways [2–20]. Botulinum toxin can also exert its analgesic effect through other mechanisms; for instance, the toxin can deactivate the sodium channels which are present in abundance on the sensory nerves [21]. These channels are known to have a pivotal role in the function of sensory nerves while conducting the pain signals. Outside of the field of Dentistry, botulinum toxins are shown to exert analgesic effect in a variety of human pain disorders described in the previous chapters of this book [22–38]. Botox is FDA approved for treatment of chronic migraine (Chap. 4) and, since 2010, is widely used for treatment of this disabling painful condition worldwide.

Botulinum Toxin Treatment for Painful Disorders in Dentistry

Temporomandibular Disorder (TMD)

Temporomandibular joint, acting as a sliding hinge connects the jawbone (mandible) to the skull (temporal bone) (Fig. 15.1).

A group of painful and non-painful conditions interrupt the function of temporomandibular joint (TMJ)—muscles of chewing (masticatory) and adjoining structures are termed as temporomandibular disorder (TMD) [39]. Approximately 33% of adults, at least once during their lifetime, experience symptoms related to TMD [40]. Close to half of the patients with TMD report persistent jaw pain [41]. Women are twice as affected as men. Association of TMD with migraine and neck pain is not uncommon. The pain of TMD is often felt in front of the ear and exaggerated by jaw movement. The jaw is stiff, and patients have difficulty to open their mouth fully. Many patients, while eating or chewing, hear a clicking sound. Both medical and surgical treatments are contemplated for management of the symptoms of TMD (especially for pain). Medical treatment consists of the use of analgesic drugs for pain, physiotherapy and the use of jaw splints (occlusal splints). When these non-pharmacological measures fail, physicians inject anesthetics, steroids and a material

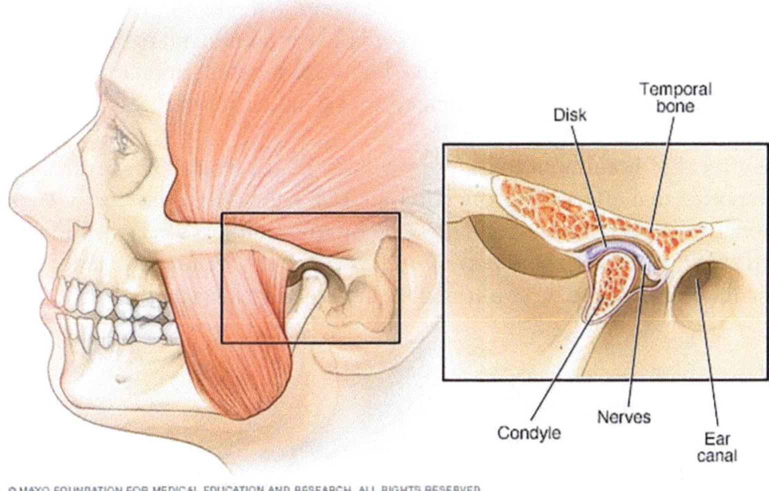

Fig. 15.1 Temporomandibular joint—with permission from Mayo clinic foundation

called hyaluronate into the affected jaw joint [42]. In recalcitrant pain caused by TMD, two surgical procedures are commonly performed: arthrocentesis and arthroscopy. Both aim to wash and clean inside the TM joint from debris and loose elements. In arthrocentesis, the procedure is done blindly through a cannula which is inserted inside the joint, whereas in arthroscopy the inserted cannula has a camera attached to it. Both procedures are effective and reduce the patients' pain and discomfort.

Botulinum Toxin Treatment of TMD

Two techniques are currently employed: 1- Injecting muscles involved with jaw closure—temporalis, and masseter muscles (two muscles shown in Fig. 15.1) only. 2- Injecting both muscles of jaw closure and jaw opening. The main muscle for jaw opening is the lateral pterygoid muscle.

The largest experience to date with the first approach comes from the experience of clinicians from Columbia University in New York and Harvard Medical School in Boston. In a joint publication these researchers presented their experience with 200 patients affected with TMD treated with BoNT injections over 20 years. A total of 50 units of Botox was injected into masseter muscles at 5 points, whereas temporalis muscles were injected at 4 points (Fig. 15.3). Sixty per cent of the patients reported significant improvement of pain and jaw function [43].

Patel et al. [44] conducted a blinded study (doctor and patient) in 20 patients with TMD. Xeomin (botulinum toxin A with an strength close to Botox) was injected into the masseter (50 units), temporalis (25 units) and lateral pterygoid (10 units) muscles bilaterally. Patients were followed every 4 weeks for 16 weeks. Pain was measured on a scale of 0–10. At 4 weeks, there was significant pain reduction (both patient's pain perception and pain evoked by local pressure upon the affected joint) in the Xeomin injected group compared to the saline injected group (statistically significant $P < 0.05$).

The effects of botulinum toxin usually lasts 12–16 weeks. However, one recent study reported that after BoNT injection for TMD, the effects lasted 33 weeks [45]. Deterioration of jawbone has been reported by some authors after injection of BoNT for TMD [46]. However, the reported studies are of low quality and the significance of these findings need to be confirmed by high quality investigations.

Technique of Injection

Injections are usually done at four to five locations into the masseter and temporalis muscles (Fig. 15.2). Patients is asked to clinch the teeth to activate the muscles of jaw closure (masseter and temporalis muscles). The anatomically complicated muscles can be identified by the use of electromyography (recording electrical activity of the muscle) or directly visualizing the muscle under ultrasound.

A recent comparative study has shown that the efficacy of botulinum toxin injections for alleviating pain of TMD is comparable with arthrocentesis and arthroscopy [47]. The toxin injection has the advantage of being less painful using thin gauge (27.5 or 30) needles and taking less time as combined temporalis and masseter injections take only 10–15 min. It requires no skin incision and does not need prior local injection of anesthetic agents.

Fig. 15.2 Botox injection sites into temporalis and masseter muscles for treatment of TMD. From Mor et al. [43]. (Method and sites of temporalis and masseter muscle injections in temporomandibular pain disorder advocated by Dr. Blitzer and his group from Columbia University Published under Creative Commons Attribution license (http://creativecommons.org/licenses/by/4.0/). Courtesy of publisher- Toxins)

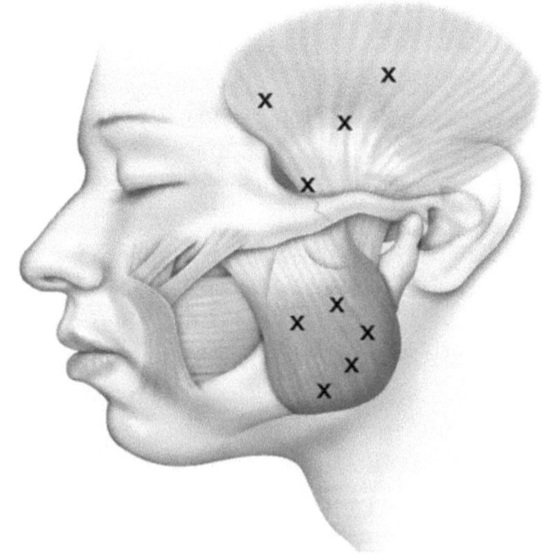

Teeth Grinding (Bruxism)

Teeth grinding can be seen in adults or children during wakefulness or sleep. Severe teeth grinding during sleep interrupts the individual and/or the bed partner's sleep. Severe teeth grinding may cause chronic pain in the jaw and lead to teeth damage. For waking and sleep teeth grinding prevalences of 22–31% and 7.4% has been reported, respectively [40].

Treatment of teeth grinding may start with non-pharmacological approaches such as biofeedback, muscle stretching, occlusal devices, and/or electrical stimulation of jaw muscles, but these approaches have questionable longstanding effectiveness [48]. Pharmacological treatment with tricyclic antidepressants or non-narcotic analgesics can offer temporary pain relief.

Botulinum Toxin Treatment of Teeth Grinding

Botulinum toxin treatment of teeth grinding is based on the premise that relaxing the jaw muscles can interrupt the grinding cycle and help the patients. Several trials have studied the utility of botulinum toxin injections in bruxism. Injections were made either in the masseter muscles alone or in both masseter and temporalis muscles (bilaterally).

A recent review (2022) on this subject has found ten clinical trials. A meta-analysis of these studies found that BoNT injection was superior to oral splints or saline (placebo injection) at 1,3 and 6 months [49]. Meta-analysis is a sophisticated method of statistical analysis can determine the efficacy of a drug for a certain indication through comparison of the result of several studies published for a given indication. The usual injected dose of the toxin for treatment of teeth grinding varied from 30 to 50 units of Botox or Xeomin (units of the two are relatively comparable) for each masseter or temporalis muscle. A recent blinded study found no difference in efficacy against pain and patient satisfaction between two protocols (masseter injection alone or masseter and temporalis combined) [50]. Another recent review found botulinum toxin injection particularly effective for reducing pain associated with sleep teeth grinding [51]. One recent study indicated that even injection of low dose botulinum toxin (20 units in each masseter and temporalis muscle) is effective in reducing pain and achieving patient satisfaction in bruxism [52].

Despite these encouraging results, BoNT therapy for teeth grinding is not yet FDA approved. Based on the volume the literature, clinicians, especially in academic centers, do use BoNT injections for management of bruxism. High quality studies are needed to assess the efficacy of repeated (usually every 3–4 months) toxin injections beyond 1 year in this disorder. A detailed review of all studies reported on botulinum toxin therapy for teeth grinding has been published by Etemad-Mogadam and co-workers in 2022 [53].

Fracture of the Jawbone (Mandible) and Cheekbone (Zygoma)

Attachment of muscles to the jawbone facilitates jaw movements, controls growth of the muscular and bony structures and dental occlusion (how teeth come together when mouth is closed). Fracture of the jawbone, depending on the severity of injury, and direction of the fracture, causes functional complications. Relaxing the muscles that move the jaw (temporalis and masseter -mouth closure; lateral pterygoid-jaw opening) by botulinum toxin injections can reduce pain and complications. Jaw fractures can involve the condyle (top of the vertical portion of the jawbone), the angle (were horizontal and vertical parts of the jaw bones meet, the symphysis (midline where the jawbone from one side meets the other) or zygoma (fracture of check bone).

For all these conditions, the limited available literature suggests that injection of botulinum toxin into muscles involved in jaw opening and jaw closure (masseter and pterygoid muscles-Fig. 15.3) alleviates pain and smooths the post- surgical outcome [54–57].

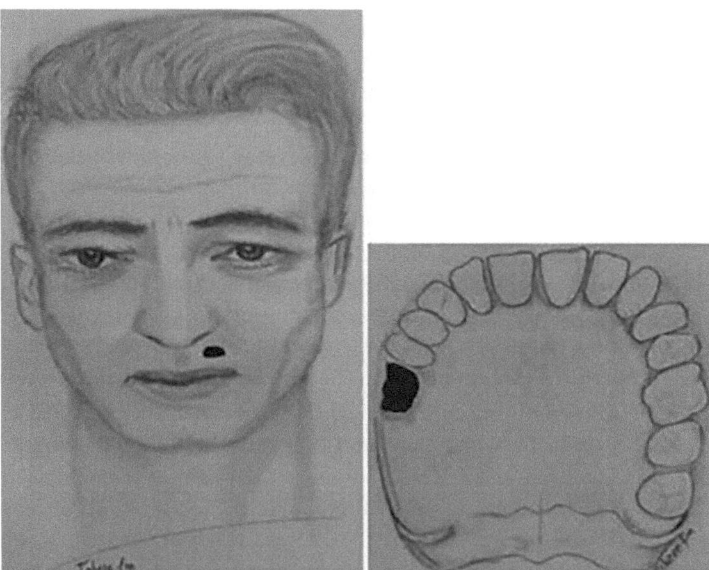

Fig. 15.3 The site of skin sensitivity and pain shown with dark ink. Botox was injected in the area of extracted tooth (painted dark). (Drawing courtesy of Dr. Damoun Safarpour)

Preventing Plate Fracture

Plates are used for fixation of bone segments after a fracture. The commonly used plates are made from titanium or are resorbable plates. Plate fracture due to contraction of masseter muscles is a common occurrence. Shin and co-worker's [54] studied 16 patients who had plate insertion after jaw fracture. Half of the patients were injected with 25 units of Botox into each masseter muscle, while the other half did not have Botox injection. After 6 months, the incidence of plate fracture was significantly lower in the patients who had received Botox injections for to relaxation of masseter muscles.

Post-extraction Pain

In this area, there are only anecdotal observations. The following case is presented from the author's experience.

Case Report

A healthy 60-year-old man presented with significant painful hypersensitivity to touch on the gums (gingiva) adjacent to extraction site of molar teeth. The allodynia (sensitivity to touch- touch perceived as pain) developed 3 years ago, following the extraction of three molars. He also described attacks of severe and jabbing pain that radiated to the upper lip on the same side. The pain attacks occurred several times a day with an intensity of 9 or 10 on a scale of 0–10. Pain prevented him from comfortable brushing. He was taking 600 mg gabapentin, four times daily without achieving satisfactory pain control. Marked sensitivity of the gums, over and anterior to the extraction site, was confirmed on examination (Fig. 15.3). He was injected with 10 U (2.5 U × 4 points) of Botox into the painful area, with a thin needle (gauge 30), 2 mm below the surface. He reported distinct improvement of gum sensitivity and cessation of pain attacks after 7 days. The effects lasted up to 6 months and a second round of treatment was administered at the patient's request, which yielded the same efficacy. On PGIC scale (patient global impression of change), he reported his pain as "very much improved".

Botulinum Toxin Treatment for Non- painful Disorders in Dentistry

Gummy Smile (Excessive Gingival Display)

Display of upper gums, more than 3 mm upon smiling, is known as gummy smile (Fig. 15.4). Hyperactivity of muscles responsible for lip elevation is one of the major factors causing gummy smile. Treatment usually involves application of orthodontic and surgical procedures to correct the elevated lip responsible for the gummy smile [58–61]. Gummy smile is more common in females [61]. A few small studies have used botulinum toxin injection to improve the gummy smile. Five units of Botox on each side is recommended. The Yonsei point is considered a good point for a single injection on each side of the face. This point is at the junction of a horizontal line drawn 1 cm from the lateral part of the nostril and a vertical line drawn 3 cm up from the lateral junction of the two lips (corner of the mouth) [61, 62]. Injection complications include asymmetric smiling and or developing difficulty in smiling.

Burning Mouth Syndrome (BMS)

International Classification of Oro-facial Pain (ICOP) defines BMS as a burning sensation inside the mouth that lacks apparent local or systemic cause and occurs more than 2 h a day with a minimum duration of 3 months [39]. BMS is three times more common among women and is more prevalent after age 50. The prevalence of BMS in North America is almost equal to Asia (1–1% versus 1.05%), whereas it is higher in Europe (5.58%) [64]. The cause(s) of BMS is not clearly defined. It is

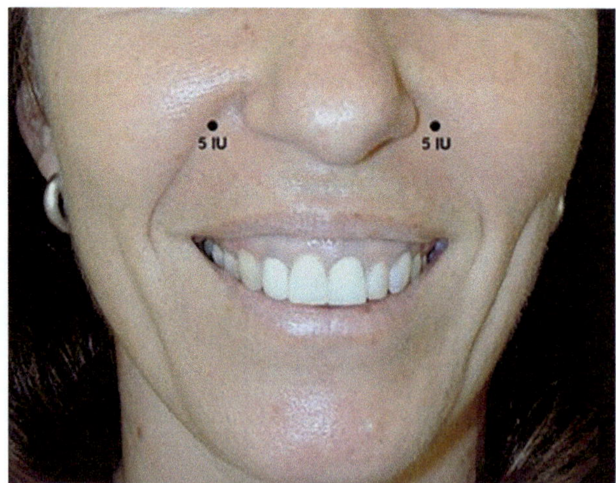

Fig. 15.4 Gummy smiles and site of injections. The toxin dose is 5 units of Dysport on each side (approximately 2 units of Botox). (From Mazzuco et al. [63] 2010, reproduced with permission from the publisher (Elsevier))

suggested that this condition is a form of sensory neuropathy affecting the sensory fibers inside the oral cavity (including the tongue) [65].

Exercise of muscles of chewing (temporalis and masseter muscles), application of hot pack, ultrasound and physical therapy offer limited success in treatment of burning mouth syndrome. The literature on botulinum toxin treatment for BTS is limited to a few single case reports and one study of 6 patients [66]. In the latter study investigators performed bilateral injection of the tongue (anterior two third) and lower lip with 16 units of botulinum toxin A (in this case Xeomin with comparable units to Botox). Three patients had diabetes. They reported a marked reduction of burning sensation from the initial value of 6–9 (on 0–10 scale) to 0 in 48 h. The effects lasted 12–20 weeks. Studies with a larger number of patients, and preferably blinded, are needed to confirm these results.

Angular Cheilitis (AC)

Angular Cheilitis (AC) refers to inflammation of the corner of the mouth presenting with redness, cracks (fissure) and, in severe cases, ulceration. In older individuals, progressive deep creases in the corner of the mouth collect saliva and bacteria leading to the development of infection. Single case reports claim injection of Botox around the mouth can improve this condition. In one report, a 60-year-old patient with 2-year history of AC improved substantially after Botox injections into face muscles close to the corner of the mouth [66].

Botulinum Toxin Treatment Before Implant Surgery

Patients with teeth clinching (bruxism) may develop problems after implant surgery. Severe teeth clinching can lead to loss of implants. As described earlier in this chapter, botulinum toxin injections into muscles involved in chewing can relax these muscles and improve teeth clinching. In one study [67], researchers investigated the number of implant loss in 13 patients injected with botulinum toxin 3 weeks before implant with 13 patients who did not receive such injections; all patients had teeth clinching. Dysport (a botulinum toxin A similar to Botox) injected into temporalis and masseter muscles (see Fig. 15.1 for locations of these muscles). The injected dose of Dysport on each side was 90 units for masseter (approximately equal to 30–40 units of Botox) and 70 units for temporalis muscle (approximately equal to 20–25 units of Botox). Patients were followed for 18 to 51 months. Each group had approximately 100 implants. During the follow up period, no implant was lost in the botulinum toxin injected group, whereas in the non-injected group, two patients demonstrated lost implants.

Tongue Trust

Forward tongue trust can interfere with speaking and eating and put pressure against the teeth. Protruded tongue intermittent or sustained, can be a complication of medications used in psychiatry. A protruded tongue can interfere with and when present can prolong dental surgery. Botulinum injection of the tongue has been suggested in conjunction with dental crib (a metal structure that protects the teeth from the protruding tongue) insertion to reduce tongue pressure [68]. Tongue injections by botulinum toxin is tricky and in unexperienced hands can lead to tongue paralysis and difficulty in swallowing. It should be performed only by experienced physicians with significant knowledge of oral anatomy.

I have injected a dozen patients with severely protruded tongue for non-dental indications. Quick Injections of 5 units of Botox on each side of the tongue with a thin short needle in my experience helped two third of the patients and did not produce any complications. In a very small tongue, however, it would be wise to reduce the dose.

References

1. Frederich Michas. Statistica; November 15, 2020.
2. Rossetto O, Pirazzini M, Fabris F, Montecucco C. Botulinum neurotoxins: mechanism of action. Handb Exp Pharmacol. 2021; 263:35–47. https://doi.org/10.1007/164_2020_355. PMID: 32277300.
3. Bach-Rojecky L, Relja M, Lacković Z. Botulinum toxin type A in experimental neuropathic pain. J Neural Transm (Vienna). 2005 Feb;112(2):215–9. https://doi.org/10.1007/s00702-004-0265-1. PMID: 15657640.
4. Matak I, Tékus V, Bölcskei K, Lacković Z, Helyes Z. Involvement of substance P in the antinociceptive effect of botulinum toxin type A: evidence from knockout mice. Neuroscience. 2017 Sep 1;358: 137–45. https://doi.org/10.1016/j.neuroscience.2017.06.040. Epub 2017 Jul 1. PMID: 28673722.
5. Marino MJ, Terashima T, Steinauer JJ, Eddinger KA, Yaksh TL, Xu Q. Botulinum toxin B in the sensory afferent: transmitter release, spinal activation, and pain behavior. Pain. 2014 Apr;155(4):674–84. https://doi.org/10.1016/j.pain.2013.12.009. Epub 2013 Dec 11. PMID: 24333775; PMCID: PMC3960322.
6. Cui M, Khanijou S, Rubino J, Aoki KR. Subcutaneous administration of botulinum toxin A reduces formalin-induced pain. Pain. 2004 Jan;107(1–2):125–33. https://doi.org/10.1016/j.pain.2003.10.008. PMID: 14715398.
7. Mika J, Rojewska E, Makuch W, Korostynski M, Luvisetto S, Marinelli S, Pavone F, Przewlocka B. The effect of botulinum neurotoxin A on sciatic nerve injury-induced neuroimmunological changes in rat dorsal root ganglia and spinal cord. Neuroscience. 2011 Feb 23;175:358–66. https://doi.org/10.1016/j.neuroscience.2010.11.040. Epub 2010 Nov 25. PMID: 21111791.
8. Bossowska A, Lepiarczyk E, Mazur U, Janikiewicz P, Markiewicz W. Botulinum toxin type A induces changes in the chemical coding of substance P-immunoreactive dorsal root ganglia sensory neurons supplying the porcine urinary bladder. Toxins (Basel). 2015 Nov 16;7(11):4797–816. https://doi.org/10.3390/toxins7114797. PMID: 26580655; PMCID: PMC4663534.

9. Safarpour Y, Jabbari B. Botulinum toxin treatment of pain syndromes -an evidence based review. Toxicon. 2018 Jun 1;147:120–8. https://doi.org/10.1016/j.toxicon.2018.01.017. Epub 2018 Feb 1. PMID: 29409817.

10. Shin MC, Wakita M, Xie DJ, Yamaga T, Iwata S, Torii Y, Harakawa T, Ginnaga A, Kozaki S, Akaike N. Inhibition of membrane Na+ channels by A type botulinum toxin at femtomolar concentrations in central and peripheral neurons. J Pharmacol Sci. 2012;118(1):33–42. https://doi.org/10.1254/jphs.11060fp. Epub 2011 Dec 10. PMID: 22156364.

11. Hong B, Yao L, Ni L, Wang L, Hu X. Antinociceptive effect of botulinum toxin A involves alterations in AMPA receptor expression and glutamate release in spinal dorsal horn neurons. Neuroscience 2017 Aug 15;357:197–207. https://doi.org/10.1016/j.neuroscience.2017.06.004. Epub 2017 Jun 10. PMID: 28606856.

12. Matak I, Bölcskei K, Bach-Rojecky L, Helyes Z. Mechanisms of botulinum toxin type A action on pain. Toxins (Basel). 2019 Aug 5;11(8):459. https://doi.org/10.3390/toxins11080459. PMID: 31387301; PMCID: PMC6723487.

13. Matak I, Riederer P, Lacković Z. Botulinum toxin's axonal transport from periphery to the spinal cord. Neurochem Int. 2012 Jul;61(2):236–9. https://doi.org/10.1016/j.neuint.2012.05.001. Epub 2012 May 8. PMID: 22580329.

14. Lacković Z. Botulinum toxin and pain. Handb Exp Pharmacol. 2021; 263:251–64. https://doi.org/10.1007/164_2019_348. PMID: 32016565.

15. Drinovac Vlah V, Filipović B, Bach-Rojecky L, Lacković Z. Role of central versus peripheral opioid system in antinociceptive and anti-inflammatory effect of botulinum toxin type A in trigeminal region. Eur J Pain. 2018 Mar;22(3):583–91. https://doi.org/10.1002/ejp.1146. Epub 2017 Nov 13. PMID: 29134730.

16. Wang W, Kong M, Dou Y, Xue S, Liu Y, Zhang Y, Chen W, Li Y, Dai X, Meng J, Wang J. Selective expression of a SNARE-cleaving protease in peripheral sensory neurons attenuates pain-related gene transcription and neuropeptide release. Int J Mol Sci. 2021 Aug 17;22(16):8826. https://doi.org/10.3390/ijms22168826. PMID: 34445536. PMCID: PMC8396265.

17. Hok P, Veverka T, Hluštík P, Nevrlý M, Kaňovský P. The central effects of botulinum toxin in dystonia and spasticity. Toxins (Basel). 2021 Feb 17;13(2):155. https://doi.org/10.3390/toxins13020155. PMID: 33671128. PMCID: PMC7922085.

18. Meng J, Ovsepian SV, Wang J, Pickering M, Sasse A, Aoki KR, Lawrence GW, Dolly JO. Activation of TRPV1 mediates calcitonin gene-related peptide release, which excites trigeminal sensory neurons and is attenuated by a retargeted botulinum toxin with anti-nociceptive potential. J Neurosci. 2009 Apr 15;29(15):4981–92. https://doi.org/10.1523/JNEUROSCI.5490-08.2009. PMID: 19369567; PMCID: PMC6665337.

19. Lacković Z. New analgesic: focus on botulinum toxin. Toxicon. 2020 May; 179:1–7. https://doi.org/10.1016/j.toxicon.2020.02.008. Epub 2020 Feb 11. PMID: 32174507.

20. Bittencourt da Silva L, Karshenas A, Bach FW, Rasmussen S, Arendt-Nielsen L, Gazerani P. Blockade of glutamate release by botulinum neurotoxin type A in humans: a dermal microdialysis study. Pain Res Manag. 2014 May–Jun;19(3):126–32. https://doi.org/10.1155/2014/410415. PMID: 24851237; PMCID: PMC4158957.

21. Meng J, Wang J, Lawrence G, Dolly JO. Synaptobrevin I mediates exocytosis of CGRP from sensory neurons and inhibition by botulinum toxins reflects their anti-nociceptive potential. J Cell Sci. 2007 Aug 15;120(Pt 16):2864–74. https://doi.org/10.1242/jcs.012211. Epub 2007 Jul 31. PMID: 17666428.

22. Aurora SK, Dodick DW, Turkel CC, et al. OnabotulinumtoxinA for treatment of chronic migraine: results from the double-blind, randomized, placebo-controlled phase of the PREEMPT 1 trial. Cephalalgia. 2010;30(7):793–803. https://doi.org/10.1177/0333102410364676.

23. Schaefer SM, Gottschalk CH, Jabbari B. Treatment of chronic migraine with focus on botulinum neurotoxins. Toxins (Basel). 2015;7(7):2615–28. Published 2015 Jul 14. https://doi.org/10.3390/toxins7072615.

24. Xiao L, Mackey S, Hui H, Xong D, Zhang Q, Zhang D. Subcutaneous injection of botulinum toxin a is beneficial in postherpetic neuralgia. Pain Med. 2010;11(12):1827–33. https://doi.org/10.1111/j.1526-4637.2010.01003.x.
25. Ranoux D, Attal N, Morain F, Bouhassira D. Botulinum toxin type A induces direct analgesic effects in chronic neuropathic pain [published correction appears in Ann Neurol. 2009 Mar;65(3):359]. Ann Neurol. 2008;64(3):274–83. https://doi.org/10.1002/ana.21427.
26. Wu CJ, Lian YJ, Zheng YK, et al. Botulinum toxin type A for the treatment of trigeminal neuralgia: results from a randomized, double-blind, placebo-controlled trial. Cephalalgia. 2012;32(6):443–50. https://doi.org/10.1177/0333102412441721.
27. Yuan RY, Sheu JJ, Yu JM, et al. Botulinum toxin for diabetic neuropathic pain: a randomized double-blind crossover trial. Neurology. 2009;72(17):1473–8. https://doi.org/10.1212/01.wnl.0000345968.05959.cf.
28. Restivo DA, Casabona A, Frittitta L, et al. Efficacy of botulinum toxin A for treating cramps in diabetic neuropathy. Ann Neurol. 2018;84(5):674–82. https://doi.org/10.1002/ana.25340.
29. Foster L, Clapp L, Erickson M, Jabbari B. Botulinum toxin A and chronic low back pain: a randomized, double-blind study. Neurology. 2001;56(10):1290–3. https://doi.org/10.1212/wnl.56.10.1290.
30. De Andrés J, Adsuara VM, Palmisani S, Villanueva V, López-Alarcón MD. A double-blind, controlled, randomized trial to evaluate the efficacy of botulinum toxin for the treatment of lumbar myofascial pain in humans. Reg Anesth Pain Med. 2010;35(3):255–60. https://doi.org/10.1097/AAP.0b013e3181d23241.
31. Babcock MS, Foster L, Pasquina P, Jabbari B. Treatment of pain attributed to plantar fasciitis with botulinum toxin A: a short-term, randomized, placebo-controlled, double-blind study. Am J Phys Med Rehabil. 2005;84(9):649–54. https://doi.org/10.1097/01.phm.0000176339.73591.d7.
32. Huang YC, Wei SH, Wang HK, Lieu FK. Ultrasonographic guided botulinum toxin type a treatment for plantar fasciitis: an outcome-based investigation for treating pain and gait changes. J Rehabil Med. 2010;42(2):136–40. https://doi.org/10.2340/16501977-0491.
33. Fishman LM, Anderson C, Rosner B. BOTOX and physical therapy in the treatment of piriformis syndrome. Am J Phys Med Rehabil. 2002;81(12):936–42. https://doi.org/10.1097/00002060-200212000-00009.
34. Wong SM, Hui AC, Tong PY, Poon DW, Yu E, Wong LK. Treatment of lateral epicondylitis with botulinum toxin: a randomized, double-blind, placebo-controlled trial. Ann Intern Med. 2005;143(11):793–7. https://doi.org/10.7326/0003-4819-143-11-200512060-00007.
35. Placzek R, Drescher W, Deuretzbacher G, Hempfing A, Meiss AL. Treatment of chronic radial epicondylitis with botulinum toxin A. A double-blind, placebo-controlled, randomized multicenter study. J Bone Joint Surg Am. 2007;89(2):255–60. https://doi.org/10.2106/JBJS.F.00401.
36. Han ZA, Song DH, Oh HM, Chung ME. Botulinum toxin type A for neuropathic pain in patients with spinal cord injury. Ann Neurol. 2016;79(4):569–78. https://doi.org/10.1002/ana.24605.
37. Gottsch HP, Yang CC, Berger RE. A pilot study of botulinum toxin A for male chronic pelvic pain syndrome. Scand J Urol Nephrol. 2011;45(1):72–6. https://doi.org/10.3109/0036559 9.2010.529820.
38. Falahatkar S, Shahab E, Gholamjani Moghaddam K, Kazemnezhad E. Transurethral intraprostatic injection of botulinum neurotoxin type A for the treatment of chronic prostatitis/chronic pelvic pain syndrome: results of a prospective pilot double-blind and randomized placebo-controlled study. BJU Int. 2015;116(4):641–9. https://doi.org/10.1111/bju.12951.
39. International Classification of Orofacial Pain, 1st edition (ICOP). Cephalalgia. 2020;40(2):129–221. https://doi.org/10.1177/0333102419893823
40. Muñoz Lora VR, Del Bel Cury AA, Jabbari B, Lacković Z. Botulinum toxin type A in dental medicine. J Dent Res. 2019 Dec;98(13):1450–7. https://doi.org/10.1177/0022034519875053. Epub 2019 Sep 18. PMID: 31553008.

41. Ettlin DA, Napimoga MH, Meira E, Cruz M, Clemente-Napimoga JT. Orofacial musculoskeletal pain: an evidence-based bio-psycho-social matrix model. Neurosci Biobehav Rev. 2021 Sep;128:12–20. https://doi.org/10.1016/j.neubiorev.2021.06.008. Epub 2021 Jun 9. PMID: 34118294.

42. Gil-Martínez A, Paris-Alemany A, López-de-Uralde-Villanueva I, La Touche R. Management of pain in patients with temporomandibular disorder (TMD): challenges and solutions. J Pain Res. 2018 Mar 16;11:571–87. https://doi.org/10.2147/JPR.S127950. PMID: 29588615; PMCID: PMC5859913.

43. Mor N, Tang C, Blitzer A. Temporomandibular myofacial pain treated with botulinum toxin injection. Toxins (Basel). 2015 Jul 24;7(8):2791–800. https://doi.org/10.3390/toxins7082791. PMID: 26213970; PMCID: PMC4549724.

44. Patel AA, Lerner MZ, Blitzer A. IncobotulinumtoxinA injection for temporomandibular joint disorder. Ann Otol Rhinol Laryngol. 2017 Apr;126(4):328–33. https://doi.org/10.1177/0003489417693013. Epub 2017 Feb 1. PMID: 28290229.

45. Sitnikova V, Kämppi A, Teronen O, Kemppainen P. Effect of botulinum toxin injection on EMG activity and bite force in masticatory muscle disorder: a randomized clinical trial. Toxins (Basel). 2022 Aug 10;14(8):545. https://doi.org/10.3390/toxins14080545. PMID: 36006207; PMCID: PMC9416064.

46. Owen M, Gray B, Hack N, Perez L, Allard RJ, Hawkins JM. Impact of botulinum toxin injection into the masticatory muscles on mandibular bone: a systematic review. J Oral Rehabil. 2022 Jun;49(6):644–53. https://doi.org/10.1111/joor.13326. Epub 2022 Apr 9. PMID: 35348239.

47. Rodrigues ALP, Cardoso HJ, Ângelo DF. Patient experience and satisfaction with different temporomandibular joint treatments: a retrospective study. J Craniomaxillofac Surg. 2023 Jan;51(1):44–51. https://doi.org/10.1016/j.jcms.2023.01.006. Epub 2023 Jan 23. PMID: 36739190.

48. Goldstein G, DeSantis L, Goodacre C. Bruxism: best evidence consensus statement. J Prosthodont. 2021 Apr;30(S1):91–101. https://doi.org/10.1111/jopr.13308. PMID: 33331675.

49. Chen Y, Tsai CH, Bae TH, Huang CY, Chen C, Kang YN, Chiu WK. Effectiveness of botulinum toxin injection on bruxism: a systematic review and meta-analysis of randomized controlled trials. Aesthetic Plast Surg. 2023 Jan 24. https://doi.org/10.1007/s00266-023-03256-8. Epub ahead of print. PMID: 36694050.

50. da Silva Ramalho JA, Palma LF, Ramalho KM, Tedesco TK, Morimoto S. Effect of botulinum toxin A on pain, bite force, and satisfaction of patients with bruxism: a randomized single-blind clinical trial comparing two protocols. Saudi Dent J. 2023 Jan;35(1):53–60. https://doi.org/10.1016/j.sdentj.2022.12.008. Epub 2022 Dec 24. PMID: 36817026; PMCID: PMC9931508.

51. Pereira IN, Hassan H. Botulinum toxin A in dentistry and orofacial surgery: an evidence-based review—part 1: therapeutic applications. Evid Based Dent. 2022 May 27. https://doi.org/10.1038/s41432-022-0256-9. Epub ahead of print. Erratum in: Evid Based Dent. 2022 Jun;23(2):47. PMID: 35624296.

52. de Lima MC, Rizzatti Barbosa CM, Duarte Gavião MB, Ferreira Caria PH. Is low dose of botulinum toxin effective in controlling chronic pain in sleep bruxism, awake bruxism, and temporomandibular disorder? Cranio. 2021 Sep 6:1–8. https://doi.org/10.1080/08869634.2021.1973215. Epub ahead of print. PMID: 34488556.

53. Etemad Moghadam S, Alaeddini M, Jabbari B. In botulinum toxin for pain disorders. Chapter 16. In: Jabbari, editor. Botulinum toxin treatment in dentistry and treatment of orofacial pain. Springer; 2022. p. 311–58.

54. Shin SH, Kang YJ, Kim SG. The effect of botulinum toxin-A injection into the masseter muscles on prevention of plate fracture and post-operative relapse in patients receiving orthognathic surgery. Maxillofac Plast Reconstr Surg. 2018 Nov 25;40(1):36. https://doi.org/10.1186/s40902-018-0174-0. PMID: 30538972. PMCID: PMC6261083.

55. Akbay E, Cevik C, Damlar I, Altan A. Treatment of displaced mandibular condylar fracture with botulinum toxin A. Auris Nasus Larynx. 2014 Apr;41(2):219–21. https://doi.org/10.1016/j.anl.2013.08.002. Epub 2013 Oct 21. PMID: 24156980.
56. Canter HI, Kayikcioglu A, Aksu M, Mavili ME. Botulinum toxin in closed treatment of mandibular condylar fracture. Ann Plast Surg. 2007 May;58(5):474–8. https://doi.org/10.1097/01.sap.0000244987.68092.6e. PMID: 17452828.
57. Kayikçioğlu A, Erk Y, Mavili E, Vargel I, Ozgür F. Botulinum toxin in the treatment of zygomatic fractures. Plast Reconstr Surg. 2003 Jan;111(1):341–6. https://doi.org/10.1097/01.PRS.0000037870.07434.D0. PMID: 12496600.
58. Hwang WS, Hur MS, Hu KS, Song WC, Koh KS, Baik HS, Kim ST, Kim HJ, Lee KJ. Surface anatomy of the lip elevator muscles for the treatment of gummy smile using botulinum toxin. Angle Orthod. 2009 Jan;79(1):70–7. https://doi.org/10.2319/091407-437.1. PMID: 19123705.
59. Polo M. Botulinum toxin type A in the treatment of excessive gingival display. Am J Orthod Dentofacial Orthop. 2005 Feb;127(2):214–8; quiz 261. https://doi.org/10.1016/j.ajodo.2004.09.013. PMID: 15750541.
60. Dilaver E, Uckan S. Effect of V-Y plasty on lip lengthening and treatment of gummy smile. Int J Oral Maxillofac Surg. 2018 Feb;47(2):184–7. https://doi.org/10.1016/j.ijom.2017.09.015. Epub 2017 Oct 16. PMID: 29042176.
61. Mazzuco R, Hexsel D. Gummy smile and botulinum toxin: a new approach based on the gingival exposure area. J Am Acad Dermatol. 2010 Dec;63(6):1042–51. https://doi.org/10.1016/j.jaad.2010.02.053.
62. Few JW Jr. Commentary on: gummy smile treatment: proposal for a novel corrective technique and a review of the literature. Aesthet Surg J. 2018 Nov 12;38(12):1339–40. https://doi.org/10.1093/asj/sjy220. PMID: 30215674.
63. Duruel O, Ataman-Duruel ET, Tözüm TF, Berker E. Ideal dose and injection site for gummy smile treatment with botulinum toxin-A: a systematic review and introduction of a case study. Int J Periodontics Restorative Dent. 2019 Jul/Aug;39(4):e167–73. https://doi.org/10.11607/prd.3580. PMID: 31226199.
64. Wu S, Zhang W, Yan J, Noma N, Young A, Yan Z. Worldwide prevalence estimates of burning mouth syndrome: a systematic review and meta-analysis. Oral Dis. 2022 Sep;28(6):1431–40. https://doi.org/10.1111/odi.13868. Epub 2021 Apr 19. PMID: 33818878.
65. Restivo DA, Lauria G, Marchese-Ragona R, Vigneri R. Botulinum toxin for burning mouth syndrome. Ann Intern Med. 2017 May 16;166(10):762–3. https://doi.org/10.7326/L16-0451. Epub 2017 Apr 11. PMID: 28395302.
66. Kwon CI, Shin YB, Jo JW, Jeong HB, Moon YS, Jung EC, Kim CY, Yoon TJ. P272: A case of angular cheilitis treated with botulinum toxin. Program Book (Old Green Collection). 2018;70(1):413.
67. Mijiritsky E, Mortellaro C, Rudberg O, Fahn M, Basegmez C, Levin L. Botulinum toxin type A as preoperative treatment for immediately loaded dental implants placed in fresh extraction sockets for full-arch restoration of patients with bruxism. J Craniofac Surg. 2016 May;27(3):668–70. https://doi.org/10.1097/SCS.0000000000002566. PMID: 27092916.
68. Taslan S, Biren S, Ceylanoglu C. Tongue pressure changes before, during and after crib appliance therapy. Angle Orthod. 2010 May;80(3):533–9. https://doi.org/10.2319/070209-370.1. PMID: 20050749; PMCID: PMC8985714.

Chapter 16
Botulinum Toxin Therapy in Veterinary Medicine

Abstract Emerging literature supports that local injection of botulinum toxins can help local pain in animals. In dogs, botulinum toxin injections have been studied for treatment of painful joints (osteoarthritis) and pain after breast removal (mastectomy) for malignant breast cancer. In horses, botulinum toxin injections have been used to improve pain resulting from bone degeneration in animal's hoofs leading to soft tissue damage (laminitis and synovitis). This chapter reviews the potential of botulinum toxin therapy for alleviation of local pain in canine and equine species.

Keywords Botulinum toxin · Botulinum neurotoxin · Canine osteoarthritis · Canine postmastectomy pain · Equine laminitis · Equine synovitis · Equine hoof pain

Introduction

Pet ownership is constantly on the rise in US with dogs being the most favored pets. According to Insurance Information Institute in 2022, 69 million American households have a pet dog versus 45.5% having a pet cat. Data from American Veterinary Association shows the highest pet ownership in the state of Wyoming (71%) closely followed by Nebraska, Arkansas and Indiana (each 70%), while the state of Rhode Island has the lowest figure (45%). Being the most common household pets, dog care- cost has risen steadily over the past two decades. The average monthly insurance for dogs is $65. Pain is a major complaint that brings dogs to the attention of veterinarians. The most common types of pain in dogs are pain related to trauma, pain of arthritis (joint pain) and pain after surgical procedures. In the novel called " traveling with Charley", the Nobel- prize winner John Steinbeck describes in detail his dog's (Charley) discomfort and pain after urinary retention while travelling widely in US. This chapter describes the potential role of local botulinum toxin injection in improving joint pain and post-surgical pain in dogs and pain issues in horses.

B. Jabbari, *Botulinum Toxin Treatment*,
https://doi.org/10.1007/978-3-031-54471-2_16

As described in the previous chapters of this book (Chaps. 2 and 5) botulinum neurotoxins can improve pain through different mechanisms. When pain is due to muscle contraction or muscle spasms (such as is seen after trauma), the injected toxin relaxes the muscle through blocking the release of acetylcholine at nerve-muscle junction. Furthermore, it has been shown that botulinum toxins can reduce the major pain transmitters (glutamate, substance P, calcitonin gene related peptide) in animal pain models both centrally and peripherally [1–22]. Inhibition of sodium channel that conducts some pain signals in another pain- relieving mechanism attributed to the analgesic function of botulinum toxins [9, 23]. Finally, local botulinum toxin injections, by influencing fine fibers within the muscles (intrafusal fibers), reduce sensory input to the spinal cord and the sensitization of central pain pathways [24] which contribute to pain maintenance in chronic pain conditions.

In human, botulinum toxins have been shown to improve several pain disorders including chronic migraine, pain after shingles (post-herpetic neuralgia), pain after trauma (post traumatic neuralgia) and a variety of facial pains (trigeminal neuralgias), as well as plantar fasciitis, piriformis syndrome, interstitial cystitis, pelvic pain, pain from diabetic neuropathy and certain types of low back pain (described in previous chapters of this book) [25–34].

Chronic pain disorders in dogs and horses are one of the most common medical conditions encountered in veterinary practice. In recent years, some veterinary researchers have explored the analgesic role of botulinum neurotoxins (BoNTs) in painful disorders of dogs and horses. In dogs, the studies have focused on osteoarthritis and post- surgical pain so far. In horses, the analgesic effects of BoNTs have been explored in soft tissue damage of the foot (laminitis, synovitis) and pain in the hoof secondary to degenerative changes of the navicular bone.

Osteoarthritis of Dogs (Canine Osteoarthritis)

Mammalian joints are made of two bones that come together, separated by cartilage (connective tissue) and surrounded by a fluid called synovial fluid (like egg white) (Fig. 16.1). Osteoarthritis is characterized by degeneration of joint cartilage associated with changes in synovial lining and synovial inflammation. The inflammatory response in osteoarthritis is often mediated by hormone like substances called cytokine prostaglandin E2 (PGe2) [35, 36]. A prevalence ranging from 2.5 to 20% has been reported in dogs for osteoarthritis [37, 38]. Osteoarthritis is one of the leading causes of canine chronic pain and disability, especially in older dogs.

Treatment plan for canine osteoarthritis includes both pharmacological and non-pharmacological approaches. Common non-pharmacological approaches include physical therapy, weight bearing physiotherapy and nutraceuticals (food that contains health-giving additives such as vitamin E, fish oil, chondroitin). Pharmacological treatment includes use of oral analgesic drugs as well as injection of drugs and hormones into the joint (intra-articular injection) [39]. Among intra-articular (IA) injections, steroids are commonly employed. Although IA injection of steroids

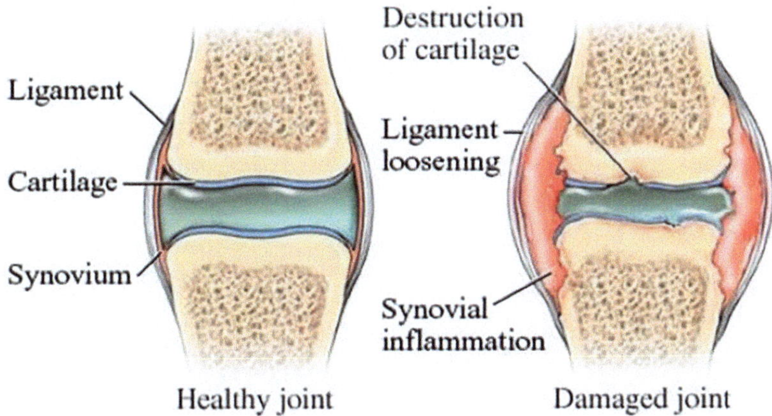

Fig. 16.1 Pathological changes in osteoarthritis

often alleviates dogs' pain, the results usually do not last more than 8 weeks [40]. Furthermore, IA injection of steroids can cause several undesirable side effects such as focal infection of the joints (septic arthritis) [41, 42]. Recently, investigators have reported that intra-articular injection of a non-steroid drug, celecoxib, improved pain and quality of life in 30 studied dogs with painful osteoarthritis [43]. Trials injection of stem cells derived from the fat (adipose) tissue of the affected dogs into the affected joint and with plasma rich platelets (blood cells important for coagulation) are ongoing in canine osteoarthritis. Some preliminary results have shown improvement of pain and quality of life lasting up to 6 months [44, 45].

Botulinum Toxin Treatment of Osteoarthritis in Dogs

Limited number of studies suggest that botulinum toxin injection into the joint can reduce or alleviate pain in dogs with painful arthritis. This literature includes one open label (no placebo) and two blinded (placebo-controlled) studies [46–48] (Table 16.1).

In 2004, Hadley and co-workers [46] reported the result of an open label study on the efficacy of Botox injections into the affected joints of five dogs with osteoarthritis. All dogs had chronic pain and their condition was stable. They were all on medications for inflammation (not steroids) and on nutraceuticals (see above). The studied dogs had lameness and pain due to elbow or hip osteoarthritis. After sedation, each dog received an injection of 25 units of Botox into the affected joint. Animals were evaluated by pressure platform gait analysis (ground pressure/ weight bearing) and owner perception of outcome (walking discomfort) at baseline and at 2,4,8 and 12 weeks post injection. All dogs, following Botox injection, demonstrated improvement of ground reaction forces. At week 12, two of five owners reported significant and one owner reported moderate improvement of dogs'

Table 16.1 Studies assessing efficacy of BoNT injections in canine osteoarthritis

Authors and date	Type of study	Study class	Number of dogs	Location of OA	Toxin type	Dose in units	Assessed scales	Results
Hadley et al, 2010 [46]	Open label (not blinded)	IV[a]	5	Elbow, hip	onaA	25	Pressure Platform Gait Analysis (PPGA), Owner Perception (OP)	PPGA improved in all dogs at week 12, OP: two dogs significantly and one dog moderately improved
Heikkila et al, 2014 [47]	Blinded, placebo-controlled	I	35	Stifle, elbow, hip	onaA	30	Helsinki Chronic Pain Index (HCPI), Ground Reaction Force (GRF)	At 12 weeks, both HCPI and GRF improved significantly ($P < 0.005$)
Nicacio et al, 2019 [48]	Blinded, placebo-controlled	II	16	Hip	aboA	25	Vet-score, Helsinki Chronic Pain Index (HCPI)	Both toxin and placebo groups improved in all measures compared to baseline

[a]Study class is defined according the guidelines of the American Academy of Neurology
onaA onabotulinumtoxinA-botox, *aboA* abobotulinumtoxinA (Dysport), *PPGA* Pressure Platform Gait Analysis, *HCPI* Helsinki Chronic Pain Index, *GRF* Ground Reaction Force, *CBPI* Canine Brief Pain Inventory, *OA* osteoarthritis

function and discomfort. Among the other two, one owner reported mild and the other reported no improvement. No side effects were reported.

In 2014, Heikkila and co-workers [47] published their study on Botox's effectiveness in osteoarthritis of 35 client owned dogs. The animals had osteoarthritis of the stifle, hip and elbow joints. The study was placebo-controlled. Each dog received intra-articular injection (into painful joint) of either Botox or placebo (saline). The injected dose of the toxin was 30 units. The primary outcome measures of the study were Helsinki Chronic Pain Index (HCPI) and changes in the ground reaction forces evaluated by a force plate. HCPI is a questionnaire for dog owners through which they rate a dog's chronic joint pain. In this scale, a score of 17 or higher denotes severe pain. Secondary outcome measures of the study consisted of the need for rescue analgesia (pain medications) and a subjective pain scale rated by a veterinarian. Dog owners were given caprofen tablets (Pfizer's Rimadyl) for pain (rescue analgesic) to be given to their dogs once daily (4 mg/Kg) if needed. They would record this rescue analgesic use as 0=not needed, 1= needed once or twice/week, 2- needed 3 to 4 times/week and 3- needed 5–6 times/week and 5- when needed every day. The duration of the study was 12 weeks. At the end of the study (12 weeks after injection), the investigators noted a significant improvement of ground force in the toxin injected group (P < 0.005). The group that was injected with Botox also demonstrated a significant reduction of HCPI score (pain score) from baseline when compared to placebo. The authors did not observe any serious side effects in the participant dogs.

In 2019, in another study, Nicacio et al [48] published their research on BoNT treatment of canine osteoarthritis. In this blinded and placebo-controlled study, the researchers injected either Dysport (another BoNT-A, like Botox) or saline into the hip joint of 16 dogs with osteoarthritis. The injected dose of Dysport was 25 units. The dogs' response to intra-articular (IA) toxin injections was evaluated over 12 weeks with a Vet-Score and an owner rating scale. The Vet-score includes 4 subsets of pain on manipulation, lameness, ability to jump and ability to climb stairs, each rated from 1 to 4. The owners were trained to use two validated pain scales to rate the level of pain change in the dogs namely, HCPI (see above) and Canine Brief Pain Inventory (CBPI). The investigators found that both Dysport and saline injections improved Vet Scores, HCPI and CBPI scores significantly, but the improvement had a higher magnitude in the saline group! The large placebo effect in this study makes any conclusions about toxin efficacy invalid. Furthermore, Furthermore, if one uses a ratio of 1:2.5 for Botox/Dysport, the dose of Dysport used in Nicacio and co-worker's study [48] would be substantially lower (almost half) that that of the toxin dose used in the study of Heikkila and co-workers who used Botox[47]. Using the efficacy criteria of Assessment and Guideline subcommittee of the American Academy of Neurology [49, 50], IA injections of Botox for canine osteoarthritis would have a level B efficacy (probably effective based on one class I study (blinded, carefully screened) [47]. Studies investigating the efficacy of botulinum toxin injection in canine osteoarthritis are illustrated in Table 16.1.

Heikkila and co-workers [51] also investigated if after Botox injection into the joint of healthy dogs, the toxin spreads to other joints and into adjacent muscles and causes any deleterious effects. Six healthy dogs were injected into a joint either by 30 units of Botox or by comparable volume of saline (same joint on the other side). The study was blinded and placebo-controlled (saline). Although by electrophysiological assessment (electromyography), there was some evidence of spread of the toxin into the adjacent muscles, none of the dogs showed muscle weakness or any other adverse effects.

BoNT Injections for Post-surgical Pain in Dogs

In human, BoNT injections can relieve local pain after neck surgery, breast pain after mastectomy and pain after breast expander surgery [52–55]. So far, in dogs, only one study has reported the results of BoNT treatment for pain after mastectomy. Vilhegas and co-workers [56] enrolled 16 studied dogs scheduled to have bilateral mastectomy for malignant tumors. The study was blinded, placebo-controlled and had a duration of 10–14 days. The study cohort was randomized into toxin and placebo groups. The dogs in the toxin group were injected with Dysport (7units/kg), 24 h before surgery. Injections were performed into the middle of the mammary glands (breasts). An identical volume of normal saline was injected into the breast of the control group. Authors assessed dogs' post-operative pain by the Visual Analogue Scale (VAS, 0–10) and by modified Glasgow Composite Measure Pain Scale (GCMPS). Rescue analgesia was prescribed during the study when deemed necessary. The authors found that pain scores evaluated by VAS and modified-GCMPS were significantly lower in the BoNT-A group compared to the control group (P < 0.05). Only two of the eight dogs injected with Dysport required strong pain medications after mastectomy compared to seven of eight dogs in the placebo group - a finding that was statistically significant (P = 0.022). The authors concluded that "pre-emptive botulinum therapy appears to be effective in reducing post-operative pain in dogs undergoing bilateral radical mastectomy." No adverse effects from botulinum toxin (Dysport) injections were noted.

BoNT Treatment in Equine Pain Disorders

Horses may suffer several ailments that cause chronic pain, leading to lameness and loss of function. The literature on the use of BoNTs as an analgesic in equine pain disorders is limited to studies on laminitis, synovitis and chronic pain in the hoof due to degeneration of navicular bone and the surrounding tissue.

Laminitis

Laminitis refers to inflammation of the soft tissue structures that attach the coffin (pedal bone of the foot) to the hoof wall. Inflammation and damage to the lamina of the horse can cause severe pain and lead to instability of the coffin bone in the horse's hoof. With progression of the disorder, the third phalanx rotates and under-goes distal displacement in the hoof capsule. In more severe cases, it can lead to complete separation and rotation of the pedal bone within the hoof wall. Recurrent attacks of laminitis after the initial attack are not uncommon. Severe laminitis can cripple the horse and may even be fatal. Since management of laminitis is difficult, prevention of laminitis is an important task in equine veterinary medicine.

The reported incidence of equine laminitis varies from 1.5% to 24%, reflecting variation in the type of horses, horses's nutritional status and their geographical location [57]. Mitchell et al [58] described five principles for treatment of acute equine laminitis: nutritional and medical management of primary disease process, cryotherapy (keeping the temperature below 10 degrees centigrade for 48 h), treat-ment of inflammation, pain control and biomechanical optimization. Among drugs used for treatment of inflammation, phenylbutazone is commonly administered with a dose of 2.2–4.4 mg/kg given by mouth or administered intravenously every 12 h [58].

For management of mild to moderate pain, amitriptyline and soluble epoxide hydrolase inhibitor may be helpful [59]. More severe cases of pain may require use of opioids or constant rate infusions of α-2 agonists, ketamine, and lidocaine [59]. In case of recalcitrant pain, deep digital tendon resection (tenotomy) may offer pain relief [60].

Botulinum Toxin Treatment in Equine Laminitis

The feasibility of denervating the deep digital flexors of the horse by BoNT injections (producing a similar effect to tenotomy) has been explored by several studies in recent years [61–63]. These studies have shown that injections of BoNTs into the deep digital flexors produce sustained denervation of these muscles with reduced electrical activity of the muscle on electromyography (EMG) and, in appropriate doses, these injections do not cause lameness or loss of function. The authors concluded that BoNT injections may offer a safe approach for treatment of laminitis, the efficacy of which needs to be confirmed by large clinical trials.

In a small open- label study, Carter and Renroe [64] investigated the effect of deep digital flexor denervation by BoNT-A for treatment of equine laminitis. Seven horses with chronic laminitis were injected by 100–200 units of Botox into the digital flexor muscles of one or both front limbs. The horses were followed for a period of 6–36 months. Six of the seven horses demonstrated improvement of pain and function; most of them becoming pressure sound. One of the six responding horses fully recovered and could ride through all gates. No adverse effects were seen after BoNT injections.

Botulinum Toxin Effect on Podotrochlear (Navicular) Pain Syndrome

In the horse's hoof, podotrochlear apparatus (navicular apparatus) includes the navicular bone, the navicular bursa, the coffin joint and suspensory ligament of the navicular bone as well as the deep digital flexor tendon (DDFT). Degenerative changes affecting navicular bone and adjacent tissue result in hoof pain and lameness. Corrective shoeing, controlled exercises, extracorporeal shock therapy as well as oral or intra-articular injection of drugs that combat inflammation are helpful, but still a majority of the horses fail to respond to these treatments [65].

In an open label study (not blinded) [65], the authors injected Myobloc (botulinum toxin B) into the navicular bursa of 7 horses with severe lameness and pain due to degeneration of podonavicular apparatus. The dose of injected toxin was 3.8 to

4.5units/kg. The response to BoNT-B injections was assessed over 14 days via study of videos by veterinarians. After Myobloc injections, investigators noted a significant decrease in the severity of lameness. However, none of the horses fully recovered from lameness which the authors attributed this to possibly the low dose of the injected toxin.

BoNT Effect on Acute Synovitis

Depuy et al [66], in a double- blind, placebo -controlled study, injected 50 units of Botox into the middle carpal joint (both limbs) of two healthy horses. Two other horses (controls) received the same volume of saline injections bilaterally. Then, all four horses were injected by interleukin 1-beta in order to induce acute inflammation (synovitis). Study veterinarians evaluated the analgesic activity of the injected Botox using a computer-assisted analysis of lameness. After interleukin injection, both saline injected horses developed lameness, whereas only one of the two horses that had received BoNT injection demonstrated lameness. All horses were euthanized at day 14 after interleukin injection. The histological evaluation of the injected joints revealed evidence of suppurative inflammation in all four horses.

Comment

The low-quality (not blinded) studies cited above, suggest that local injection of Botox into the joint of horses affected by painful lameness due to inflammation of the synovial fluid and soft tissue can relief pain and improve equine lameness. The proof of utility of Botox in equine pain disorders awaits the results of well-designed, blinded and placebo-controlled studies. Since horses are known to be more sensitive than many other species (including man) to the effects of botulinum toxins [67], future studies need to monitor and titrate the injected doses of the toxin carefully in order to avoid inducing botulism. A detailed and up to date review of BoNT toxin treatment in veterinary medicine has been published recently (2020) by Helga Heikkila PhD, DVM [68].

References

1. Matak I, Tékus V, Bölcskei K, Lacković Z, Helyes Z. Involvement of substance P in the antinociceptive effect of botulinum toxin type A: evidence from knockout mice. Neuroscience. 2017;358:137–45. https://doi.org/10.1016/j.neuroscience.2017.06.040.
2. Rossetto O, Pirazzini M, Fabris F, Montecucco C. Botulinum neurotoxins: mechanism of action. Handb Exp Pharmacol. 2021;263:35–47. https://doi.org/10.1007/164_2020_355.

3. Marino MJ, Terashima T, Steinauer JJ, Eddinger KA, Yaksh TL, Xu Q. Botulinum toxin B in the sensory afferent: transmitter release, spinal activation, and pain behavior. Pain. 2014;155(4):674–84. https://doi.org/10.1016/j.pain.2013.12.009.

4. Bach-Rojecky L, Relja M, Lacković Z. Botulinum toxin type A in experimental neuropathic pain. J Neural Transm (Vienna). 2005;112(2):215–9. https://doi.org/10.1007/s00702-004-0265-1.

5. Cui M, Khanijou S, Rubino J, Aoki KR. Subcutaneous administration of botulinum toxin A reduces formalin-induced pain. Pain. 2004;107(1-2):125–33. https://doi.org/10.1016/j.pain.2003.10.008.

6. Mika J, Rojewska E, Makuch W, Korostynski M, Luvisetto S, Marinelli S, Pavone F, Przewlocka B. The effect of botulinum neurotoxin A on sciatic nerve injury-induced neuroimmunological changes in rat dorsal root ganglia and spinal cord. Neuroscience. 2011;175:358–66. https://doi.org/10.1016/j.neuroscience.2010.11.040.

7. Bossowska A, Lepiarczyk E, Mazur U, Janikiewicz P, Markiewicz W. Botulinum toxin type A induces changes in the chemical coding of substance P-immunoreactive dorsal root ganglia sensory neurons supplying the porcine urinary bladder. Toxins (Basel). 2015;7(11):4797–816. https://doi.org/10.3390/toxins7114797.

8. Safarpour Y, Jabbari B. Botulinum toxin treatment of pain syndromes – an evidence based review. Toxicon. 2018;147:120–8. https://doi.org/10.1016/j.toxicon.2018.01.017.

9. Shin MC, Wakita M, Xie DJ, Yamaga T, Iwata S, Torii Y, Harakawa T, Ginnaga A, Kozaki S, Akaike N. Inhibition of membrane Na+ channels by A type botulinum toxin at femtomolar concentrations in central and peripheral neurons. J Pharmacol Sci. 2012;118(1):33–42. https://doi.org/10.1254/jphs.11060fp.

10. Hong B, Yao L, Ni L, Wang L, Hu X. Antinociceptive effect of botulinum toxin A involves alterations in AMPA receptor expression and glutamate release in spinal dorsal horn neurons. Neuroscience. 2017;357:197–207. https://doi.org/10.1016/j.neuroscience.2017.06.004.

11. Matak I, Bölcskei K, Bach-Rojecky L, Helyes Z. Mechanisms of botulinum toxin type A action on pain. Toxins (Basel). 2019;11(8):459. https://doi.org/10.3390/toxins11080459.

12. Lacković Z. Botulinum toxin and pain. Handb Exp Pharmacol. 2021;263:251–64. https://doi.org/10.1007/164_2019_348.

13. Matak I, Riederer P, Lacković Z. Botulinum toxin's axonal transport from periphery to the spinal cord. Neurochem Int. 2012;61(2):236–9. https://doi.org/10.1016/j.neuint.2012.05.001.

14. Drinovac Vlah V, Filipović B, Bach-Rojecky L, Lacković Z. Role of central versus peripheral opioid system in antinociceptive and anti-inflammatory effect of botulinum toxin type A in trigeminal region. Eur J Pain. 2018;22(3):583–91. https://doi.org/10.1002/ejp.1146.

15. Wang W, Kong M, Dou Y, Xue S, Liu Y, Zhang Y, Chen W, Li Y, Dai X, Meng J, Wang J. Selective expression of a SNARE-cleaving protease in peripheral sensory neurons attenuates pain-related gene transcription and neuropeptide release. Int J Mol Sci. 2021;22(16):8826. https://doi.org/10.3390/ijms22168826.

16. Hok P, Veverka T, Hluštík P, Nevrlý M, Kaňovský P. The central effects of botulinum toxin in dystonia and spasticity. Toxins (Basel). 2021;13(2):155. https://doi.org/10.3390/toxins13020155.

17. Meng J, Ovsepian SV, Wang J, Pickering M, Sasse A, Aoki KR, Lawrence GW, Dolly JO. Activation of TRPV1 mediates calcitonin gene-related peptide release, which excites trigeminal sensory neurons and is attenuated by a retargeted botulinum toxin with anti-nociceptive potential. J Neurosci. 2009;29(15):4981–92. https://doi.org/10.1523/JNEUROSCI.5490-08.2009.

18. Li X, Ye Y, Zhou W, Shi Q, Wang L, Li T. Anti-inflammatory effects of BoNT/A against complete freund's adjuvant-induced arthritis pain in rats: transcriptome analysis. Front Pharmacol. 2021;12:735075. https://doi.org/10.3389/fphar.2021.735075.

19. Lacković Z. New analgesic: focus on botulinum toxin. Toxicon. 2020;179:1–7. https://doi.org/10.1016/j.toxicon.2020.02.008.

20. Meng J, Wang J, Lawrence G, Dolly JO. Synaptobrevin I mediates exocytosis of CGRP from sensory neurons and inhibition by botulinum toxins reflects their anti-nociceptive potential. J Cell Sci. 2007;120(Pt 16):2864–74. https://doi.org/10.1242/jcs.012211.
21. Waskitho A, Yamamoto Y, Raman S, Kano F, Yan H, Raju R, Afroz S, Morita T, Ikutame D, Okura K, Oshima M, Yamamoto A, Baba O, Matsuka Y. Peripherally administered botulinum toxin type A localizes bilaterally in trigeminal ganglia of animal model. Toxins (Basel). 2021;13(10):704. https://doi.org/10.3390/toxins13100704.
22. Vacca V, Marinelli S, Eleuteri C, Luvisetto S, Pavone F. Botulinum neurotoxin A enhances the analgesic effects on inflammatory pain and antagonizes tolerance induced by morphine in mice. Brain Behav Immun. 2012;26(3):489–99. https://doi.org/10.1016/j.bbi.2012.01.002.
23. Rosales RL, Arimura K, Takenaga S, Osame M. Extrafusal and intrafusal muscle effects in experimental botulinum toxin-A injection. Muscle Nerve. 1996;19(4):488–96. https://doi.org/10.1002/(SICI)1097-4598(199604)19:4<488::AID-MUS9>3.0.CO;2-8.
24. Aoki KR, Francis J. Updates on the antinociceptive mechanism hypothesis of botulinum toxin A. Parkinsonism Relat Disord. 2011;17(Suppl 1):S28–33. https://doi.org/10.1016/j.parkreldis.2011.06.013.
25. Dodick DW, Turkel CC, DeGryse RE, Aurora SK, Silberstein SD, Lipton RB, Diener HC, Brin MF, PREEMPT Chronic Migraine Study Group. OnabotulinumtoxinA for treatment of chronic migraine: pooled results from the double-blind, randomized, placebo-controlled phases of the PREEMPT clinical program. Headache. 2010;50(6):921–36. https://doi.org/10.1111/j.1526-4610.2010.01678.x.
26. Wu CJ, Lian YJ, Zheng YK, Zhang HF, Chen Y, Xie NC, Wang LJ. Botulinum toxin type A for the treatment of trigeminal neuralgia: results from a randomized, double-blind, placebo-controlled trial. Cephalalgia. 2012;32(6):443–50. https://doi.org/10.1177/0333102412441721.
27. Xiao L, Mackey S, Hui H, Xong D, Zhang Q, Zhang D. Subcutaneous injection of botulinum toxin a is beneficial in postherpetic neuralgia. Pain Med. 2010;11(12):1827–33. https://doi.org/10.1111/j.1526-4637.2010.01003.x.
28. Yuan RY, Sheu JJ, Yu JM, Chen WT, Tseng IJ, Chang HH, Hu CJ. Botulinum toxin for diabetic neuropathic pain: a randomized double-blind crossover trial. Neurology. 2009;72(17):1473–8. https://doi.org/10.1212/01.wnl.0000345968.05959.cf.
29. Babcock MS, Foster L, Pasquina P, Jabbari B. Treatment of pain attributed to plantar fasciitis with botulinum toxin A: a short-term, randomized, placebo-controlled, double-blind study. Am J Phys Med Rehabil. 2005;84(9):649–54. https://doi.org/10.1097/01.phm.0000176339.73591.d7.
30. Childers MK, Wilson DJ, Gnatz SM, Conway RR, Sherman AK. Botulinum toxin type A use in piriformis muscle syndrome: a pilot study. Am J Phys Med Rehabil. 2002;81(10):751–9. https://doi.org/10.1097/00002060-200210000-00006.
31. Foster L, Clapp L, Erickson M, Jabbari B. Botulinum toxin A and chronic low back pain: a randomized, double-blind study. Neurology. 2001;56(10):1290–3. https://doi.org/10.1212/wnl.56.10.1290.
32. Giannantoni A, Gubbiotti M, Bini V. Botulinum neurotoxin A intravesical injections in interstitial cystitis/bladder painful syndrome: a systematic review with meta-analysis. Toxins (Basel). 2019;11(9):510. https://doi.org/10.3390/toxins11090510.
33. Abbott JA, Jarvis SK, Lyons SD, Thomson A, Vancaille TG. Botulinum toxin type A for chronic pain and pelvic floor spasm in women: a randomized controlled trial. Obstet Gynecol. 2006;108(4):915–23. https://doi.org/10.1097/01.AOG.0000237100.29870.cc.
34. Ranoux D, Attal N, Morain F, Bouhassira D. Botulinum toxin type A induces direct analgesic effects in chronic neuropathic pain. Ann Neurol. 2008;64(3):274–83. https://doi.org/10.1002/ana.21427.
35. Lyn-Jones S, Palmer AJ, Agricola R, Price AJ, Vincent TL, Weinans H, Carr AJ. Osteoarthritis. Lancet. 2015;386:376–87. https://doi.org/10.1016/S0140-6736(14)60802-3.
36. Hugle T, Geurts J. What drives osteoarthritis? – synovial versus subchondral bone pathology. Rheumatology. 2017;56:1461–71.

37. Johnston SA. Osteoarthritis. Joint anatomy, physiology, and pathobiology. Vet Clin North Am Small Anim Pract. 1997;27(4):699–723. https://doi.org/10.1016/s0195-5616(97)50076-3.

38. Anderson KL, O'Neill DG, Brodbelt DC, Church DB, Meeson RL, Sargan D, Summers JF, Zulch H, Collins LM. Prevalence, duration and risk factors for appendicular osteoarthritis in a UK dog population under primary veterinary care. Sci Rep. 2018;8(1):5641. https://doi.org/10.1038/s41598-018-23940-z.

39. Heikkila H. Botulinum toxin treatment in veterinary medicine: clinical implications (chapter 17). In: Jabbari B, editor. Botulinum toxin treatment in surgery, dentistry and veterinary medicine. Springer; 2020. p. 337–57.

40. Bellamy N, Campbell J, Robinson V, Gee T, Bourne R, Wells G. Intraarticular corticosteroid for treatment of osteoarthritis of the knee. Cochrane Database Syst Rev. 2006;2:CD005328.

41. Huscher D, Thiele K, Gromnica-Ihle E, Hein G, Demary W, Dreher R, Zink A, Buttgereit F. Dose-related patterns of glucocorticoid-induced side effects. Ann Rheum Dis. 2009;68:1119–24. https://doi.org/10.1136/ard.2008.092163.

42. Xing D, Yang Y, Ma X, Ma J, Ma B, Chen Y. Dose intraarticular steroid injection increase the rate of infection in subsequent arthroplasty: grading the evidence through a meta-analysis. J Orthop Surg Res. 2014;9:107-014-0107-2. https://doi.org/10.1186/s13018-014-0107-2.

43. Tellegen AR, Rudnik-Jansen I, Utomo L, Versteeg S, Beukers M, Maarschalkerweerd R, van Zuilen D, van Klaveren NJ, Houben K, Teske E, van Weeren PR, Karssemakers-Degen N, Mihov G, Thies J, Eijkelkamp N, Creemers LB, Meij BP, Tryfonidou MA. Sustained release of locally delivered celecoxib provides pain relief for osteoarthritis: a proof of concept in dog patients. Osteoarthr Cartilage. 2022;S1063-4584(22):00934–7. https://doi.org/10.1016/j.joca.2022.11.008.

44. Sanghani-Kerai A, Black C, Cheng SO, Collins L, Schneider N, Blunn G, Watson F, Fitzpatrick N. Clinical outcomes following intra-articular injection of autologous adipose-derived mesenchymal stem cells for the treatment of osteoarthritis in dogs characterized by weight-bearing asymmetry. Bone Joint Res. 2021;10(10):650–8. https://doi.org/10.1302/2046-3758.1010.BJR-2020-0540.R1.

45. Alves JC, Santos A, Jorge P. Platelet-rich plasma therapy in dogs with bilateral hip osteoarthritis. BMC Vet Res. 2021;17(1):207. https://doi.org/10.1186/s12917-021-02913-x.

46. Hadley HS, Wheeler JL, Petersen SW. Effects of intra-articular botulinum toxin type A (Botox) in dogs with chronic osteoarthritis. Vet Comp Orthop Traumatol. 2010;23(4):254–8. https://doi.org/10.3415/VCOT-09-07-0076.

47. Heikkilä HM, Hielm-Björkman AK, Morelius M, Larsen S, Honkavaara J, Innes JF, Laitinen-Vapaavuori OM. Intra-articular botulinum toxin A for the treatment of osteoarthritic joint pain in dogs: a randomized, double-blinded, placebo-controlled clinical trial. Vet J. 2014;200(1):162–9. https://doi.org/10.1016/j.tvjl.2014.01.020.

48. Nicácio GM, Luna SPL, Cavaleti P, Cassu RN. Intra-articular botulinum toxin A (BoNT/A) for pain management in dogs with osteoarthritis secondary to hip dysplasia: a randomized controlled clinical trial. J Vet Med Sci. 2019;81(3):411–7. https://doi.org/10.1292/jvms.18-0506.

49. French J, Gronseth G. Lost in a jungle of evidence: we need a compass. Neurology. 2008;71(20):1634–8. https://doi.org/10.1212/01.wnl.0000336533.19610.1b.

50. Gronseth G, French J. Practice parameters and technology assessments: what they are, what they are not, and why you should care. Neurology. 2008;71(20):1639–43. https://doi.org/10.1212/01.wnl.0000336535.27773.c0.

51. Heikkilä HM, Jokinen TS, Syrjä P, Junnila J, Hielm-Björkman A, Laitinen-Vapaavuori O. Assessing adverse effects of intra-articular botulinum toxin A in healthy Beagle dogs: a placebo-controlled, blinded, randomized trial. PLoS One. 2018;13(1):e0191043. https://doi.org/10.1371/journal.pone.0191043.

52. Alvandipour M, Tavallaei M, Rezaei F, Khodabakhsh H. Postoperative outcomes of intra-sphincteric botox injection during hemorrhoidectomy: a double-blind clinical trial. J Res Med Sci. 2021;26:53. https://doi.org/10.4103/jrms.JRMS_612_18.

53. Blaha L, Chouliaras K, White A, McNatt S, Westcott C. Intraoperative botulinum toxin chemodenervation and analgesia in abdominal wall reconstruction. Surg Innov. 2020:1553350620975253. https://doi.org/10.1177/1553350620975253.
54. Shandilya S, Mohanty S, Sharma P, Chaudhary Z, Kohli S, Kumar RD. Effect of preoperative intramuscular injection of botulinum toxin A on pain and mouth opening after surgical intervention in temporomandibular joint ankylosis cases: a controlled clinical trial. J Oral Maxillofac Surg. 2020;78(6):916–26. https://doi.org/10.1016/j.joms.2020.02.011.
55. Gabriel A, Champaneria MC, Maxwell GP. The efficacy of botulinum toxin A in post-mastectomy breast reconstruction: a pilot study. Aesthet Surg J. 2015;35(4):402–9. https://doi.org/10.1093/asj/sjv040.
56. Vilhegas S, Cassu RN, Barbero RC, Crociolli GC, Rocha TL, Gomes DR. Botulinum toxin type A as an adjunct in postoperative pain management in dogs undergoing radical mastectomy. Vet Rec. 2015;177(15):391. https://doi.org/10.1136/vr.102993.
57. Wylie CE, Collins SN, Verheyen KL, Richard NJ. Frequency of equine laminitis: a systematic review with quality appraisal of published evidence. Vet J. 2011;189(3):248–56. https://doi.org/10.1016/j.tvjl.2011.04.014.
58. Mitchell CF, Fugler LA, Eades SC. The management of equine acute laminitis. Vet Med (Auckl). 2014;6:39–47. https://doi.org/10.2147/VMRR.S39967.
59. Hopster K, Driessen B. Pharmacology of the equine foot: medical pain management for laminitis. Vet Clin North Am Equine Pract. 2021;37(3):549–61. https://doi.org/10.1016/j.cveq.2021.08.004.
60. Eastman TG, Honnas CM, Hague BA, Moyer W, von der Rosen HD. Deep digital flexor tenotomy as a treatment for chronic laminitis in horses: 35 cases (1988–1997). J Am Vet Med Assoc. 1999;214(4):517–9.
61. Hardeman LC, van der Meij BR, Oosterlinck M, Veraa S, van der Kolk JH, Wijnberg ID, et al. Effect of Clostridium botulinum toxin type A injections into the deep digital flexor muscle on the range of motion of the metacarpus and carpus, and the force distribution underneath the hooves, of sound horses at the walk. Veter J. 2013;198:e152–6.
62. Wijnberg ID, Hardeman LC, van der Meij BR, Veraa S, Back W, van der Kolk JH. The effect of Clostridium botulinum toxin type A injections on motor unit activity of the deep digital flexor muscle in healthy sound Royal Dutch sport horses. Veter J. 2013;198:e147–51.
63. Hardeman LC, van der Meij BR, Back W, van der Kolk JH, Wijnberg ID. The use of electromyography interference pattern analysis to determine muscle force of the deep digital flexor muscle in healthy and laminitic horses. Veter Quart. 2015;36(1):10–5.
64. Carter DW, Renfroe BJ. A novel approach to the treatment and prevention of laminitis: botulinum toxin type A for the treatment of laminitis. J Equine Veter Sci. 2009;29(7):595–600.
65. Nibeyro SDG, White Na II, Wepy NM. Outcome of medical treatment for horses with foot pain: 56 cases. Equine Veter J. 2010;42(8):680–5.
66. DePuy T, Howard R, Keegan K, Wilson D, Kramer J, Cook JL, et al. Effects of intra-articular botulinum toxin type A in an equine model of acute synovitis: a pilot study. Am J Phys Med Rehabil. 2007;86(10):777–83.
67. Bakheit AM, Ward CD, McLellan DL. Generalised botulism-like syndrome after intramuscular injections of botulinum toxin type A: a report of two cases. J Neurol Neurosurg Psy. 1997;62(2):198. https://doi.org/10.1136/jnnp.62.2.198.
68. Heikkila H. Chapter 17. In: Jabbari B, editor. Botulinum toxin treatment in surgery, dentistry and veterinary medicine. Cham: Springer-Nature; 2020. p. 337–57.

Chapter 17
Cost and Insurance Issues in Botulinum Toxin Therapy

Abstract Botulinum toxin therapy is now an established mode of treatment for a large number of medical problems. It is FDA approved for treatment of migraine, spasticity (stiff and painful muscles) due to stroke, brain and spinal cord trauma, cerebral palsy, involuntary movements of the neck and face as well as certain bladder disorders. For these indications and for cosmetic use, it is now one of the leading therapeutic approaches used in millions of people worldwide. Botulinum toxin therapy is expensive. This chapter discusses the venues that are available to the patients through the manufacturing companies to defray some of the cost of botulinum toxin therapy. The role of patient and treating physician in facilitating co-pays is also discussed. Finally, data from the literature for certain indications, showing cost-effectiveness of botulinum toxin therapy (despite its high cost) is provided.

Keywords Botulinum toxin · Botulinum neurotoxin · Insurance · Cost · Cost efficiency, migraine, spasticity, cerebral palsy, overactive bladder

Introduction

Botulinum toxin therapy is now an established mode of treatment for a large number of medical problems. It is FDA approved for treatment of migraine, spasticity (stiff and painful muscles) caused by stroke, brain and spinal cord trauma, cerebral palsy, involuntary movements such as cervical dystonia and facial involuntary movements as well as certain bladder disorders. These medical disorders involve millions of people in the US and more than 100 million worldwide.

The six FDA approved botulinum toxins in the US are distributed under the trade names of Botox (Allergan Inc), Xeomin (Merz Pharmaceutical), Dysport (Ipsen), Jeuveau (Evolus), Daxxify (Revance) and Myobloc (Solstice Neuroscience). The first five are type A and the last (Myobloc) is a type B toxin. Of eight distinctly defined serotypes of botulinum toxins in nature (A, B, C, D, E, F, G, X), only types A and B are currently approved for clinical use (partly due to their long duration of action). FDA has a long propriety name for each of these toxins that is usually used in research and publications; onabotulinumtoxinA, incobotulinumtoxinA, abobotulinumtoxinA, probobotulinumtoxinA, DaxibotulinumtoxinA and rimabotulinumtoxinB, respectively. The reader is referred to Chaps. 2 and 3 of this book for further definition of these toxins including their molecular structure, physical properties and mechanisms of action. There are also two other well-known toxins (both type A) with trade names of Prosigne (Lanzhou Institute-China) and Meditox (Korea) that are widely used in Asia, but are not approved by FDA for use in the US.

Due to the expense of botulinum toxin therapy, programs have been established by the manufacturing companies to defray some of the cost to the patients.

For enrollment into botulinum toxin patient assistant programs, patients have to meet certain eligibility criteria. These eligibility criteria are more or less the same for all companies that produce the FDA approved toxins. The eligibility criteria consist of:

1. Age of 18 years or older.
2. Medical condition must be FDA approved for botulinum toxin therapy.
3. The patient should have either no insurance or a private insurance coverage.
4. The patient should not be enrolled in a federally insured program such as Medicare, Medicaid or Tricare.

Some exceptions exists. For instance Merz program covers ages 2–64 years and, in Dysport's program patients can have medicare.

The total amount of medical aid ranges from $4000 (for Xeomin,Dysport and Botox) to $5000 per year. The limit for each treatment is up to $500 per session and it can be repeated several times per year as repeat injection sessions are indicated. The aid covers both cost of the vials and payment to doctor's office for medical assessment and botulinum toxin injection. It may cover the cost of ancillary diagnostic techniques such as ultrasound that visualizes the targeted muscle (for instance in spasticity), or electromyography that locates muscle activity by recording the electrical activity of the muscle.

In case of patients who have insurance, the patient informs the physician's office regarding being enrolled in the patient-assisted program. The physician's office then submits a bill to the insurance company for patient assessment and procedure cost. If the patient receives an invoice asking payment for part of the bill not covered by patient's insurance, he/she can submit a copy of that bill to the patient assisted program that is geared to cover up to $500 of the unpaid bill for each treatment.

The cost of botulinum toxins varies among the states. In 2005, the price was higher in the northern states compared to western states in pharmacies and hospitals provided the toxin by the whole sale organizations. The current whole sale acquisition cost (WAC) for the three widely used botulinum toxins in the US are as follows:

- Botox vials: 50 units ($300), 100 units ($600), 200 units ($1200)
- Xeomin vials: 50 units ($253), 100 units ($482), 200 units ($964)
- Dysport vials: 300 units: $491

Although the units of the toxins are not truly interchangeable, each one unit of Botox approximates one unit of Xeomin and 2.5 units of Dysport.

Various strategies are used by physicians to lower the price of toxin used per patient. Some of these practices are inappropriate such as an injection arrangement called "Botox parties." Usually, practiced for cosmetic purposes that require much fewer units of Botox than that used for spasticity or dystonia; a physician injects a large number of patients (20 or more) in a rapid sequence. Although somewhat cheaper for the patient, such a practice is not sound and safe since rushed injections may jeopardize the accuracy of the procedure and could potentially interrupt maintenance of full sterility.

Patients and Insurance Companies

Insurance companies use a list of different diagnoses with designated diagnostic codes that reflect indications that a particular company has approved for botulinum toxin therapy. This list varies somewhat among different companies. In consultations with experts in the field, the companies often update this list annually or biannually. Although the list(s) are somewhat rigid, there is often some room for negotiation. In each region of the country, insurance companies have physicians in their payroll who deal with insurance issues with medical providers. If your insurance company refuses to approve you for botulinum toxin treatment of your condition, you may ask your physician if he can call the insurance company and present your case for you. Sometimes, a very informed nurse can do as well as the treating physician but usually the process works better when the issue is discussed between the treating and the company physician. The medical conditions considered for insurance approval do not always have to be FDA approved indications. For several non-approved clinical conditions, there is now ample literature to support effectiveness of botulinum toxin therapy. Some of these off-label conditions include injection of Botox and other neurotoxins into the skin for alleviating the pain associated with shingles (post-herpetic neuralgia) or the pain in the distal part of the limbs resulting from nerve damage from diabetes or local trauma. Your treating physician can provide the company's physician, before their telephonic communication, the relevant literature that strongly supports the use of botulinum toxin injection for your medical condition. In busy practices, many physicians may not find the time to do this but I know, from personal experience, that treating physicians' calls to insurance company's physician, in many cases succeeds in gaining treatment approval for patients.

One of the reasons for disapproval for some disorders is an insurance company policy that requires evidence for failure of other medications before botulinum toxin therapy. A brief request for approval submitted to the insurance company by the clinic staff may not provide convincing information on this issue. Again, a call from treating physician or an informed nurse is helpful. In many instances, specific medications asked by insurance companies to be used before botulinum toxin therapy may not be compatible with the patient's age or it may interfere with other medications essential for patient's health. It is the treating physician who can best discuss and document these issues or, even better, explain it over the phone.

Contact Information for Patient Support and Co-pay Programs in the US

Dysport (Ipsen Inc): Ipsen Care Program

Telephone: 1-866-435-5677- 8 am to 8 pm (ET)
Website: Ipsencares.com

Botox (Allergan Inc): Reimbursement Solutions Patient Assistance Programs

The programs assists uninsured and underinsured patients with their treatment through donation of Botox.

https://www.botoxone.com/ Download program application instructions. Out of pocket costs of patients' for treatment of cervical dystonia may be covered through National Organization of Rare Diseases (NORD-rarediseases.org).

Telephone: 1-855-864-4024
Website: Cervicaldystonia@rarediseases.org

Xeomin (Merz Pharma): Xeomin Patient Co-pay Program

Telephone: 888-493-6646- 8 am to 8 pm (ET)
Website: Xeomin.com

Myobloc (Solstice Neuroscience): Myobloc Co-pay Program

Telephone: 888-461-2255- 8 am to 8 pm (ET).
Website: www.myobloc-reimbursement.com

Jeuveau (Evolus): Evolus reward program. 949-284-4555 (PT)

Daxxify (Revance) Telephone: 877-373-8669 (ET) hcp.doxxifytherapy.com, find Daxxify near me. Currently (as of Dec 2023), Revance company is in the process of developing saving programs for patients who use Daxxify.

Several other botulinum toxin type As are currently in use in the Far East and China. The Chinese toxin (form Lanzhou Institute) and the South Korean Toxin (Meditoxin) have some similarity to Botox with their units closely approximating that of Botox. Neither of these two toxins are currently approved by FDA for use in the US (Table 17.1).

Cost-effectiveness

Botulinum toxin therapy is expensive. Depending on the indications, the effect of botulinum toxin injection into the muscle lasts 3–9 months. The need for repeat injections to maintain long-term efficacy adds to long-term expense of botulinum toxin therapy over time. The high cost of botulinum toxin therapy is balanced by its long-term effect that reduces the need for taking medications daily. Furthermore, it has been shown that utilization of botulinum toxin therapy for its major indications (chronic migraine, spasticity, bladder dysfunction) clearly reduces emergency room visits and the frequency of hospitalizations. For these reasons, investigators began to assess the cost efficacy of botulinum toxin therapy compared with other modes of therapy. They also studied the cost-effectiveness of botulinum toxin therapy, comparing some of the FDA approved toxins with each other. The cost efficacy studies have been published for both adult and childhood indications of botulinum toxin therapy. The results of some of these studies are presented below.

Dr. Visco and his colleagues compared the cost of Botox treatment with standard oral medications (anticholinergics) in 231 women with bladder dysfunction causing urgency and incontinence. Botox injection into the bladder wall (see Chap. 10) was as effective as the use of oral medications. Interestingly, The cost for Botox treatment was lower after 6 months of treatment, averaging $207/month versus $305/month for oral medications [1]. These findings were supported by a subsequent British study of 101 patients with bladder problems, in whom the cost savings in favor of Botox treatment was found to be 617 pounds per patients per year [2].

In his publication of 2006 [3], Dr. Squenazi, a knowledgeable and well published physician in the fields of neurology and toxicology discusses why intramuscular botulinum toxin injections, in the long-term, are more cost effective for patients suffering from stroke, spinal cord injury and multiple sclerosis. Such patients are affected by spasticity, a condition of heightened muscle tone and stiffness (and sometimes jerkiness of the limbs), that limits their daily activities and impairs their quality of life. Botulinum toxin injection into the muscle reduces the muscle tone and improves spasticity. This allows patients to reduce, and in many instances, stop anti-spasticity medications which in many cases are poorly tolerated, especially by elderly patients. Furthermore, relief from spasticity reduces associated muscle pain, and in some patients, prevents falls resulting from poor balance due to stiff and jerky legs (see Chaps. 7 and 8 on stroke and multiple sclerosis).

In a study of a large cohort of patients from US based hospitals, Dr. Hepp and coworkers found positive gains in patients with chronic migraine after Botox

Table 17.1 FDA approved botulinum toxins in the USA

Trade name	Proprietary name given by FDA	Manufacturer	Medical condition	Year of FDA approval
Botox	OnabotulinumtoxinA	Allergan/Abbvie Irvine, Ca	Blepharospasm Hemifacial spasm Strabismus (crossed eyes) Cervical dystonia Armpit sweating Chronic migraine Upper limb spasticity Bladder (NDO)[a] Bladder (OAB)[a] Lower limb spasticity (adult) Esthetics(forehead wrinkles) Upper limb spasticity (child)	1989 1989 1989 2000 2004 2010 2010 2011 2013 2014 2017 2019
Xeomin	IncobotulinumtoxinA	Merz Pharma Frankfurt, Germany	Cervical dystonia Blepharospasm Excessive sweating Esthetics (glabellar lines) Upper limb spasticity(adult) Excessive drooling	2010 2010 2010 2011 2015 2018
Dysport	AbobotulinumtoxinA	Ipsen Pharma-UK	Cervical dystonia Esthetics (glabellar lines) Upper limb spasticity (adult) Lower limb spasticity (child) Loewr limb spasticity adult	2009 2009 2015 2016 2017
Jeuveau	Probobotulinum toxinA	Evolus, InC Santa Barbara, CA	Esthetics (wrinkles)	2019
Daxxify	Daxibotulinum toxinA	Revance; Nashville, TN	Esthetics Cervical dystonia	2022 2023
Myobloc	RimabotulinumtoxinB	Solstice Neuroscience	Cervical dystonia Excessive drooling	2009 2010

[a]*NDO* neurogenic detrusor over-activity. Detrusser is the main muscle of the bladder wall. *OAB* overactive bladder (see Chap. 10)

treatment [4]. The Botox treated group had significantly lower visits to emergency room at 6, 9 and 12 months; the visits were 21%, 10% and 20% less, respectively. The figures for reduced hospitalizations over those three time lines were 47%, 48% and 56%, respectively. In 2020, Dr. Hansson-Headblom and co-workers also found that Botox treatment was cost effective for migraine in Sweden and Norway by reducing headache days, the main driver of indirect cost [5]. In a recent report [6], Dr. Murry and his coworkers compared the cost of Botox treatment with several modes of treatment in overactive bladder. Botox was most cost effective compared to current oral medications (anticholinergics and adrenoreceptor agonist) as well as electrical stimulation of the spinal cord and sacrum. Finally, in a recently published article from Spain [7] authors found that combined treatment of Dysport with physiotherapy was less costly that physiotherapy alone in a group of patients with post-stroke spasticity.

Few studies have compared two or more toxins for cost-effectiveness. Drs Kazerooni and Broadhead compared cost-effectiveness of Botox, Dysport and Xeomin in cervical dystonia [8]. Cervical dystonia is a late onset movement disorder characterized by posturing and twisting of the neck as well as neck pain. It responds very well to Botox or other toxin injections into the neck and shoulder muscles (see Chap. 8 of this book). Kazerooni and Broadhead found Xeomin to be the most cost effective of the three toxins followed by Dysport. In another study of a large number of patients with cervical dystonia (Chap. 8) who received several cycles of injections (into neck and shoulder), treatment with dysport was 37% cheaper than treatment with Botox [9]. Drs Tilden and Guanierie also found Xeomin superior to Botox in terms of cost-effectiveness when they studied patients in the Australian Health System [10].

In children with upper limb spasticity, Dr. Danchench and colleague compared the cost of treatment with Botox and Dysport in 6 clinical trials [11]. In regard to cost-effectiveness analysis, Dysport was more economical. "The cost per responder at 1 year was estimated to be £39,056 for Dysport vs. £54,831 for Botox". In another study comparing Botox injection for bladder over activity (see Chap. 10), Botox was more cost effective than the new expensive drug oxibutinin used for control of bladder symptoms [12]. Oxybutinin is also hard to tolerate by the patients over time. In a Swedish study, Dr. Tedroff and her colleagues treated 159 children with cerebral palsy(CP) and spasticity with Botox and Dysport over 18 months. Treatment of CP children with spasticity turned out to be 41% cheaper with Dysport than Botox [13]. In another study of patients with facial movement disorders, blepharospasm and hemifacial spasm (see Chap. 8), authors compared the price of Botox with Xeomin (another type A toxin similar to Botox). Both toxins were equally effective for treatment of these conditions but Botox was 33% more costly than Xeomin [14].

Conclusion

Cost issues are important to the patients who receive expensive botulinum toxin therapy for management of their symptom(s). Patient co-pay programs are available through manufacturers of botulinum toxins to defray some of patients' out of pocket costs. There is evidence from published literature that despite the apparent high cost, botulinum toxin therapy is cost effective compared to other modes of therapy in management of chronic migraine, spasticity associated with stroke, multiple sclerosis, spinal cord injury and chronic bladder disorders. A limited published literature from comparative studies suggests that Botox is the least cost effective compared to Dysport and Xeomin when used for the same indications.

References

 1. Visco AG, Zyczynski H, Brubaker L. Cost-effectiveness analysis of anticholinergics versus Botox for urgency urinary incontinence: results from the anticholinergic versus Botox comparison randomized trial. Female Pelvic Med Reconstr Surg. 2016;22(5):311–6.
 2. Kalsi V, Popat RB, Apostolidis A, et al. Cost-consequence analysis evaluating the use of botulinum neurotoxin-a in patients with detrusor overactivity based on clinical outcomes observed at a single UK centre. Eur Urol. 2006;49(3):519–27.
 3. Esquenazi. Improvement in health care and cost benefits associated with botulinum toxin treatment of spasticity and muscle overactivity. Eur J Neurol. 2006;13(Suppl 4):27–34.
 4. Hepp Z, Rosen NL, Gillard PG. Comparative effectiveness of onabotulinumtoxinA versus oral migraine prophylactic medications on headache-related resource utilization in the management of chronic migraine: retrospective analysis of a US-based insurance claims database. Cephalalgia. 2016;36(9):862–74.
 5. Hansson-Hedblom A, Axelsson I, Jacobson L, Tedroff J, Borgström F. Economic consequences of migraine in Sweden and implications for the cost-effectiveness of onabotulinumtoxinA (Botox) for chronic migraine in Sweden and Norway. J Headache Pain. 2020;21(1):99. https://doi.org/10.1186/s10194-020-01162-x.
 6. Murray B, Miles-Thomas J, Park AJ, Nguyen VB, Tung A, Gillard P, Lalla A, Nitti VW, Chermansky CJ. Cost-effectiveness of overactive bladder treatments from a US commercial and payer perspective. J Comp Eff Res. 2023;12(2):e220089. https://doi.org/10.2217/cer-2022-0089.
 7. Errea Rodríguez M, Fernández M, Del Llano J, Nuño-Solinís R. Systematic review and cost-effectiveness analysis of the treatment of post-stroke spasticity with abobotulinumtoxinA compared to physiotherapy. Farm Hosp. 2023;47(5):T201–9. https://doi.org/10.1016/j.farma.2023.06.008.
 8. Kazerooni R, Broadhead C. Cost-utility analysis of botulinum toxin type a products for the treatment of cervical dystonia. Am J Health Syst Pharm. 2015;72(4):301–7.
 9. Trosch RM, Shillington AC, English ML, Marchese D. A retrospective, single-center comparative cost analysis of onabotulinumtoxina and abobotulinumtoxina for cervical dystonia treatment. J Manag Care Spec Pharm. 2015;21(10):854–60. https://doi.org/10.18553/jmcp.2015.21.10.854.
10. Tilden D, Guanierie C, Value health. Cost-effectiveness of incobotulinumtoxin-a with flexible treatment intervals compared to onabotulinumtoxin-a in the management of blepharospasm and cervical. Dystonia. 2016;19(2):145–52.
11. Danchenko N, Johnston KM, Haeussler K, Whalen J. Comparative efficacy, safety, and cost-effectiveness of abobotulinumtoxinA and onabotulinumtoxinA in children with upper limb spasticity: a systematic literature review, indirect treatment comparison, and economic evaluation. J Med Econ. 2021;24(1):949–61. https://doi.org/10.1080/13696998.2021.1957582.

12. Shabir H, Hashemi S, Al-Rufayie M, Adelowo T, Riaz U, Ullah U, Alam B, Anwar M, de Preux L. Cost-utility analysis of oxybutynin vs. OnabotulinumtoxinA (Botox) in the treatment of overactive bladder syndrome. Int J Environ Res Public Health. 2021;18(16):8743. https://doi.org/10.3390/ijerph18168743.
13. Tedroff K, Befrits G, Tedroff CJ, et al. To switch from Botox to Dysport in children with CP, a real world, dose conversion, cost-effectiveness study. Eur J Paediatr Neurol. 2018;22(3):412–8.
14. Bladen JC, Favor M, Litwin A, Malhotra R. Switchover study of onabotulinumtoxinA to incobotulinumtoxinA for facial dystonia. Clin Experiment Ophthalmol. 2020;48(9):1146–51. https://doi.org/10.1111/ceo.13829.

Chapter 18
Is Botulinum Toxin Treatment Safe?

Abstract The issue of safety is often raised with botulinum toxin therapy due to the lethal potential of these toxins if used improperly. In this chapter, safety issues regarding recognized indications of botulinum toxin therapy are reviewed and discussed. These topics include, migraine, spasticity in adults and children, bladder problems, pain from neuropathy (diabetes, singles), osteoarthritis and movement disorders as well as the area of aesthetic use.

Keywords Botulinum toxin · Botulinum neurotoxin · Migraine · Spasticity · Neurogenic bladder · Overactive bladder · Cervical dystonia · Neuropathic pain

Introduction

Botulinum toxins are one of the most potent toxins in nature. Severe toxicity with these toxins can lead to botulism, a disease that can lead to paralysis of respiratory (breathing) muscles. Although in the era of modern medicine with early diagnosis and advanced respiratory support, most patients ultimately recover (toxin induced paralysis usually does not last more than 3 months), botulism is a life- threatening medical emergency. For these reasons, over the past 20 years, a large volume of literature has been published addressing the safety of botulinum toxin therapy.

In the previous chapters of this book, I have discussed mainly the utility of botulinum toxin therapy in several disease conditions (Chaps. 4–16) with the exception of Chap. 13 (aesthetics) which has been prepared by Drs. Noland and Dennis and address the use of botulinum toxin in aesthetics. In the current chapter, the safety issues of botulinum toxin therapy will be discussed. The format will include a summary of safety issues in several different medical indications followed by a brief discussion and conclusion for each condition. The presented data will also include safety information on vulnerable and special categories of patients such as children and pregnant women.

© The Author(s), under exclusive license to Springer Nature Switzerland AG 2024   285
B. Jabbari, *Botulinum Toxin Treatment*,
https://doi.org/10.1007/978-3-031-54471-2_18

Safety Issues

Migraine

Botox was approved for treatment of chronic migraine by FDA for use in US based on two large carefully crafted multicenter studies [1, 2]. Subsequent studies have shown that the effect after repeated injections (every 3–4 months) is sustained and is associated with improvement of quality of life [3]. The technique of injections and recommended dose(s) has been described in Chap. 4. To date, millions of people worldwide have received Botox injections for treatment of chronic migraine.

Over the past 10 years, several reviews attesting to the safety of botulinum toxin therapy in migraine have appeared in the literature. In a very recent published review [4], authors carefully studied the issue of safety in all reported clinical trials that used Botox for treatment of chronic migraine and then performed a meticulous statistical analysis (meta-analysis) on the collected data. The conclusion of this review was that Botox is safe for management of migraine [4]. Side effects are mild and usually confined to transient pain at the site of injection and minor bleeding. More serious side effects such as drooping of the eyelids or weakness of the facial muscle can be avoided by adherence to recommended injection site(s) while avoiding overdosing.

In a comparison study of Botox with Topiramate, over time, Botox dropout rate was 8% compared to 68% for Topiramate. Furthermore, one study found that combination of Botox with erenumab, one of the newer drugs for treatment of migraine, reduced the migraine attacks by 50% or more in 58% of the patient. The findings suggested that Botox may be more effective in reducing migraine attacks than erenumab, a myoclonal antibody widely used drug for treatment of migraine, currently [5].

The data on botulinum toxin therapy in children (ages 11–18) with migraine is also promising and indicates no occurrence of serious safety issues if the injections are carried out by experienced injectors following the recommended site and dose guidelines [6–8]. The side effects are similar to those in adults and include pain at the site of injection, minor, transient bleeding and mild transient muscle weakness.

Spasticity

A significant increase in muscle tone encountered after stroke, brain or spinal injury is a disabling phenomenon that interferes with activities of daily life and impairs patients' quality of life. Furthermore, severe spasticity makes physical therapy and ambulation difficult. One of the major contributions of botulinum toxin therapy to the field of medicine has been its use in treatment of spasticity (see Chaps. 6 and 7 on Stroke and multiple sclerosis). Botulinum toxin injections into the muscles, by inhibiting the release of acetylcholine (muscle stimulator released from nerve endings), is very effective in substantially reducing the muscle tone. Spasticity is now a major indication for botulinum toxin therapy worldwide. Botulinum toxins (Botox and other similar toxins) are now approved by FDA for treatment of both adults and children's spasticity [9, 10].

Muscles involved in spasticity are much larger than those involved in involuntary movement of the face, eyelid or neck (other common indications of Botox), and hence, need hundreds of units to relax. This raises the question that what is the safe total dose of the toxin that can be injected in one session? Although FDA approval recommends 500–600 units/session for limb spasticity, recent data from American and European investigators strongly suggest that in an average size person, Botox doses of up to 800 units/session are safe and do not cause botulism [11, 12].

In stroke related spasticity, there is another issue of concern. After stroke, many patients are kept on blood thinners (anticoagulants) in order to prevent occlusion of blood vessels; as a side effect, these drugs can cause bleeding or prolong the bleeding time. Since local injections of botulinum toxins may cause minor bleeding, the question arises as to whether toxin injections are safe for patients who are on blood thinners?

In a study that pooled the data from several investigations, the authors found that the incidence of bleeding in patients who were on blood thinners and received botulinum toxin injections was comparable and statistically not different from those who were on blood thinners and did not receive botulinum toxin injections (0.9% versus 1.4%) [13]. The authors, therefore, concluded that toxin injections are safe in patients who are taking blood thinners.

Spasticity in children arises from several different pathological conditions, some of which are similar to the cause of spasticity in adults such as brain and spinal cord trauma. A major cause of spasticity in children is cerebral palsy. Cerebral palsy arises from unfortunate conditions before or at the time of birth that deprive the brain of oxygen. The affected children are often mentally challenged, and over time, develop severe spasticity of the limbs confining many of them to the wheelchair. For the past 10 years, botulinum toxin therapy has been a major mode of treatment for spasticity in cerebral palsy, reducing its severity and preventing development of more severe spasticity.

Gromley and co-workers [14] recently published a review on the efficacy and safety of botulinum toxin treatment in children with cerebral palsy (CP). The data showed that a total dose of 8 units of Botox /kg body of weight /session is safe. Like adults with spasticity, side effects of botulinum toxin therapy in children were minor and there was no clinical evidence of spread of the toxin from the site of injection to distant regions. In another recent review (2023), Yang and co-workers [15] looked at the efficacy and safety of botulinum toxin injection in 656 children with CP involved in 12 clinical trials (two performed on children, younger than 2 years). Botox injections were found to be safe in children younger than 2 years of age when appropriate doses were used.

Movement Disorders

Movement disorders are another major area where botulinum toxin therapy is used in clinical medicine (see Chap. 8). Spasms of facial muscles such as blepharospasm (spasm of eyelids), hemifacial spasm (spasm of muscles on one side of the face) and cervical dystonia (twisting and twitching of neck muscles) are major indications and received the earliest FDA approval for use of botulinum toxin therapy in the US. The toxin safety is not usually an issue with blepharospasm and hemifacial spasm since the applied dose is small. The side effects of botulinum toxin therapy for these indications such as drooping of the eyelids and weakness of facial muscles can be usually avoided by careful selection of the sites of injection and by avoiding overdosing the involved muscles.

Cervical dystonia gradually twists and turns the head to one side and is often associated with severe neck stiffness and pain. Botulinum toxin injection into the involved neck muscles is now considered the first line of treatment [16]. Toxin therapy improves neck posture, stiffness, and reduces pain significantly (Chap. 8). Since neck muscles are larger and more powerful than face and eyelid muscles, patients with cervical dystonia require larger doses of botulinum toxins. For Botox the dose range is usually between 150 and 400 units. Most side effects of toxin therapy in CD are subtle and insignificant. One side effect of concern is difficulty in swallowing (dysphagia). In the experience of this author, very few patients voluntarily complain of dysphagia. However, in clinical drug trials, when patients are specifically asked about it, 10–15% of the patients report transient dysphagia following botulinum toxin injections (both type A and type B toxin) [17, 18]. Most clinicians experienced with botulinum toxin injections (including this author) believe that dysphagia can be avoided by not injecting large units of toxins into anterior neck muscles (especially sternocleidomastoid—see location in Chap. 8) bilaterally. Long-term studies on the use of botulinum toxin therapy in cervical dystonia have noted its safety and sustained efficacy after repeated injections [17–19].

Facial Rejuvenation and Aesthetics

Safety of botulinum toxin injections in facial rejuvenation was reviewed in a recent publication that evaluated the data from 32 clinical trials including 96,555 patients [20]. No serious side effects were reported. Reported side effects included mild transient facial weakness, transient elevation of the lateral part of eyebrow and, in some cases, transient headaches.

Osteoarthritis

Osteoarthritis is a common human ailment. According to the World Health Organization (WHO), in 2015, 18% of women and 9.6% of men, 60 years or older were affected by osteoarthritis [21]. Several studies have shown that Botulinum toxin injections into the affected joint can alleviate joint pain and reduce inflammation (Chap. 12). A recent review of the efficacy and safety of botulinum toxin injections in knee osteoarthritis (pooled data from 6 clinical trials, 466 patients) [22] indicated that toxin injections (into the joint) significantly reduced joint pain (both under and over 4 weeks) as well as improved the scores of WOMAC assessment (pain, physical activity, joint stiffness). No serious side effects were reported in any of the assessed studies.

Excessive Drooling (Sialorrhea)

Both botulinum toxin type A (Botox, Dysport and Xeomin) and type B (Myobloc) effectively reduce drooling when injected through a thin needle into the glands that produce saliva (parotid, submaxillary) (Chap. 14). A recent review of literature including 17 studies and 981 patients [23] concluded that both type A and B are effective in reducing excessive saliva; side effects were uncommon and, when occurred were mild to moderate in intensity.

Botulinum Toxins Treatment of Neurogenic and Overactive Bladder (NB and OAB)

Injection of botulinum toxins into the bladder wall can significantly reduce frequency and urgency of urination in patients affected by NB and OAB (Chap. 10). Botulinum toxin therapy for these indications is approved for use in the US by FDA and is now widely utilized by urologists. A recent review of world's literature on 24 clinical trials including 1187 patients concluded that botulinum toxin injections were effective in reducing the symptoms of OAB, but was considered as third line of treatment [24]. The main side effect of botulinum toxin injection for alleviation of symptoms related to OAB and NB found in these studies, was a need for increased self-catheterization. However, it should be noted that many of the patients affected by NB and OAB, especially those with advanced multiple sclerosis, do perform self- catheterization daily.

Neuropathic Pain

Botulinum toxins (type A and type B) inhibit the function of pain transmitters and, hence, have been found useful in alleviating neuropathic pain (burning pain associated with diabetic neuropathy, shingles, trauma to peripheral nerves) (see Chap. 5). Dr. Hary and co-workers [25], recently published a review of this subject assessing the efficacy and safety of botulinum toxin injections on neuropathic pain. The review extracted data from 10 clinical trials including 505 patients. Subcutaneous (under the skin) injections of botulinum toxins were effective in reducing the NP at 1- and 3-months post-injection. There was no significant difference between placebo and botulinum toxins as to the adverse effects.

Safety Data in Pregnancy

The issue of safety of botulinum toxin in pregnancy has been a focus of research since the early days of botulinum toxin therapy 30 years ago. Recently, Brin and co-workers published a cumulative 29-Year Safety Update on the use of Botox in pregnant women. Of 397 pregnancies, 13 had major fetal abnormalities amounting to an incidence of 0.7% [26]. This was comparable and not higher than that reported in general population. For comparison, Brin and co-workers cited the following data from published literature for birth anomalies in general population: The Center for Disease Control (CDC): 3% of US births [27], The Texas Birth Defects Registry-4.3% of live births [28], Registry data from the United Kingdom- 1.7–2.0% of children younger than 1 year [29], and The March of Dimes Foundation—6% of total births world -wide [30].

None of the pregnant women in these clinical trials delivered a child with fetal botulism. These data are encouraging and suggests safety of Botox in pregnancy. The author of this chapter, however, believes that specific safety data are still needed on pregnant women who have been injected with high doses of Botox during pregnancy for conditions such as severe spasticity caused by multiple sclerosis or brain/spinal cord trauma.

References

1. Diener HC, Dodick DW, Aurora SK, Turkel CC, DeGryse RE, Lipton RB, Silberstein SD, Brin MF. PREEMPT 2 chronic migraine study group. OnabotulinumtoxinA for treatment of chronic migraine: results from the double-blind, randomized, placebo-controlled phase of the PREEMPT 2 trial. Cephalalgia. 2010;30(7):804–14. https://doi.org/10.1177/0333102410364677.
2. Dodick DW, Turkel CC, RE DG, Aurora SK, Silberstein SD, Lipton RB, Diener HC, Brin MF, PREEMPT Chronic Migraine Study Group. OnabotulinumtoxinA for treatment of

chronic migraine: pooled results from the double-blind, randomized, placebo-controlled phases of the PREEMPT clinical program. Headache. 2010;50(6):921–36. https://doi.org/10.1111/j.1526-4610.2010.01678.x.

3. Lipton RB, Rosen NL, Ailani J, DeGryse RE, Gillard PJ, Varon SF. OnabotulinumtoxinA improves quality of life and reduces impact of chronic migraine over one year of treatment: pooled results from the PREEMPT randomized clinical trial program. Cephalalgia. 2016;36(9):899–908. https://doi.org/10.1177/0333102416652092.

4. Corasaniti MT, Bagetta G, Nicotera P, Tarsitano A, Tonin P, Sandrini G, Lawrence GW, Scuteri D. Safety of onabotulinumtoxin a in chronic migraine: a systematic review and meta-analysis of randomized clinical trials. Toxins (Basel). 2023;15(5):332. https://doi.org/10.3390/toxins15050332.

5. Rothrock JF, Adams AM, Lipton RB, Silberstein SD, Jo E, Zhao X, Blumenfeld AM. FORWARD study investigative group. FORWARD study: evaluating the comparative effectiveness of OnabotulinumtoxinA and Topiramate for headache prevention in adults with chronic migraine. Headache. 2019;59(10):1700–13. https://doi.org/10.1111/head.13653.

6. Santana L, Liu C. Experience of botulinum toxin a injections for chronic migraine headaches in a pediatric chronic pain clinic. J Pediatr Pharmacol Ther. 2021;26(2):151–6. https://doi.org/10.5863/1551-6776-26.2.151.

7. Kabbouche M, O'Brien H, Hershey AD. OnabotulinumtoxinA in pediatric chronic daily headache. Curr Neurol Neurosci Rep. 2012;12(2):114–7. https://doi.org/10.1007/s11910-012-0251-1.

8. Peck J, Zeien J, Patel M, Cornett EM, Berger AA, Hasoon J, Kassem H, Jung JW, Ramírez GF, Fugueroa PC, Singhal NR, Song J, Kaye AM, Kaye AD, Koushik SS, Strand NH, Ganti L. Review of interventional therapies for refractory pediatric migraine. Health Psychol Res. 2023;10(5):67853. https://doi.org/10.52965/001c.67853.

9. Safarpour D, Jabbari B. Botulinum toxin for motor disorders. Handb Clin Neurol. 2023;196:539–55. https://doi.org/10.1016/B978-0-323-98817-9.00003-X.

10. Simpson DM, Hallett M, Ashman EJ, Comella CL, Green MW, Gronseth GS, Armstrong MJ, Gloss D, Potrebic S, Jankovic J, Karp BP, Naumann M, So YT, Yablon SA. Practice guideline update summary: botulinum neurotoxin for the treatment of blepharospasm, cervical dystonia, adult spasticity, and headache: report of the guideline development Subcommittee of the American Academy of neurology. Neurology. 2016;86(19):1818–26. https://doi.org/10.1212/WNL.0000000000002560.

11. Baricich A, Grana E, Carda S, Santamato A, Cisari C, Invernizzi M. High doses of onabotulinumtoxinA in post-stroke spasticity: a retrospective analysis. J Neural Transm (Vienna). 2015;122(9):1283–7. https://doi.org/10.1007/s00702-015-1384-6.

12. Wissel J, Bensmail D, Ferreira JJ, Molteni F, Satkunam L, Moraleda S, Rekand T, McGuire J, Scheschonka A, Flatau-Baqué B, Simon O, Rochford ET, Dressler D, Simpson DM. TOWER study investigators. Safety and efficacy of incobotulinumtoxinA doses up to 800 U in limb spasticity: the TOWER study. Neurology. 2017;88(14):1321–8. https://doi.org/10.1212/WNL.0000000000003789.

13. Dimitrova R, James L, Liu C, Orejudos A, Yushmanova I, Brin MF. Safety of OnabotulinumtoxinA with concomitant antithrombotic therapy in patients with muscle spasticity: a retrospective pooled analysis of randomized double-blind studies. CNS Drugs. 2020;34(4):433–45. https://doi.org/10.1007/s40263-020-00709-5.

14. Gormley M, Chambers HG, Kim H, Leon J, Dimitrova R, Brin MF. Treatment of pediatric spasticity, including children with cerebral palsy, with Botox (onabotulinumtoxinA): development, insights, and impact. Medicine (Baltimore). 2023;102(S1):e32363. https://doi.org/10.1097/MD.0000000000032363.

15. Yang H, Chen S, Shen J, Chen Y, Lai M, Chen L, Fang S. Safety and efficacy of botulinum toxin type a in children with spastic cerebral palsy aged <2 years: a systematic review. J Child Neurol. 2023;38(6–7):454–65. https://doi.org/10.1177/08830738231183484.

16. Bledsoe IO, Comella CL. Botulinum toxin treatment of cervical dystonia. Semin Neurol. 2016;36(1):47–53. https://doi.org/10.1055/s-0035-1571210.
17. Jost WH, Kaňovský P, Hast MA, Hanschmann A, Althaus M, Patel AT. Pooled safety analysis of IncobotulinumtoxinA in the treatment of neurological disorders in adults. Toxins (Basel). 2023;15(6):353. https://doi.org/10.3390/toxins15060353.
18. Petracca M, Lo Monaco MR, Ialongo T, Di Stasio E, Cerbarano ML, Maggi L, De Biase A, Di Lazzaro G, Calabresi P, Bentivoglio AR. Efficacy and safety of long-term botulinum toxin treatment for acquired cervical dystonia: a 25-year follow-up. J Neurol. 2023;270(1):340–7. https://doi.org/10.1007/s00415-022-11343-0.
19. Marsili L, Bologna M, Jankovic J, Colosimo C. Long-term efficacy and safety of botulinum toxin treatment for cervical dystonia: a critical reappraisal. Expert Opin Drug Saf. 2021;20(6):695–705. https://doi.org/10.1080/14740338.2021.1915282.
20. Gostimir M, Liou V, Yoon MK. Safety of botulinum toxin a injections for facial rejuvenation: a meta-analysis of 9,669 patients. Ophthalmic Plast Reconstr Surg. 2023;39(1):13–25. https://doi.org/10.1097/IOP.0000000000002169.
21. Zhang Y, Niu J. Editorial: shifting gears in osteoarthritis research toward symptomatic osteoarthritis. Arthritis Rheumatol. 2016;68(8):1797–800. https://doi.org/10.1002/art.39704.
22. Ismiarto YD, Prasetiyo GT. Efficacy and safety of intra-articular botulinum toxin a injection for knee osteoarthritis: a systematic review, meta-analysis, and meta-regression of clinical trials. JBJS Open Access. 2023;8(1):e22.00121. https://doi.org/10.2106/JBJS.OA.22.00121.
23. Yu YC, Chung CC, Tu YK, Hong CT, Chen KH, Tam KW, Kuan YC. Efficacy and safety of botulinum toxin for treating sialorrhea: a systematic review and meta-analysis. Eur J Neurol. 2022;29(1):69–80. https://doi.org/10.1111/ene.15083.
24. De Nunzio C, Brucker B, Bschleipfer T, Cornu JN, Drake MJ, Fusco F, Gravas S, Oelke M, Peyronnet B, Tutolo M, van Koeveringe G, Madersbacher S. Beyond antimuscarinics: a review of pharmacological and interventional options for overactive bladder management in men. Eur Urol. 2021;79(4):492–504. https://doi.org/10.1016/j.eururo.2020.12.032.
25. Hary V, Schitter S, Martinez V. Efficacy and safety of botulinum a toxin for the treatment of chronic peripheral neuropathic pain: a systematic review of randomized controlled trials and meta-analysis. Eur J Pain. 2022;26(5):980–90. https://doi.org/10.1002/ejp.1941.
26. Brin MF, Kirby RS, Slavotinek A, Adams AM, Parker L, Ukah A, Radulian L, Elmore MRP, Yedigarova L, Yushmanova I. Pregnancy outcomes in patients exposed to OnabotulinumtoxinA treatment: a cumulative 29-year safety update. Neurology. 2023;101(2):e103–13. https://doi.org/10.1212/WNL.0000000000207375.
27. Centers for Disease Control and Prevention (CDC). Update on overall prevalence of major birth defects—Atlanta, Georgia, 1978-2005. MMWR Morb Mortal Wkly Rep. 2008;57(1):1–5.
28. Texas Department of State Health Services. Birth defects among 1999–2011 deliveries: summary and key findings from the texas birth defects registry's report of birth defects among 1999–2011 deliveries. Texas Department of State Health Services; 2016.
29. Sokal R, Fleming KM, Tata LJ. Potential of general practice data for congenital anomaly research: comparison with registry data in the United Kingdom. Birth Defects Res A Clin Mol Teratol. 2013;97(8):546–53. https://doi.org/10.1002/bdra.23150.
30. Christianson A, Howson CP, Modell B. March of dimes global report on birth defects. March of Dimes Birth Defects Foundation; 2006.

Chapter 19
Botulinum Toxin Therapy-Future Perspectives

Abstract New potential applications for botulinum neurotoxin (BoNT) therapy are constantly emerging through the expanding literature in the field of clinical toxicology. In this chapter, we discuss potential indications for botulinum neurotoxin treatment in five major fields of medicine: Psychiatry (depression), cardiology (irregular heartbeats, atrial fibrillation), cancer related disorders (cancer related pain, prevention of post-surgical and post radiation pain, prevention of esophageal narrowing after surgery for esophagal cancer, prevention of parotid gland fistula and cyst formation after parotid cancer surgery and alleviating excessive face sweating and severe jaw pain after first bite following parotid gland surgery). In dermatology, there is evidence that local botulinum toxin injections can help psoriasis and recalcitrant itch as well as palm pain and vascular palm problems associated with Raynaud syndrome. In pain medicine, botulinum toxin injections can help to reduce teeth grinding and associated pain, jaw pain from temporomandibular disorder, pain and discomfort of anal fissure.

Keywords Botulinum toxin · Botulinum neurotoxin · Cancer related pain · Post-surgical pain · Post radiation pain · Neuropathic pain · Atrial fibrillation · Depression · Raynaud syndrome

Introduction

In the preceding chapters, we have discussed clinical conditions in which high quality studies have shown the efficacy of botulinum neurotoxins (BoNTs) in improving the symptoms of various medical disorders. There are many other important clinical conditions in which the preliminary results of BoNT therapy are encouraging, but the proof of efficacy for most of these conditions requires the availability of positive results from well- designed, and high quality clinical trials. These potential indications pertain to medical disorders for which current medical management is challenging and often provides unsatisfactory results. The challenged clinicians, therefore, would welcome alternative treatment approaches, that in addition to efficacy, do not require daily use of oral medications or surgery, while producing fewer side effects.

The list of potential indications for BoNT therapy is long and is growing. For this chapter, we have selected potential indications in five major fields of medicine: Psychiatry, cardiology, cancer related disorders and dermatology and pain medicine. Since the first edition of this book which was published 5 years ago, there have been more publications supporting BoNT therapy for these indications. In psychiatry, we will address treatment of depression with botulinum neurotoxins and the possible mechanisms of its effectiveness. In cardiology, there is evidence that careful and titrated injection of botulinum toxins into the surface of the heart (where heart's nerves are located) can improve irregular heartbeats caused by atrial fibrillation. Potential indications in cancer related disorders include treatment of pain after cancer surgery and/or radiation, prevention of esophageal narrowing (stricture) after removal of esophageal cancer, prevention of parotid gland fistula and cyst formation after parotid cancer surgery, as well as excessive face sweating after parotid surgery. In dermatology botulinum toxin injections into the skin may abort recalcitrant itch, improve psoriasis and alleviate palm pain and skin changes in Raynaud syndrome.

Psychiatry: Depression

Severe depression, a major depressive disorder (MDD), is a common disease that affects 5–10% of men and 10–25% of women [1]. Lack of interest and severe depressive mood of the affected patients often lead to an impaired quality of life and ultimately to the patients' functional disability. Medical treatment of depression includes application of several different categories of medication and is beyond the scope of this chapter; this information is available in recent extensive reviews [2]. Although antidepressive medications are effective, their side effects (some severe) limit their use in many patients and it may take 6 weeks before seeing results [2]. Therefore, availability of a mode of treatment that has less side effects, acts faster and does not require daily consumption of medications is highly desirable for treatment of chronic depression.

Following earlier observations that botulinum toxin injections into the forehead muscles for cosmetic reasons, significantly improved mood in some patients [3, 4], researchers began to methodically study the effect of botulinum toxin therapy on severe depression. Over the past 20 years, 6 high quality studies [5–10] have been conducted on the subject of botulinum toxin therapy in depression (Table 19.1). These studies were double—blind and placebo-controlled, i.e. the effect of the injected toxin into the forehead and, in some cases, with additional injections into the muscles over the corner of the eyes was compared with injection of placebo (salt water). Double- blind means that both the injecting physician and the patient were not aware whether the injected material was Botox or salt water in any of the injection sessions. In all studies, the glabellar muscles were included in the plan of injection. Glabella is the forehead region above the nose and between the two eyebrows.

Table 19.1 High quality, double-blind, placebo- controlled studies reported on safety and efficacy of Botox and other type A botulinum toxin injections into the glabellar and forehead muscles of depressed patients

Author and date	#pts	Study design	Toxin type, total dose	Assessment	Results
Vollmer et al. [5]	30	DB, PC	Botox, 26 units	Hamilton depression rating scale-21 (HDRS) at week 6	Significant improvement Botox: 47.1% vs placebo:9.2%
Finzi and Rosenthal [6]	74	DB, PC	Botox, 29–40 units	50% reduction in Montgomery-Asberg depression scale at week 6	Significant improvement Botox: 52% vs placebo: 15%
Magid et al. [7]	30	DB, PC	Botox, 29–30 units	Beck depression scale at week 6	Significant improvement Botox: 55% vs placebo: 5%
Brin et al. [8]	255	DB, PC	Botox, 30 units	Montgomery-Asberg (MA) depression scale assessed every 3 weeks up to 24 weeks	M-A depression scores consistently and significantly improved in Botox group compared to placebo group over 24 weeks (Fig. 19.2)
Zhang et al. [9] Comparing Botox with sertraline	76	DB	Botulinum toxin A from Lanshou-China.:100 units, Sertarline: 50–100 mg	Hamilton depression (HD) scale and Hamilton anxiety (HA) scale-at 12 weeks	In both groups botulinum toxin and sertraline reduced HD and HA scores significantly. Onset of Botox effect was earlier and Botox injections had less side effects
Li et al. [10]	88	DB, PC	Botulinum toxin A from Lanshou institute in China: 100	Hamilton depression scale and Hamilton anxiety scale-12 weeks	Both Hamilton scores improved significantly over 12 weeks compared to placebo

DB double blind, *PC* placebo controlled

It covers a single muscle (procerus) located at midline between the two eyebrows and the two corrugator muscles—one on each side above the most medial part (closest to the nose) of the eyebrows (Fig. 19.1). These muscles are also called frown line muscles as their contraction leads to frowning and pulls the eyebrows together. As can be seen in Table 19.1, Botox injection into the forehead muscles (and in some studies combined with injection at corner of the eyes) significantly improved depression scores in patients who received Botox. This effect was much less noted in the placebo-injected patients. The total dose of Botox used in these studies varied from 30 to 100 units. Each injection site received a small dose of 5 units.

The largest of these six double- blind, placebo- controlled studies on efficacy of botulinum toxins in depression was performed by Brin and coworkers [8]; they

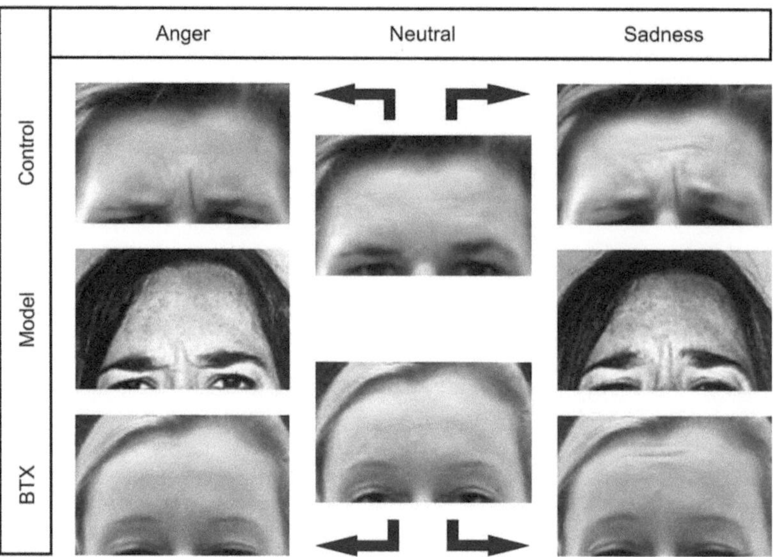

Fig. 19.1 The function of glabellar muscles: frowning during volition (not shown) and during anger and sadness. Lower part of the figure shows the effect after Botox treatment. (From Hennenlotter et al. [4]. Courtesy of Oxford Academic Press)

studied 225 patients. This study was designated as a Phase II clinical trial study (for definition of clinical trials and phases see Chap. 2). A phase II clinical study aims mainly to establish the safety of a new drug, but also to some extent investigates the drug's efficacy. This study demonstrated that repeated Botox injections into the forehead area of depressed patients over 24 weeks was safe and devoid of serious side effects. It also showed that over the period of 24 weeks, at each assessment point (every 3 weeks) (Fig. 19.2). Botox injection of 30 units (total dose) was superior to placebo in improving the patients' depression. A positive Phase II study is a requirement for proceeding to a phase III study, upon the positive results of which, FDA usually approves the drug for clinical use in the US. Phase III studies are large multi-center studies conducted under more stringent regulations.

The positive data from the above mentioned studies (Table 19.1) are supported by further positive data from literature that have shown botulinum toxin therapy can also alleviate depression associated with chronic migraine and Parkinson disease [11, 12]. The theories that how BoNT injection into skin and thin muscles of the forehead (glabellar region) can relieve depression are presented later in this chapter.

Technical Points

Injections are performed with a small needle (gauge 27.5 orvv30) into thin muscles of glabellar and low forehead. Injections are quick and all can be completed within 4–5 min. In very sensitive individuals, the skin may be numbed before injections

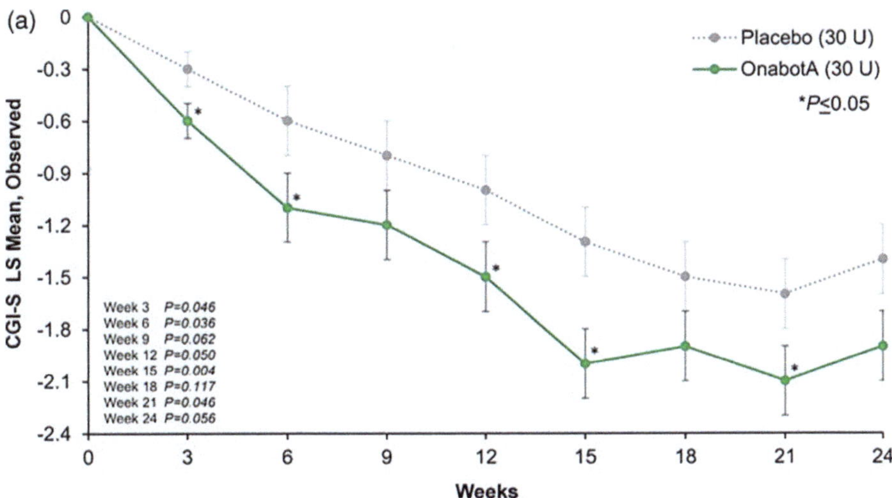

Fig. 19.2 On each assessment point after injections (Botox or placebo), Botox improved the depression scores more than the placebo (green line). (From Brin et al. [8]. Printed with permission from publisher, Wolters Kluwer)

with a topical anesthetic cream an hour before injection (for example, Emla cream). In most patients, however, numbing the injection sites is not necessary. Most studies have used 5–8 injection sites limited to glabellar region(procerus and corrugator muscles) and lower forehead [5–8] (Fig. 19.3). Some investigators include additional injection sites, for instance three additional injections at the corner of each eye [9].

Zhang and co-investigators compared the result of BoNT-A injections (Chinese toxin with units comparable to Botox) with the oral use of antidepressive drug sertraline in 78 patients with depression [9]. The total dose of BoNT-A was 100 units and the total dose of daily sertraline was 50–100 mg/day. BoNT-A was injected into 20 points at the glabellar and low frontal regions as well as both corner of the eyes (5 units/site). Both modes of treatment improved depression with comparable magnitude. The onset of botulinum toxin effect however was earlier. Also, botulinum toxin treatment of depressed patient caused less side effects compared to sertraline therapy (15.4% versus 33%).

Schultze and coworkers [12] performed a meta-analysis of the published data on the role of botulinum toxins in alleviating depression. Meta-analysis is defined as a quantitative, formal, epidemiological study design used to systematically assess previous research studies to derive conclusions about that body of research. The authors concluded that despite some methodological limitations, botulinum toxin treatment has shown to be effective for treatment of depression and the road seems to be paved for its use in the field of psychiatry.

How injection of Botox into low frontal region and glabellar muscles (procerus and corrugator) leads to improvement of major depression is difficult to explain.

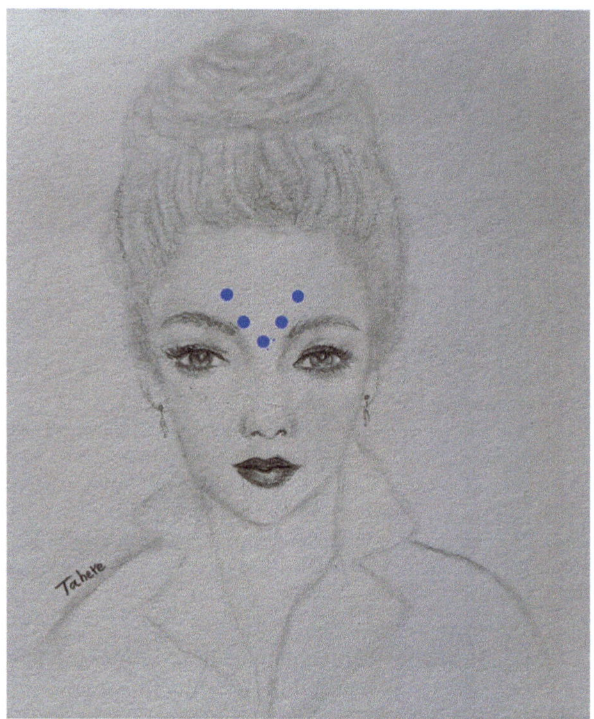

Fig. 19.3 Recommended injection sites of Botox d for treatment of depression per Finzi and Rosenthal, 2014. The injection between two eyebrows is into the procerus muscle that pulls the skin between two eyebrows down. The two infections at the medial border of eyebrows are into the corrugator muscles that bring eyebrows together. Upper injections are into frontalis muscles. (Drawing courtesy of Dr. Tahere Safarpour)

One simple explanation is that improvement of frown lines makes the patients happier and happier patients are less depressed.

Finzi and Rosenthal [6] have proposed that glabellar muscles, as muscles of facial expression, influence the activity of the brain cells in those areas of the brain that are involved in emotions such as temporal lobe and part of frontal lobe (prefrontal cortex -PFC). Another area of the brain which is involved in emotions is called amygdala. Amygdala (meaning almond in Greek) is an almond shape structure that consists of a group of nerve cells located deep in the brain with connections to other areas of the brain that are concerned with emotions. Functional MRI (fMRI) studies have shown frowning, following observing an unpleasant picture is associated with decreased activity in pre-frontal cortex (PFC) and increased activity in amygdala [13]. Antidepressant medications (drugs used for treatment of depression) like paroxetine increase activity of PFC and decrease the activity of amygdala in fMRI. Studies of the brain activity with fMRI have shown that the same thing happens with Botox injection into the glabellar muscles which decreases the tone of glabellar muscles and flattens the frown lines [14] (Fig. 19.2).

Using the criteria of American Academy of Neurology (see Chap. 3 of this book for definition of AAN criteria, study class and efficacy levels), and based on the current published literature that includes one class I [8] and 5 class II [5–7, 9, 10] studies in this area, the efficacy level of Botox therapy for depression would be "B", i.e. probably effective (a definitely effective designation requires two class I studies) .

So far, most of the reported patients in the high quality studies (Table 19.1) have been women. There is a need for similar studies in male patients. Furthermore, Botox and Chinese toxin (another type A toxin) have been the only two botulinum toxins investigated in high quality studies. It remains to be seen if the same positive response can be duplicated with the use of other major FDA approved botulinum type A toxins such as Xeomin, Dysport and Diddify or with the type B toxin, Myobloc.

Cardiology: Treatment of Atrial Fibrillation (Irregular Heart Beats)

The human heart is a marvel of function and engineering. It has four chambers; two small ones called atriums with thin walls, and two large ones called ventricles with thick walls. The two atriums (atria) are located above the ventricles and each atrium has an opening into the ventricle below, on the same side. There are valves between atria and ventricles which control the blood flow through them. The mitral valve is located on the left and the aortic valve is located on the right side (Fig. 19.4).

Human heart beats approximately 10,000 times/24 h. Its continuous beating is maintained through the function of a conglomeration of sympathetic and parasympathetic nerve cells called nodes (located in the left atrium) and networks of nerve cells and fibers called ganglionic plexi (GP) located inside the fat pads on the surface of the heart (epicardium) around the atria. The two nodes sinoatrial and atrioventricular (AV) work as a pacemaker for the heart; electrical impulses generated in the AV node travel through nerve bundles along the wall of the ventricles exciting the heart muscles. The electrical activity generated by the AV node contracts the atria and the ventricles.

In recent years, the importance of GP as an extensive combinations of nerve cells and fibers has been emphasized with some authors describing it as a "little brain sitting over the heart" (Fig. 19.5).

Five locations for ganglionic plexi (GP) containing sympathetic and parasympathetic cells and fibers have been identified around left and right atria embedded in the small fat pads. These overlie the surface of the right atrium, superior surface of the left atrium, posterior surface of the right atrium, posterior medial surface of the left atrium and inferiolateral aspects of the posterior left atrium. Abnormal electrical activity in these sites which are often located close to the pulmonary veins, can cause a condition called atrial fibrillation.

Atrial fibrillation (AF) affects 2.5% of the general population (9% or higher after age 75) and is associated with an annual stroke incidence of 5% [16]. About 1 out of 4 adults develop atrial fibrillation during their life time [17]. With increase in our aging population, the incidence and prevalence of atrial fibrillation is on the rise (17.8% after age 85), imposing a growing cost on the health care budget [18].

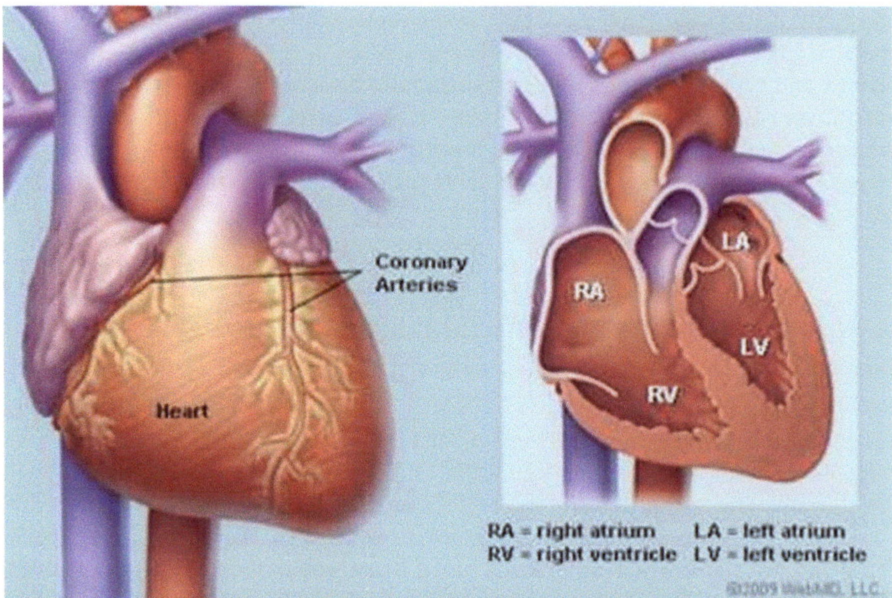

Fig. 19.4 Right: chambers of the heart and large blood vessels. Left: coronary arteries that feed the heart muscle. (Courtesy of Dr. Poonan Sachdev and WebMD editorial contributors)

Atrial fibrillation is characterized by irregular, fast and somewhat chaotic beating of the upper two chambers (atria) of the heart. Several factors can cause atrial fibrillation; most notable among them are high blood pressure, damage to the heart structure from coronary artery disease (vessels that feed the heart muscle), myocardial infarction (heart attack), abnormal thyroid function, diabetes, kidney disease and a congenital heart anomaly. Atrial fibrillation is a frequent complication of Coronary Artery Bypass Grafting (CABG) surgery that replenishes blood supply to parts of the heart that lack sufficient blood supply. Experimentally, researchers have produced atrial fibrillation in animals by electrical stimulation of the vagus nerve which supplies parasympathetic innervation to the heart (the nerve that slows the heart beat).

The symptoms of AF include shortness of breath, palpitation (rapid heartbeat) and fatigue. However, AF can be asymptomatic and may suddenly present itself with a stroke (due to the travel of a small blood clot to the brain). Beta-blocker medications, calcium channel blocking agents, digoxin and drugs that thin the blood (anticoagulants) are commonly used in patients with AF for normalization of the heart rate and prevention of stroke. Currently used medications for control of atrial fibrillation are effective but often require careful titration. Side effects of these medications are not infrequent including bleeding that can be sometimes serious) as a side effect of anticoagulants. Severe and recalcitrant cases of AF may respond to ablation of the AV node by high energy radio frequency pulse. Ablation of the atrioventricular (AV) node helps a large number of patients with AF, but the procedure requires insertion of a permanent heart pacemaker.

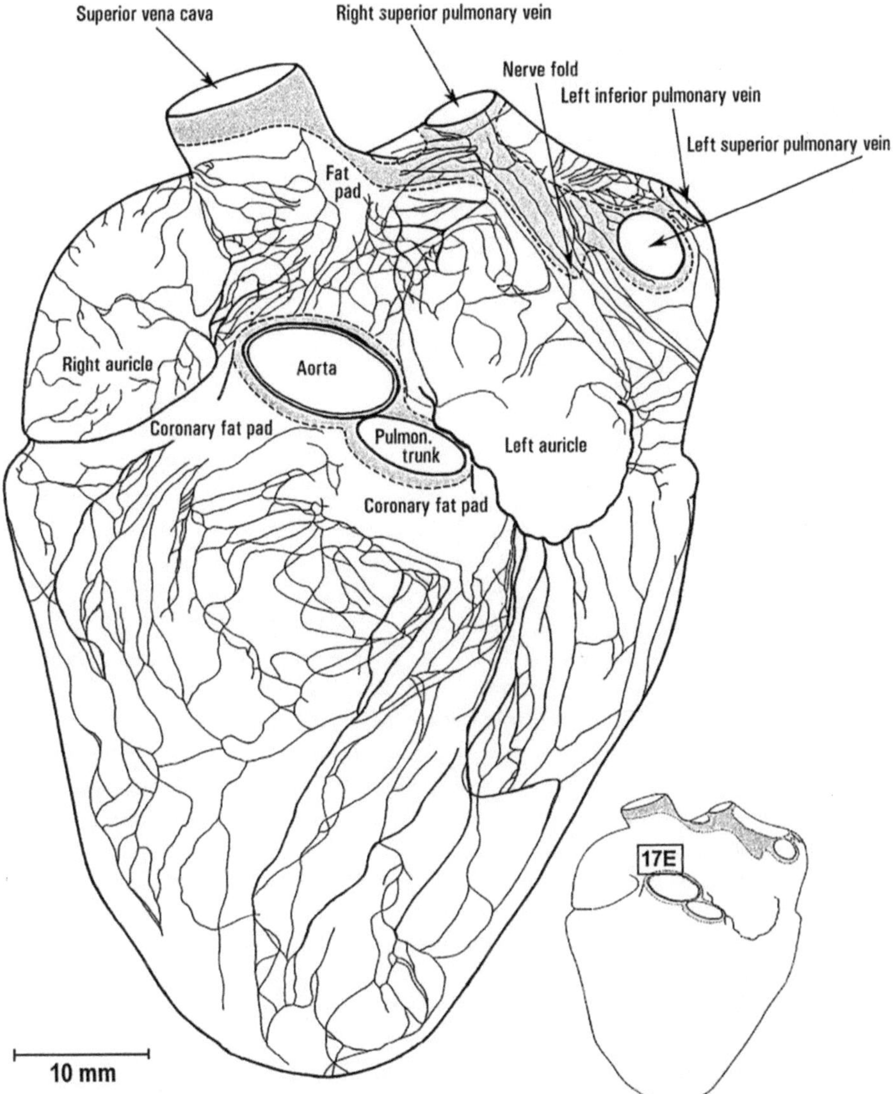

Fig. 19.5 Ganglionic plexus of the heart with nerve cells innervating the heart located in fat pads close to large vessels of the heart and diffuse nerve fibers that excites the heart. (From Pauza et al. [15]. Courtesy of the publisher, Wiley and Sons)

Since injection of botulinum toxins inhibits the activity of acetylecholine (see previous chapters), the chemical that is the neurotransmitter for parasympathetic nerve (vagus nerve), researchers began to explore the potential role of botulinum toxin therapy in atrial fibrillation. It has been shown that injection of botulinum toxin A (Botox) into the ganglionic plexus (GP) of dog's heart can suppress AF caused by electrical stimulation of the dog's vagus nerve [19]. Similar results were found in electrical stimulation induced atrial fibrillation of sheep following injection of Botox (25 units) units into different surface fat pads (containing GP) of the sheep's heart [20].

Pukoshalov and coworkers [21] first investigated the effect of botulinum toxin injections into the GP of human heart in a double- blind, placebo-controlled study. Prior to cardiac bypass surgery, 60 surgery candidates were randomized into toxin and saline groups (30 each). After opening the chest wall (thoracotomy), 50 units of Xeomin or 1 cc of normal saline (placebo) was injected into each of four pericardial fat pads containing GP. During the first 30 days after surgery, 2 of 30 patients (7%) in the botulinum toxin group and 9 of 30 patients (30%) in the placebo group experienced recurrence of atrial fibrillation (statistically significant difference, P = 0.024). Over the next 12 months, none of the patients in the Xeomin group experienced recurrence of AF, while 7 of the 30 (27%) subjects in the placebo group had recurrences (also statistically significant, P = 0.002). No patient reported any side effects. Xeomin is a Botulinum toxin type A like Botox, with units comparable to Botox.

In another study published 4 years later in 2019, a group of investigators assessed the effect of injection of 50 units of Xeomin into each 4 GPs around the heart of 60 patients with AF and compared the results with placebo injection (saline) at 36 months postinjection [22]. The results showed that while in the saline injected group, 50% still had AF, in the BoNT injected group only 23.3% still had AF at 36 months post injection. The number of hospitalizations was also reduced in the toxin injected group compared to saline injected group (2 patients versus 10 patients). In another study, fewer patients with Botox injections (50 units into each GP) prior to cardiac surgery developed AF after cardiac surgery compared to those who had received placebo injections (36.5% versus 47.8%), but the difference was not statistically significant [23]. The latter study, however, also included patients who underwent valve replacement surgery, whereas the surgery in the first two studies was coronary artery bypass grafting (CABG). In all three studies, side effects after BoNT injection were comparable with the side effects in the placebo group who were injected with saline; all side effects were defined as insignificant. These studies strongly suggest that for recalcitrant AF caused by CABG surgery, BoNT injection into GP would be a good alternative to AV node ablation; BoNT injection, unlike AV node ablation, does not require the patient to be placed on permanent pacemaker. Nevertheless, there is a need for further well-designed studies to carefully investigate the efficacy of preventive value of BoNT injection into heart's fat pads in patients undergoing cardiac surgery. These studies should control for potential confounding factors such as type of surgery, left atrial size, dose and site of injection of botulinum toxin as well as other relevant factors [24].

Cancer Associated Disorders

Cancer–Related Pain

Over the past 25 years, it has been shown that injection of botulinum toxins (A or B) into muscle or skin can relieve pain. This is due to the fact that Botox and other toxins deactivate the function of pain transmitters (glutamate, substance P, others) both in the peripheral nerves and in the central nervous system [25–27]. The palliative role of BoNTs in a large number of pain disorders [28–32] has been discussed in detail in Chap. 6 of this book.

Cancer can cause pain through several different mechanisms. The most commonly reported and best-studied type of pain associated with cancer is the pain felt at the site of surgery and radiation in patients with head and neck cancer (throat, tonsils, etc.). This form of pain can be severe and disabling and may significantly impair the quality of life as noted in the case described below from the author's experience.

Patient Example

A 48- year-old man had bilateral surgery on the neck (neck dissection), followed by neck radiation and chemotherapy for cancer of the larynx (beginning of the wind pipe in the throat). Two years later, he developed severe pain in the left side of the neck and painful spasms of the shoulder muscle (trapezius) close to the neck. The pain was present almost every day and impaired his quality of life significantly. Treatment with pain killers including potent agents (opioids and fentanyl), at best, provided modest relief. He was referred by his physician to the Yale Botulinum Toxin Clinic for management of his neck pain. Injection of the anterior neck region on the left, in the areas of scar and keloid formation, and left shoulder muscle with Botox resulted in marked reduction of pain and improvement of the patient's quality of life. The dose for the neck injection was 10–20 units/site (Fig. 19.6, areas marked by x) and for the shoulder it was 30–40 units/site. Over a follow- up period of 3 years, patient received injections every 4–5 months and, each time, reported satisfaction. There were no side effects.

During the years 2005–2015, the author of this chapter and his colleagues at Yale University studied the effect of botulinum toxin therapy in cancer related pain. The results were published in two small clinical trials, one on 7 and the other on 12 patients [33, 34]. In these studies, the investigators used Botox or Xeomin (another botulinum toxin type A with units comparable to Botox) to relieve neck pain in patients with history of surgery and/or radiation for laryngeal, throat or tongue cancer. A total of 80–120 units of Botox or Xeomin was injected into painful scars and indurated keloids and, sometimes additionally, into the adjacent painful muscles of the neck in order to relieve the chronic pain (Fig. 19.6). The patients' level of pain

Fig. 19.6 Sites of Botox injection in a patient with persistent neck and shoulder pain after surgery and radiation for throat cancer. (Drawing courtesy of Dr. Damoun Safarpour. From Mittal and Jabbari [43]. Courtesy of Toxins. https://creativecommons.org/licenses/by/4.0/)

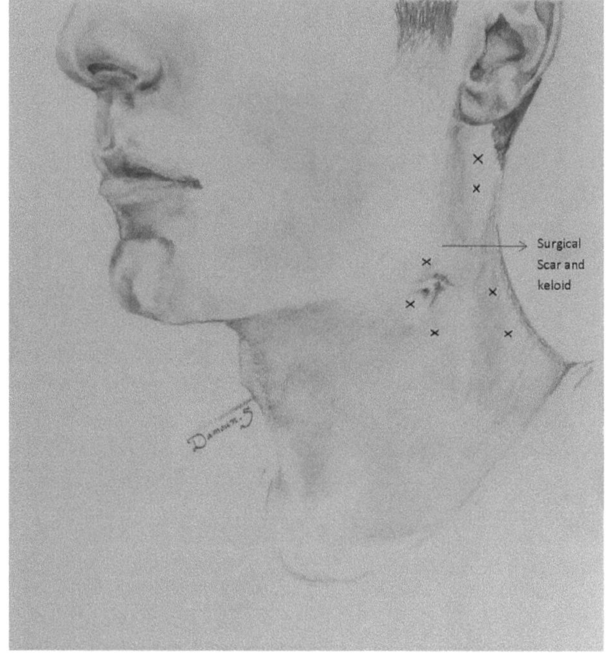

and quality of life was assessed at baseline, and after injection every 4 weeks for 3 months. In 80% of the patients, local injection of Botox or Xeomin resulted in marked reduction of local pain. Approximately half of the patients reported significant improvement of their quality of life. In recent years, several authors also reported improvement of cancer associated pain following local botulinum toxin injections in small series of patients [35–42].

Pain Due to Metastasis by Cancer

Patient Example

A 62- year old female, an intelligent and accomplished writer with history of lung cancer, experienced severe jaw pain and stiffness of the jaw muscles that gradually locked her jaw and prevented her from eating solid food. An MRI of the head showed an enlarged right masseter muscle (the masseter muscle raises the lower jaw and closes the mouth- Fig. 19.7) presumably due to metastatic cancer.

Pain killers and muscle relaxants offered little help. The jaw gradually locked and prevented her from eating solid food. She lost 15 pounds of weight over 3 months and suffered from severe depression. Patient also complained of severe jaw pain that she rated as 8 on a scale of 0–10.

Fig. 19.7 MRI showing an enlarged masseter muscle on the right side of the image (right masseter) due to invasion by tumor tissue. (From Safarpour and Jabbari 2023. Courtesy of toxins https://creativecommons.org/licenses/by/4.0/)

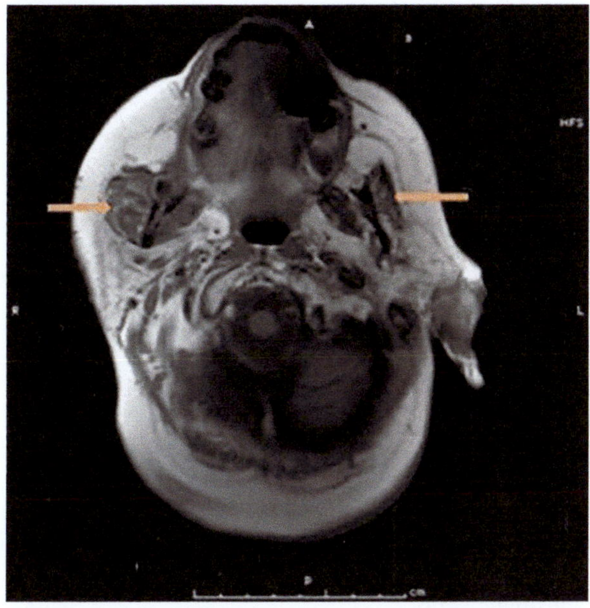

Under an approved hospital protocol and with patient's consent, Botox was injected into the masseter muscles (overlying the jaw), 70 units on the right and 30 units on the left side. Within 3–4 days after Botox injection, the contracted masseter muscles relaxed, and the jaw was unlocked allowing the patient to eat solid food. She also reported significant reduction of her jaw pain within days following the Botox injections. The effect of botulinum toxin injections lasted for 2–3 months. She experienced no side effects following injections into the masseter muscles. Repeated Botox treatment every 2–3 months had the same effect and made the patient comfortable during the last 18 months of her life.

Neuropathic Pain Caused by Chemotherapy for Cancer

Immune modifying drugs or drugs that are used for chemotherapy of cancer are toxic and often cause systemic complications. Peripheral neuropathy is common among these side effects. This form of damage to the peripheral nerves is painful and involves mainly the distal part of the limbs with the symptoms presenting most notably in the feet.

The pain is a neuropathic type of pain characterized by its sharp nature and burning quality. It can be constant and can disturb sleep. The author of this chapter observed that injection of Botox into or under the skin at multiple sites with a thin needle (gauge 30) may relieve pain in patients with this type of neuropathy. Botox injections themselves are painful in these patients since their skin is sensitive, but

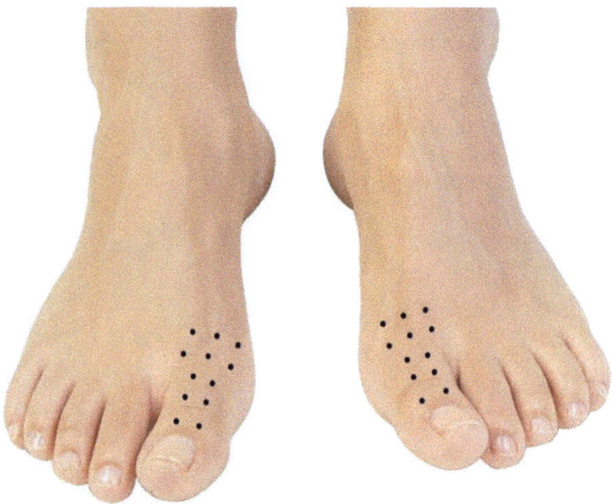

Fig. 19.8 The sites of Botox injections in the patient with cancer and neuropathic pain caused by immune modifying drugs. (From author's personal collection)

the subsequent pain relief that lasts for months makes it acceptable to most patients. Before the injections, the skin can be numbed by Emla cream and, additionally, by anesthetic spray.

Patient Example

A 64- year-old man complained of severe burning pain involving the top of his feet (mainly in the front and above the big toes) during treatment with immune modifying agents tacrolimus and cellcept which were prescribed for management of cancer of the bone morrow. He had been diagnosed with a myeloclastic syndrome (a form of bone morrow cancer) a year earlier. The pain was described as sharp, burning and unbearable at night. The most painful areas were above the big toes, on the dorsal aspect of the feet. Pain killers provided no relief. A week after injection of Botox into 10–12 sites of each affected foot (Fig. 19.8), the patient reported significant pain relief that lasted for months. The Botox dose was 1.5–2 units/site.

Botulinum Toxin Injections Help Complications That Follow Esophageal Cancer Surgery

Removal of esophageal cancer can cause significant narrowing (stricture) of esophagus impairing the passage of food. Wen and coworker [44], in a double- blind, placebo-controlled study, have shown that injection of Botox into the esophagus before tumor resection can significantly reduce development of post-surgical stricture (Botox: 6.1% versus placebo 32.4%, statistically significant P = 0.02). Another complication after esophageal cancer surgery is development of gastroparesis (weakness of stomach muscles) which leads to a delay in passage of food from stomach into the gut for absorption. Investigators have shown that injection of botulinum toxins (Botox and others) into pylorus (the circular muscle ring between stomach and first part of the gut) by relaxing this muscle ring (sphincter) and promote passage of the food into the gut [45–47].

Botulinum toxin injections are shown to be helpful in preventing or resolving complication that arise from parotid gland surgery. Parotid glands are located under the skin at the region of the jaw close to masseter muscles (muscles used for chewing). They secrete saliva. After removal of cancerous parotid glands a fistula or cyst (sialocele may develop at the site of surgery. Investigators have shown that injection of botulinum toxins into the parotid glands prevents development of fistula or cyst in a substantial number of patients [48, 49]. This function is accomplished through drying the saliva via inhibiting release of acetylcholine, the nerve transmitter that excites the parotid glands.

Another complication of parotid surgery for cancer is development of unpleasant and excessive facial sweating while chewing food (gustatory hyperhidrosis). Since the nerve transmitter for sweat glands is also acetylcholine, injection of Botox with a small and thin needle over the sweating region (multiple injections) can dry the skin for several months. The effectiveness of Botox injections for treatment of gustatory hyperhidrosis after parotidectomy has been reported in several publications [50, 51].

Dermatology

Psoriasis

Psoraias is a chronic skin disease characterized by red plaques (plaque psoriasis) covered by silvery scales that can affect any part of the body (skin, nail, scalp). Psoriasis is an autoimmune disease causing skin lesions through inflammation. It affects 3% of the adult US population and 0.1% of US children [52]. Intense itch associated with psoriatic skin lesions impairs the patients' quality of life. Most affected patients have plaque psoriasis (raised plaques as described above); additionally, approximately 30% have inverse psoriasis where the lesions are in body folds (axilla, groin, genitals) and usually have no scales. As psoriasis is a systemic inflammatory disease; patients with severe psoriasis are prone to develop cardiovascular complications and diabetes.

Treatment of psoriasis is aimed at alleviation of patients' symptoms and healing the lesions as well as controlling the basic immunological problem in order to prevent development of new lesions and spread of the disease. The first line of treatment is using phototherapy (exposure to ultraviolet light) and application of topical creams such as those containing steroids to heal skin lesions. Careful removal of the scales also promotes healing. In case of severe psoriasis involving large parts of the body, use of drugs that strengthen immunity and reduce inflammation are recommended. In the past 10 years, several of these drugs have been approved by FDA for use in the US. For example, Skyrizi (Risankizumab) selectively binds to the inflammatory agent interleukin 23 and prevents its action. These drugs are not however, free of serious side effects and should be used under supervision of specialized physicians. Since the treatment of milder forms of plaque or inverse psoriasis by phototherapy and steroid creams is not always successful, a search for new modes of therapy continues in the field of dermatology.

Botulinum Toxin Treatment

After noting that local injection of botulinum toxins decreases local inflammation in animal models [53], investigators began to explore the effectiveness of local injections of botulinum toxins in improvement of psoriatic skin lesions. In 2008, Zanchi and co-workers [54] treated 15 patients with plaque or inverse psoriasis (psoriasis affecting folded areas like axilla) with botulinum toxin injections. Botox, 50–100 units, was injected into multiple areas of the lesions. After 12 weeks, all patients reported improvement of itch (using VAS score) and. in 87% of the patients' skin lesions (redness and induration) improved. This observation was seconded by several others over publications in the past 15 years (Table 19.2).

The mostly positive data from these studies are supported by several case reports graphically demonstrating the healing of psoriasis lesions after Botox injection (Fig. 19.9).

The negative conclusion of Todberg's study (Table 19.2) is at odds with the rest of the reports in the above table that have found botulinum toxin injections useful in treatment of psoriasis. However, the toxin dose in the Todberg study (using Dysport) was much smaller than the dose used in the above described Botox studies (each Botox unit is equal to 2.5–3 Dysport units). Since success in botulinum toxin therapy is highly dependent on the applied dose, the conclusion expressed in the Todberg's study has to be considered with caution.

Recalcitrant Itch

Itch is a common human complaint, experienced often by patients affected by different skin disorders. Recalcitrant itch is a major physical and psychological nuisance and impairs patients' quality of life. Certain chemicals seem to be involved in sustenance of itch such as histamine and calicitonin gene related peptide (CGRP). The latter is a well-known pain transmitter which is inhibited by botulinum toxin injection. Sensation of itch is believed to be transmitted to the brain through the very same thin sensory nerve fibers (C fibers) that convey neuropathic pain (sharp,

Table 19.2 Reports of botulinum toxin efficacy in treatment of psoriasis

Author and date	#pts., Study type	Type of psoriasis	Type of toxin and total dose (units)	Assessment methods, clinical features	Results
Zanchi et al. [54]	15, OL	Plaque and inverse	Botox, 50–100	VAS for itch, redness; color assessed by observation	At 12 weeks, itch improved in 87%; redness and duration improved in all patients
Saber et al. [55]	1, OL	Inverse, affecting axilla	Botox, 100	Redness and color assessed by observation	At 4 weeks, extensive skin lesions were reduced to small areas of pale redness
Gilbert et al. [56]	1	Inverse, single plaque	Dysport, 30	Redness, induration	Improvement noted at 3 weeks. Total healing over succeeding weeks
Todberg et al. [57]	8, Db-PC	Plaque psoriasis	Dysport, 36	Clinical assessment of redness and induration	No patient showed improvement of lesions
Botsali et al. [58]	2, OL	Nail psoriasis	Dysport, 30	Nail improvement and clearing	Significant improvement 4 months post-injection
Gonzalez et al. [59]	8, OL	Plaque psoriasis	Dysport, 50	Redness, infiltration	Significant improvement of redness and infiltration, 2 patients reported significant improvement in itch
Khattab and Samir [60]	35, NSP	Plaque psoriasis	Refinex (Chinese toxin) 100	Redness, induration TSI	85% of the patients showed improvement of TSI with improvement of redness and induration

TSI psoriasis severity index, *OL* open label, *Db-PC* double blind, placebo controlled, *NS* blinding not specified (toxin injection was compared with fluoroucil injection)

burning) [61]. Treatment of recalcitrant itch includes use of drugs that inhibit the function of histamine (antihistaminic drugs), as well as drugs that are used for treatment of neuropathic pain such as gabapentin. Unfortunately, in many patients results do not meet patients' satisfaction.

Animal studies and studies on human volunteers have shown that local injection of botulinum toxin can inhibit the function of CGRP and histamine [62, 63]. These observations encouraged researchers to look at the effect of botulinum toxin injections into recalcitrant itchy skin lesions. They found that intense itch associated with different skin lesions improves with injection of botulinum toxin into the affected area (Table 19.3).

The data in the Table 19.3 show that although high quality studies are not yet available for this indication, botulinum toxin injection has a significant potential to suppress recalcitrant itch caused by different disorders.

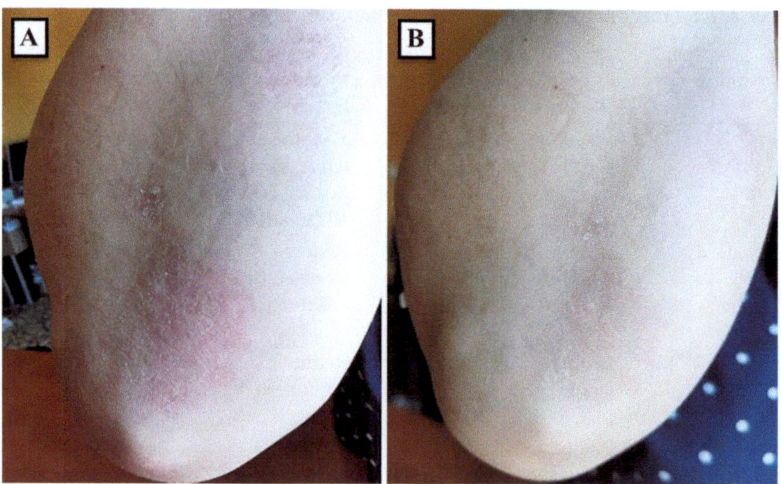

Fig. 19.9 (**a**) Psoriasis of the elbow and extensor surface of the forearm a month before Botulinum toxin injection (**b**) significant improvement of psoriatic lesion following injection of 1000 units of Dysport (approximately 300–350 units of Botox) for treatment of elbow spasticity (see Chaps. 6 and 7 for spasticity treatment in stroke and multiple sclerosis with botulinum toxins). (Courtesy of Dr. Popescu and colleagues 2022. Reproduced under Creative Commons Attribution (CC BY) license (https://creativecommons.org/licenses/by/4.0/))

Raynaud's Syndrome (RS)

Described by Maurice Raynaud in 1862 (part of his thesis), this is a disabling clinical condition characterized by poor circulation of the digits causing significant skin changes (blue or red discoloration) and pain in the hand and fingers. The condition worsens after exposure to cold and emotional stress [73]. In severe cases, poor circulation may cause intolerable pain associated with gangrene of the fingers. Raynaud's syndrome (RS) is classified into primary and secondary types [74]. In primary RS, the cause is unknown. Secondary RS is usually associated with diseases caused by failure of immune system such as scleroderma and cancer. Excessive smoking and excessive use of certain drugs (especially anti-cancer drugs) are also major contributing factors. Several modes of treatment have been tried in RS with limited success. Among drugs, gabapentin and serotonin uptake inhibitors offer analgesic effect. Laser therapy and acupuncture are also partially effective.

The reason for considering botulinum toxin therapy for alleviating the symptoms of RS is based on two premises: (1) vascular tone in the fingers is maintained by the sympathetic nervous system using acetylecholine as nerve transmitter. Botox and similar toxins are known to inhibit the release of acetylcholine from nerve endings (see Chap. 2 of this book). (2) Botulinum toxin injections into muscle and skin can alleviate pain due to inhibition of known pain transmitters [75]. The data from clinical trials and on this subject are presented in Table 19.4. Single case reports are not included in this table.

Table 19.3 Reports of itch responding to local injection of botulinum toxins into the affected region

Author and date	# pts.	Associated disease	Itch location	Toxin type and total dose in units	Method of assessment	Results
Heckmann et al. [64]	4	Lichen simplex, 5 skin lesions	Two spots, lower limbs	Dysport, 20–80	VAS for itch 0–10 scale	Itch subsided in 3–7 days. Skin lesions cleared in 2–4 weeks
Zanchi et al. [54]	15	Psoriasis	Different places: Armpits, groin,	Botox, 50–100	VAS for itch 0–10 scale	Itch improved in 87% of the patients
Salardini et al. [65]	1	Post-surgical scar	Right frontal region	Botox, 15	Patient report	"Marked reduction of itch in a few days"
Kavanagh and Tidman [66]	1	Notalgia paresthetica[a]	Posterior aspect of the arms	Botox, 100,	Patient report	Marked reduction of itch for months reproduced with repeat injections
Akhter and Brooks [67]	9	Burns	Different parts of the body	Botox, dose not specified	VAS for itch 0–10 scale	Itch intensity of 8–10 dropped to 0–4. Most patients to 0
Gonzalez et al. [59]	8	Psoriasis	Not specified	Dysport, 50	Patient report	Significant improvement of itch in two patients
Datta et al. [68]	1	Notalgia paresthetica	Not specified	Botox dose not specified	Not specified	Marked reduction of itch
Gharib et al. [69]	32	Burn scar, shingles, psoriasis,other skin lesions	Different parts of body	Botox, 50–100	VAS for itch 0–10 scale	Statistically significant decrease in intensity in all patients
Klager et al. [70]	1	Fox-Fordyce[b] disease	Right armpit	Botox, 50	VAS for itch, 0–10 scale	Initial itch:10 Itch level dropped to 3 after Botox injection
Alam et al. [71]	9	Post-surgical scar region	Face cancer	Type E toxin, 2.5 nanogram	VAS for itch 0–10 scale, scar scale	At days 2 and 8 post- surgery no patient in toxin group had itch compared to 75% and 50% in the placebo group
Mineroff et al. [72]	1	Shingles	Left upper neck	Botox, 50	Patient report	Marked reduction of itch for 3 months

VAS visual analogue scale

[a]Notalgiaparesthetica: chronic itch over the lower part of shoulder blade more common in elderly female

[b]Fox-Fordyse disease: a medical condition characterized by pathological changes in the sweat glands and chronic itch

A review and meta-analysis of data published in 2023 concluded that the reported data in the literature (Table 19.4) support the efficacy of botulinum toxin treatment to reduce the symptoms of RS [89]. However, this conclusion was challenged by a very recent double-blind, placebo-controlled study that did not find any difference between placebo and Botox in improving the symptoms of RS [90]. Yin and co-workers [91] stated that the negative results of that study [90] could be due to several factors such as longer duration of the disease in the Botox group, poor training of patients to report RP episodes, ignoring skin color changes and not reporting ethnicity of the patients which could influence the results. More high quality studies are necessary to support or refute the effectiveness of botulinum toxin treatment in Raynuad's syndrome.

Teeth Grinding (Bruxism)

Teeth grinding is a common medical problem that can affect children and adults and may present during wakefulness or sleep. It affects up to 31% of adults [92]. Severe teeth grinding can destroy teeth, cause jaw pain and headaches. Teeth grinding during sleep interrupts sleep of both patient and the bed partner. Medications like clonazepam (clonopin) provide modest relief, but may cause significant daytime sedation. Several high quality studies (double- blind and placebo- controlled), though small in number, have demonstrated that injection of Botox into the temporalis and masseter muscles (Fig. 19.10) can improve teeth grinding. These two muscles close the jaw.

A placebo-controlled study published in 2018 assessed 23 patients with teeth grinding during sleep and compared the outcome in 13 patients assigned randomly to Botox with 10 patients assigned to the placebo group (blinded study) [93]. Botox was injected into temporalis muscles (40 units on each side) and masseter muscles (60 units on each side). Authors concluded that injection of Botox into those muscles safely improves teeth grinding during sleep with no significant side effects. Two patients reported transient cosmetic change in their smile.

Two more recent blinded and placebo-controlled studies [94, 95], one investigating a larger number of patients [93] with bruxism compared the effect of Botox treatment with placebo. These studies provided results similar to the two above-mentioned studies and came to a similar conclusion. One of the two [95] found that injecting even small units of Botox into the masseter muscle only (10 units) can improve pain and discomfort associated with night time teeth grinding. These encouraging data indicate that Botox injections into muscles of mastication can improve teeth grinding during sleep and wakefulness without causing major or persistent side effects.

Table 19.4 Botulinum toxin effect on the symptoms of Raynaud's Syndrome

Author and date	Type of study	#pts	Toxin type and total dose in units	Method(s) of assessment	Results
Uppal et al. [76]	Pros	20	Botox, 100	Pain (VAS), skin color change, disability (dash score)	Reduction pain, color and disability in 85%, 75%, and 85% of the patients, respectively
Fregene et al. [77]	Retro	26	Botox, average 77	Pain (VAS), digit oxygen, healing finger ulcers	Pain, digital oxygen saturation and finger ulcers improved in 75%, 57% and 48% of the patients, respectively
Neumeister et al. [78]	Retro	33	Botox 40/hand; 4 injections	Pain(VAS), healing of ulcers	Reduction of pain: 86%; healing of ulcers: All patients
Goldbeg et al. [79]	Retro	20	Botox, 10–20/ finger	Pain(VAS), disability (dash score),	Pain: In 86% of pts.; dash score for disability: Reduced over 14 points at 6 weeks; clinical success in 84% of pts
Shanavandeh et al. [80]	Pros	26	Botox, 20 injected at the base of each involved finger	Healing of ulcer, pain(VAS), local small bleeds	Healing of ulcers: 95%; pain: Improved in all; reduced number of small bleeds
Medina et al. [81]	Retro, 3 years follow up	15	Botox, 4–8 injected into the base and lateral aspect of all fingers	Pain (VAS). Weekly episodes of RP, finger ulcers	At week 8 post injection: Pain and RP episodes markedly reduced, ulcers healed in 5 of 7 patients
Motegi et al. [82]	Pros, blinded, dose comparison	45	Myobloc 3 groups, 250, 1000 and 2000	Number of ulcers, skin temperature, RP score and pain (VAS_)	At week 4 after injection: All outcomes significantly improved in 1000 and 2000 dose groups
Bello et al. [83]	DB-PC, all had scleroderma	40	Botox, 5–10 into 7 hand areas	Blood flow to the hands, VAS for pain, RP episodes	No significant difference between groups. At 4 weeks VAS score was lower in Botox group
Quintana-castanedo et al. [84]	Pros	8	Botox. 36/ hand, base of all fingers, 7 injections	Pain (VAS), RP episodes	At 4 weeks post-injection: 6 patients had no pain;6 had significant reduction of RP episodes
Dhaliwal et al. [85]	Pros	40	Botox, 100	Pain(VAS), hand swelling, change in color	All parameters markedly improved in 48% of the patients

(continued)

Table 19.4 (continued)

Author and date	Type of study	#pts	Toxin type and total dose in units	Method(s) of assessment	Results
Du et al. [86]	Pros,	32	Botox 10 vs no Botox, injected into 2+3rd and 3rd and 4th fingers	Pain(VAS), RP episodes, microscopic parameters	VAS: No improvement; RP episodes significantly lessened, microscopic parameters improved
Seyed-mardani et al. [87]	Pors	11	Botulinum toxin A 50/hand	Raynaud score, skin color, pain(VAS)	All significantly improved at two months
Motegi et al. [88]	Pros	10	Botox, 10/hand	Pain: Measured by VAS, RP frequency and intensity	Both pain and RP frequency/intensity improved after Botox injection

DB-PC double blind placebo controlled, *Pros* prospective, *Retro* retrospective, *VAS* visual analogue scale for pain (0–10), *RP* Raynaud phenomenon episodes, Myobloc is a type B toxin (Botox is type A)

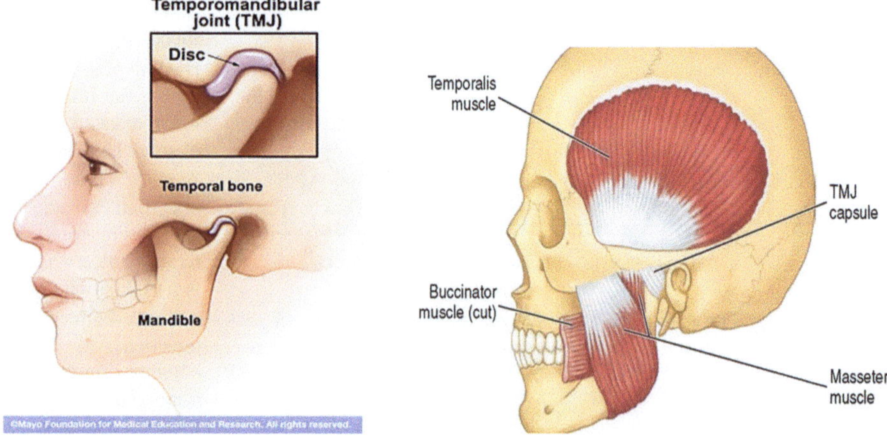

Fig. 19.10 Temporalis and masseter muscles. (Printed with permission from Mayo Foundation)

Rectal Pain Associated with Hemorrhoidectomy

Local muscle pain along the line of excision, after hemorrhoidectomy, is a common complaint. In some patients, the pain can be severe and disabling and may persist for months despite use of potent analgesics. Over the past 20 years, researchers have explored the effectiveness of botulinum toxin injections into the anal sphincter (the circular muscle that opens and closes the anus) before, during and after hemorrhoidectomy in order to prevent post-hemorrhoidectomy pain.

Davies and coworkers conducted a careful, double- blind (both physician and patient blinded to the type of injection) study of 50 patients who had undergone hemorrhoidectomy [96]. Injection of 20 units of Botox into the anal sphincter prior to removal of the hemorrhoids, markedly reduced postsurgical painful spasms of the anal sphincter, an effect which was statistically significant compared to placebo (saline) injection. The peak pain relief was at the sixth or seventh day after surgery. In another high quality study (blinded and compared with placebo), Dr. Alavandipour and her colleagues [97] have shown that injection of Botox during surgery into the anal sphincter significantly reduced pain after surgery compared to placebo injection as assessed at 12 and 48 h, as well as 7 and 14 days after operation. In addition, in the Botox injected group, the post-operative wound healed much faster than the group that had placebo (salt water) injection. Two other high quality investigations published in 2020 and 2022 [98, 99] also found similar results by injecting Botox shortly after surgery. A comparative study of Botox with local application of glycerine nitrate found botulinum toxin injections more effective than glycerine nitrate for relief of post-surgical pain [100].

The Role of Botulinum Toxin Injections in Complex Midline Abdominal Hernia Repair

The abdominal wall muscles consist of two major components: the front muscles of abdominal wall engulfing the belly button (called rectus abdominalis) and oblique lateral muscles. The existing tone in lateral abdominal oblique muscles tends to pull the anterior wall muscles laterally and to the side. This causes a problem after the repair of a large midline abdominal hernia since the pulling power of lateral oblique muscles delays healing after hernia repair surgery. Several studies have shown that relaxing lateral abdominal oblique muscles by Botox injections prior to surgery can expedite healing of the abdominal wall after hernia repair surgery [101–103].

Conclusion

Emerging literature shows potential new indications for botulinum toxin therapy in several medical conditions: depression, atrial fibrillation, cancer related pain, post-surgical pain (hemorrhoidectomy, hernia repair), teeth grinding (bruxism), psoriasis, recalcitrant itch, jaw pain in temporomandibular disorder and in Raynaud's syndrome.

References

1. Kessler RC, Berglund P, Demler O, et al. The epidemiology of major depressive disorder: results from the National Comorbidity Survey Replication (NCS-R). JAMA. 2003;18(289):3095–105.
2. Marwaha S, Palmer E, Suppes T, Cons E, Young AH, Upthegrove R. Novel and emerging treatments for major depression. Lancet. 2023;401(10371):141–53. https://doi.org/10.1016/S0140-6736(22)02080-3.
3. Lewis MB, Bowler PJ. Botulinum toxin cosmetic therapy correlates with a more positive mood. J Cosmet Dermatol. 2009;8(1):24–6. https://doi.org/10.1111/j.1473-2165.2009.00419.x.
4. Hennenlotter A, Dresel C, Castrop F, Ceballos-Baumann AO, Wohlschläger AM, Haslinger B. The link between facial feedback and neural activity within central circuitries of emotion—new insights from botulinum toxin-induced denervation of frown muscles. Cereb Cortex. 2009;19(3):537–42.
5. Wollmer MA, de Boer C, Kalak NT, et al. Facing depression with botulinum toxin: a randomized controlled trial. J Psychiatr Res. 2012;46:574–81.
6. Finzi E, Rosenthal NE. Treatment of depression with onabotulinumtoxinA: a randomized, double-blind, placebo- controlled trial. J Psychiatr Res. 2014;52:1–6.
7. Magid M, Reichenberg JS, Poth PE, et al. Treatment of major depressive disorder using botulinum toxin a: a 24-week randomized, double-blind, placebo-controlled study. Clin Psychiatry. 2014;75:837–44.
8. Brin MF, Durgam S, Lum A, James L, Liu J, Thase ME, Szegedi A. OnabotulinumtoxinA for the treatment of major depressive disorder: a phase 2 randomized, double-blind, placebo-controlled trial in adult females. Int Clin Psychopharmacol. 2020;35(1):19–28. https://doi.org/10.1097/YIC.0000000000000290.
9. Zhang Q, Wu W, Fan Y, Li Y, Liu J, Xu Y, Jiang C, Tang Z, Cao C, Liu T, Chen LH, Hu H, Luo W. The safety and efficacy of botulinum toxin A on the treatment of depression. Brain Behav. 2021;11(9):e2333. https://doi.org/10.1002/brb3.2333.
10. Li Y, Zhu T, Shen T, Wu W, Cao J, Sun J, Liu J, Zhou X, Jiang C, Tang Z, Liu T, Chen L, Hu H, Luo W. Botulinum toxin A (BoNT/A) for the treatment of depression: a randomized, double-blind, placebo, controlled trial in China. J Affect Disord. 2022;1(318):48–53. https://doi.org/10.1016/j.jad.2022.08.097.
11. Zhang H, Zhang H, Wei Y, Lian Y, Chen Y, Zheng Y. Treatment of chronic daily headache with comorbid anxiety and depression using botulinum toxin A: a prospective pilot study. Int J Neurosci. 2017;127(4):285–90. https://doi.org/10.1080/00207454.2016.1196687.
12. Zhu C, Wang K, Yu T, Liu H. Effects of botulinum toxin type a on mood and cognitive function in patients with parkinson's disease and depression. Am J Transl Res. 2021;13(4):2717–23.
13. Schulze J, Neumann I, Magid M, Finzi E, Sinke C, Wollmer MA, Krüger THC. Botulinum toxin for the management of depression: an updated review of the evidence and meta-analysis. J Psychiatr Res. 2021;135:332–40. https://doi.org/10.1016/j.jpsychires.2021.01.016.
14. Kim MJ, Neta M, Davis FC, Ruberry EJ, Dinescu D, Heatherton TF, Stotland MA, Whalen PJ. Botulinum toxin-induced facial muscle paralysis affects amygdala responses to the perception of emotional expressions: preliminary findings from an A-B-A design. Biol Mood Anxiety Disord. 2014;31(4):11. https://doi.org/10.1186/2045-5380-4-11.
15. Pauza DH, Skripka V, Pauziene N, Stropus R. Morphology, distribution, and variability of the epicardiac neural ganglionated subplexuses in the human heart. Anat Rec. 2000;259(4):353–82.
16. Go AS, Hylek EM, Phillips KA. Prevalence of diagnosed atrial fibrillation in adults: national implications for rhythm management and stroke prevention: the nTicoagulation and risk factors in atrial fibrillation (ATRIA) study. JAMA. 2001;285:2370–5.
17. Baman JR, Passman RS. Atrial Fibrillation. JAMA. 2021;325(21):2218. https://doi.org/10.1001/jama.2020.23700.

18. Boriani G, Bonini N, Imberti JF. The epidemiology and mortality of patients with atrial fibrillation: a complex landscape. J Cardiovasc Med (Hagerstown). 2023;24(11):798–801. https://doi.org/10.2459/JCM.0000000000001552.

19. Lo LW, Chang HY, Scherlag BJ, Lin YJ, Chou YH, Lin WL, Chen SA, Po SS. Temporary suppression of cardiac Ganglionated Plexi leads to long-term suppression of atrial fibrillation: evidence of early autonomic intervention to break the vicious cycle of "AF begets AF". J Am Heart Assoc. 2016;5(7):e003309. https://doi.org/10.1161/JAHA.116.003309.

20. Nazeri A, Ganapathy AV, Massumi A, Massumi M, Tuzun E, Stainback R, Segura AM, Elayda MA, Razavi M. Effect of botulinum toxin on inducibility and maintenance of atrial fibrillation in ovine myocardial tissue. Pacing Clin Electrophysiol. 2017;40(6):693–702. https://doi.org/10.1111/pace.13079.

21. Pokushalov E, Kozlov B, Romanov A, et al. Long-term suppression of atrial fibrillation by botulinum toxin injection into Epicardial fat pads in patients undergoing cardiac surgery: one-year follow-up of a randomized pilot study. Circ Arrhythm Electrophysiol. 2015;8(6):1334–41.

22. Romanov A, Pokushalov E, Ponomarev D, Bayramova S, Shabanov V, Losik D, Stenin I, Elesin D, Mikheenko I, Strelnikov A, Sergeevichev D, Kozlov B, Po SS, Steinberg JS. Long-term suppression of atrial fibrillation by botulinum toxin injection into epicardial fat pads in patients undergoing cardiac surgery: three-year follow-up of a randomized study. Heart Rhythm. 2019;16(2):172–7. https://doi.org/10.1016/j.hrthm.2018.08.019.

23. Waldron NH, Cooter M, Haney JC, Schroder JN, Gaca JG, Lin SS, Sigurdsson MI, Fudim M, Podgoreanu MV, Stafford-Smith M, Milano CA, Piccini JP, Mathew JP. Temporary autonomic modulation with botulinum toxin type A to reduce atrial fibrillation after cardiac surgery. Heart Rhythm. 2019;16(2):178–84. https://doi.org/10.1016/j.hrthm.2018.08.021.

24. Fatahian A. Botulinum toxin injection into Epicardial fat pads: a promising potential modality for prevention of postoperative atrial fibrillation after cardiac surgery. Braz J Cardiovasc Surg. 2019;34(5):643. https://doi.org/10.21470/1678-9741-2019-0309.

25. Matak I, Tékus V, Bölcskei K, Lacković Z, Helyes Z. Involvement of substance P in the antinociceptive effect of botulinum toxin type A: evidence from knockout mice. Neuroscience. 2017;1(358):137–45. https://doi.org/10.1016/j.neuroscience.2017.06.040.

26. Zhang Y, Lian Y, Zhang H, Xie N, Chen Y. CGRP plasma levels decrease in classical trigeminal neuralgia patients treated with botulinum toxin type A: a pilot study. Pain Med. 2020;21(8):1611–5. https://doi.org/10.1093/pm/pnaa028.

27. Lacković Z. Botulinum toxin and pain. Handb Exp Pharmacol. 2021;263:251–64. https://doi.org/10.1007/164_2019_348.

28. Dodick DW, Turkel CC, De Gryse RE, Aurora SK, Silberstein SD, Lipton RB, Diener HC, Brin MF, PREEMPT Chronic Migraine Study Group. OnabotulinumtoxinA for treatment of chronic migraine: pooled results from the double-blind, randomized, placebo-controlled phases of the PREEMPT clinical program. Headache. 2010;50(6):921–36. https://doi.org/10.1111/j.1526-4610.2010.01678.x.

29. Babcock MS, Foster L, Pasquina P, Jabbari B. Treatment of pain attributed to plantar fasciitis with botulinum toxin a: a short-term, randomized, placebo-controlled, double-blind study. Am J Phys Med Rehabil. 2005;84(9):649–54. https://doi.org/10.1097/01.phm.0000176339.73591.d7.

30. Yuan RY, Sheu JJ, Yu JM, Chen WT, Tseng IJ, Chang HH, Hu CJ. Botulinum toxin for diabetic neuropathic pain: a randomized double-blind crossover trial. Neurology. 2009;72(17):1473–8. https://doi.org/10.1212/01.wnl.0000345968.05959.cf.

31. Xiao L, Mackey S, Hui H, Xong D, Zhang Q, Zhang D. Subcutaneous injection of botulinum toxin a is beneficial in postherpetic neuralgia. Pain Med. 2010;11(12):1827–33. https://doi.org/10.1111/j.1526-4637.2010.01003.x.

32. Attal N, de Andrade DC, Adam F, Ranoux D, Teixeira MJ, Galhardoni R, Raicher I, Üçeyler N, Sommer C, Bouhassira D. Safety and efficacy of repeated injections of botulinum toxin A in peripheral neuropathic pain (BOTNEP): a randomised, double-blind, placebo-controlled trial. Lancet Neurol. 2016;15(6):555–65. https://doi.org/10.1016/S1474-4422(16)00017-X.

33. Mittal S, Machado DG, Jabbari B. OnabotulinumtoxinA for treatment of focal cancer pain after surgery and/or radiation. Pain Med. 2012;13:1029–33.

34. Rostami R, Mittal SO, Radmand R, Jabbari B. Incobotulinum toxin-A improves post-surgical and post-radiation pain in cancer patients. Toxins (Basel). 2016;8(1):pii: E22. https://doi.org/10.3390/toxins8010022.

35. Van Daele DJ, Finnegan EM, Rodnitzky RL, Zhen W, McCulloch TM, Hoffman HT. Head and neck muscle spasm after radiotherapy: management with botulinum toxin A injection. Arch Otolaryngol Head Neck Surg. 2002;128(8):956–9. https://doi.org/10.1001/archotol.128.8.956.

36. Vasan CW, Liu WC, Klussmann JP, Guntinas-Lichius O. Botulinum toxin type A for the treatment of chronic neck pain after neck dissection. Head Neck. 2004;26(1):39–45. https://doi.org/10.1002/hed.10340.

37. Wittekindt C, Liu WC, Preuss SF, Guntinas-Lichius O. Botulinum toxin A for neuropathic pain after neck dissection: a dose-finding study. Laryngoscope. 2006;116(7):1168–71. https://doi.org/10.1097/01.mlg.0000217797.05523.75.

38. Hartl DM, Cohen M, Juliéron M, Marandas P, Janot F, Bourhis J. Botulinum toxin for radiation-induced facial pain and trismus. Otolaryngol Head Neck Surg. 2008;138(4):459–63. https://doi.org/10.1016/j.otohns.2007.12.021.

39. Stubblefield MD, Levine A, Custodio CM, Fitzpatrick T. The role of botulinum toxin type A in the radiation fibrosis syndrome: a preliminary report. Arch Phys Med Rehabil. 2008;89(3):417–21. https://doi.org/10.1016/j.apmr.2007.11.022.

40. Chuang YC, Kim DK, Chiang PH, Chancellor MB. Bladder botulinum toxin A injection can benefit patients with radiation and chemical cystitis. BJU Int. 2008;102(6):704–6. https://doi.org/10.1111/j.1464-410X.2008.07740.x.

41. Vuong T, Waschke K, Niazi T, Richard C, Parent J, Liberman S, Mayrand S, Loungnarath R, Stein B, Devic S. The value of Botox-A in acute radiation proctitis: results from a phase I/II study using a three-dimensional scoring system. Int J Radiat Oncol Biol Phys. 2011;80(5):1505–11. https://doi.org/10.1016/j.ijrobp.2010.04.017.

42. Bach CA, Wagner I, Lachiver X, Baujat B, Chabolle F. Botulinum toxin in the treatment of post-radiosurgical neck contracture in head and neck cancer: a novel approach. Eur Ann Otorhinolaryngol Head Neck Dis. 2012;129(1):6–10. https://doi.org/10.1016/j.anorl.2011.07.002.

43. Mittal SO, Jabbari B. Botulinum neurotoxins and cancer-a review of the literature. Toxins (Basel). 2020;12(1):32. https://doi.org/10.3390/toxins12010032.

44. Wen J, Lu Z, Linghu E, Yang Y, Yang J, Wang S, Yan B, Song J, Zhou X, Wang X, Meng K, Dou Y, Liu Q. Prevention of esophageal strictures after endoscopic submucosal dissection with the injection of botulinum toxin type A. Gastrointest Endosc. 2016;84(4):606–13. https://doi.org/10.1016/j.gie.2016.03.1484.

45. Cerfolio RJ, Bryant AS, Canon CL, Dhawan R, Eloubeidi MA. Is botulinum toxin injection of the pylorus during Ivor Lewis [corrected] esophagogastrectomy the optimal drainage strategy? J Thorac Cardiovasc Surg. 2009;137(3):565–72. https://doi.org/10.1016/j.jtcvs.2008.08.049. Erratum in: J Thorac Cardiovasc Surg. 2009 Jun;137(6):1581

46. Martin JT, Federico JA, McKelvey AA, Kent MS, Fabian T. Prevention of delayed gastric emptying after esophagectomy: a single center's experience with botulinum toxin. Ann Thorac Surg. 2009;87(6):1708–14. https://doi.org/10.1016/j.athoracsur.2009.01.075.

47. Bagheri R, Fattahi SH, Haghi SZ, Aryana K, Aryanniya A, Akhlaghi S, Riyabi FN, Sheibani S. Botulinum toxin for prevention of delayed gastric emptying after esophagectomy. Asian Cardiovasc Thorac Ann. 2013;21(6):689–92. https://doi.org/10.1177/0218492312468438.

48. Steffen A, Hasselbacher K, Heinrichs S, Wollenberg B. Botulinum toxin for salivary disorders in the treatment of head and neck cancer. Anticancer Res. 2014;34(11):6627–32.

49. Melville JC, Stackowicz DJ, Jundt JS, Shum JW. Use of Botox (OnabotulinumtoxinA) for the treatment of parotid Sialocele and fistula after extirpation of buccal squamous cell carcinoma with immediate reconstruction using microvascular free flap: a report of 3 cases. J Oral Maxillofac Surg. 2016;74(8):1678–86. https://doi.org/10.1016/j.joms.2016.01.038.

50. Jansen S, Jerowski M, Ludwig L, Fischer-Krall E, Beutner D, Grosheva M. Botulinum toxin therapy in Frey's syndrome: a retrospective study of 440 treatments in 100 patients. Clin Otolaryngol. 2017;42(2):295–300. https://doi.org/10.1111/coa.12719.
51. Eckardt A, Kuettner C. Treatment of gustatory sweating (Frey's syndrome) with botulinum toxin A. Head Neck. 2003;25(8):624–8. https://doi.org/10.1002/hed.10262.
52. Rachakonda TD, Schupp CW, Armstrong AW. Psoriasis prevalence among adults in the United States. J Am Acad Dermatol. 2014;70(3):512–6. https://doi.org/10.1016/j.jaad.2013.11.013.
53. Ward NL, Kavlick KD, Diaconu D, Dawes SM, Michaels KA, Gilbert E. Botulinum neurotoxin A decreases infiltrating cutaneous lymphocytes and improves acanthosis in the KC-Tie2 mouse model. J Invest Dermatol. 2012;132(7):1927–30. https://doi.org/10.1038/jid.2012.60.
54. Zanchi M, Favot F, Bizzarini M, Piai M, Donini M, Sedona P. Botulinum toxin type-A for the treatment of inverse psoriasis. J Eur Acad Dermatol Venereol. 2008;22(4):431–6. https://doi.org/10.1111/j.1468-3083.2007.02457.x.
55. Saber M, Brassard D, Benohanian A. Inverse psoriasis and hyperhidrosis of the axillae responding to botulinum toxin type A. Arch Dermatol. 2011;147(5):629–30. https://doi.org/10.1001/archdermatol.2011.111.
56. Gilbert E, Ward NL. Efficacy of botulinum neurotoxin type A for treating recalcitrant plaque psoriasis. J Drugs Dermatol. 2014;13(11):1407–8.
57. Todberg T, Zachariae C, Bregnhøj A, Hedelund L, Bonefeld KK, Nielsen K, Iversen L, Skov L. The effect of botulinum neurotoxin A in patients with plaque psoriasis—an exploratory trial. J Eur Acad Dermatol Venereol. 2018;32(2):e81–2. https://doi.org/10.1111/jdv.14536.
58. Botsali A, Erbil H. Management of nail psoriasis with a single injection of abobotulinum toxin. J Cosmet Dermatol. 2021;20(5):1418–20. https://doi.org/10.1111/jocd.13633.
59. González C, Franco M, Londoño A, Valenzuela F. Breaking paradigms in the treatment of psoriasis: use of botulinum toxin for the treatment of plaque psoriasis. Dermatol Ther. 2020;33(6):e14319. https://doi.org/10.1111/dth.14319.
60. Khattab FM, Samir MA. Botulinum toxin type-A versus 5-fluorouracil in the treatment of plaque psoriasis: comparative study. J Cosmet Dermatol. 2021;20(10):3128–32. https://doi.org/10.1111/jocd.14306.
61. Dhand A, Aminoff MJ. The neurology of itch. Brain. 2014;137(Pt 2):313–22. https://doi.org/10.1093/brain/awt158.
62. Rapp DE, Turk KW, Bales GT, Cook SP. Botulinum toxin type a inhibits calcitonin gene-related peptide release from isolated rat bladder. J Urol. 2006;175(3 Pt 1):1138–42. https://doi.org/10.1016/S0022-5347(05)00322-8.
63. Gazerani P, Pedersen NS, Drewes AM, Arendt-Nielsen L. Botulinum toxin type A reduces histamine-induced itch and vasomotor responses in human skin. Br J Dermatol. 2009;161(4):737–45. https://doi.org/10.1111/j.1365-2133.2009.09305.x.
64. Heckmann M, Heyer G, Brunner B, Plewig G. Botulinum toxin type A injection in the treatment of lichen simplex: an open pilot study. J Am Acad Dermatol. 2002;46(4):617–9. https://doi.org/10.1067/mjd.2002.120455.
65. Salardini A, Richardson D, Jabbari B. Relief of intractable pruritus after administration of botulinum toxin A (botox): a case report. Clin Neuropharmacol. 2008;31(5):303–6. https://doi.org/10.1097/WNF.0b013e3181672225.
66. Kavanagh GM, Tidman MJ. Botulinum A toxin and brachioradial pruritus. Br J Dermatol. 2012;166(5):1147. https://doi.org/10.1111/j.1365-2133.2011.10749.x.
67. Akhtar N, Brooks P. The use of botulinum toxin in the management of burns itching: preliminary results. Burns. 2012;38(8):1119–23. https://doi.org/10.1016/j.burns.2012.05.014.
68. Datta S, Mahal S, Bhagavan SM, Govindarajan R. Use of botulinum toxin type A in a patient with refractory itch from Notalgia Paresthetica. J Clin Neuromuscul Dis. 2020;21(4):243–4. https://doi.org/10.1097/CND.0000000000000276.
69. Gharib K, Mostafa A, Elsayed A. Evaluation of botulinum toxin type A injection in the treatment of localized chronic pruritus. J Clin Aesthet Dermatol. 2020;13(12):12–7.

70. Klager S, Kumar MG. Treatment of pruritus with botulinum toxin in a pediatric patient with Fox-Fordyce disease. Pediatr Dermatol. 2021;38(4):950–1. https://doi.org/10.1111/pde.14552.

71. Alam M, Vitarella D, Ahmad W, Abushakra S, Mao C, Brin MF. Botulinum toxin type E associated with reduced itch and pain during wound healing and acute scar formation following excision and linear repair on the forehead: a randomized controlled trial. J Am Acad Dermatol. 2023;89:1317–9. https://doi.org/10.1016/j.jaad.2023.08.072.

72. Mineroff J, Uwakwe LN, Mojeski J, Jagdeo J. Using botulinum toxin A to treat postherpetic itch. Arch Dermatol Res. 2023;315(10):2971–2. https://doi.org/10.1007/s00403-023-02726-y.

73. Temprano KK. A review of Raynaud's disease. Mo Med. 2016;113(2):123–6.

74. Fardoun MM, Nassif J, Issa K, Baydoun E, Eid AH. Raynaud's phenomenon: a brief review of the underlying mechanisms. Front Pharmacol. 2016;16(7):438. https://doi.org/10.3389/fphar.2016.00438.

75. Jabbari B. Botulinum toxin treatment of pain disorders. 2nd ed. Springer Publication; 2022.

76. Uppal L, Dhaliwal K, Butler PE. A prospective study of the use of botulinum toxin injections in the treatment of Raynaud's syndrome associated with scleroderma. J Hand Surg Eur. 2014;39(8):876–80. https://doi.org/10.1177/1753193413516242.

77. Fregene A, Ditmars D, Siddiqui A. Botulinum toxin type A: a treatment option for digital ischemia in patients with Raynaud's phenomenon. J Hand Surg Am. 2009;34(3):446–52. https://doi.org/10.1016/j.jhsa.2008.11.026.

78. Neumeister MW. Botulinum toxin type A in the treatment of Raynaud's phenomenon. J Hand Surg Am. 2010;35(12):2085–92. https://doi.org/10.1016/j.jhsa.2010.09.019.

79. Goldberg SH, Akoon A, Kirchner HL, Deegan J. The effects of botulinum toxin A on pain in ischemic vasospasm. J Hand Surg Am. 2021;46(6):513.e1–513.e12. https://doi.org/10.1016/j.jhsa.2020.11.005.

80. Shenavandeh S, Sepaskhah M, Dehghani S, Nazarinia M. A 4-week comparison of capillaroscopy changes, healing effect, and cost-effectiveness of botulinum toxin-A vs prostaglandin analog infusion in refractory digital ulcers in systemic sclerosis. Clin Rheumatol. 2022;41(1):95–104. https://doi.org/10.1007/s10067-021-05900-7.

81. Medina S, Gómez-Zubiaur A, Valdeolivas-Casillas N, Polo-Rodríguez I, Ruíz L, Izquierdo C, Guirado C, Cabrera A, Trasobares L. Botulinum toxin type A in the treatment of Raynaud's phenomenon: a three-year follow-up study. Eur J Rheumatol. 2018;5(4):224–9. https://doi.org/10.5152/eurjrheum.2018.18013.

82. Motegi SI, Uehara A, Yamada K, Sekiguchi A, Fujiwara C, Toki S, Date Y, Nakamura T, Ishikawa O. Efficacy of botulinum toxin B injection for Raynaud's phenomenon and digital ulcers in patients with systemic sclerosis. Acta Derm Venereol. 2017;97(7):843–50. https://doi.org/10.2340/00015555-2665.

83. Bello RJ, Cooney CM, Melamed E, Follmar K, Yenokyan G, Leatherman G, Shah AA, Wigley FM, Hummers LK, Lifchez SD. The therapeutic efficacy of botulinum toxin in treating scleroderma-associated Raynaud's phenomenon: a randomized, double-blind, placebo-controlled clinical trial. Arthritis Rheumatol. 2017;69(8):1661–9. https://doi.org/10.1002/art.40123.

84. Quintana Castanedo L, Feito Rodríguez M, Nieto Rodríguez D, Maseda Pedrero R, Chiloeches Fernández C, de Lucas LR. Botulinum toxin A treatment for primary and secondary Raynaud's phenomenon in teenagers. Dermatologic Surg. 2021;47(1):61–4. https://doi.org/10.1097/DSS.0000000000002397.

85. Dhaliwal K, Griffin MF, Salinas S, Howell K, Denton CP, Butler PEM. Optimisation of botulinum toxin type a treatment for the management of Raynaud's phenomenon using a dorsal approach: a prospective case series. Clin Rheumatol. 2019;38(12):3669–76. https://doi.org/10.1007/s10067-019-04762-4.

86. Du W, Zhou M, Zhang C, Sun Q. The efficacy of botulinum toxin A in the treatment of Raynaud's phenomenon in systemic sclerosis: a randomized self-controlled trial. Dermatol Ther. 2022 Jul;35(7):e15529. https://doi.org/10.1111/dth.15529.

87. Seyedmardani SM, Aghdashi MA, Soltani S, Zonouz GK. Evaluation of botulinum toxin type A and its potential effect on exacerbated Raynaud's phenomenon in hospitalized scleroderma patients. Curr Rheumatol Rev. 2022;18(1):48–57. https://doi.org/10.2174/1573397117666211012105611.

88. Motegi S, Yamada K, Toki S, Uchiyama A, Kubota Y, Nakamura T, Ishikawa O. Beneficial effect of botulinum toxin A on Raynaud's phenomenon in Japanese patients with systemic sclerosis: a prospective, case series study. J Dermatol. 2016;43(1):56–62. https://doi.org/10.1111/1346-8138.13030.

89. Zhou Y, Yu Y, Bi S, Cen Y. Botulinum toxins for the treatment of Raynaud phenomenon: a systematic review with meta-analysis. J Clin Rheumatol. 2023;29(5):e92–9. https://doi.org/10.1097/RHU.0000000000001965.

90. Senet P, Maillard H, Diot E, Lazareth I, Blaise S, Arnault JP, Pistorius MA, Boulon C, Cogrel O, Warzocha U, Rivière S, Malloizel-Delaunay J, Servettaz A, Sassolas B, Viguier M, Monfort JB, Janique S, Vicaut E, BRASS collaborators. Efficacy and safety of botulinum toxin in adults with Raynaud's phenomenon secondary to systemic sclerosis: a Multicenter, randomized, double-blind, placebo-controlled study. Arthritis Rheumatol. 2023;75(3):459–67. https://doi.org/10.1002/art.42342.

91. Yin H, Liu B, Li Q, Yan Q, Lu L. Botulinum toxin for Raynaud's phenomenon associated with systemic sclerosis: comment on the article by Senet et al. Arthritis Rheumatol. 2023;75(3):486. https://doi.org/10.1002/art.42379.

92. Mesko ME, Hutton B, Skupien JA, et al. Therapies for bruxism: a systematic review and network meta-analysis (protocol). Syst Rev. 2017;6:4. https://doi.org/10.1186/s13643-016-0397-z.

93. Ondo WG, Simmons JH, Shahid MH, Hashem V, Hunter C, Jankovic J. Onabotulinum toxin-A injections for sleep bruxism: a double-blind, placebo-controlled study. Neurology. 2018;90(7):e559–64. https://doi.org/10.1212/WNL.0000000000004951.

94. Cruse B, Dharmadasa T, White E, Hollis C, Evans A, Sharmin S, Kalincik T, Kiers L. Efficacy of botulinum toxin type a in the targeted treatment of sleep bruxism: a double-blind, randomised, placebo-controlled, cross-over study. BMJ Neurol Open. 2022;4(2):e000328. https://doi.org/10.1136/bmjno-2022-000328.

95. Shehri ZG, Alkhouri I, Hajeer MY, Haddad I, Abu Hawa MH. Evaluation of the efficacy of low-dose botulinum toxin injection into the masseter muscle for the treatment of nocturnal bruxism: a randomized controlled clinical trial. Cureus. 2022;14(12):e32180. https://doi.org/10.7759/cureus.32180.

96. Davies J, Duffy D, Boyt N, et al. Botulinum toxin (botox) reduces pain after hemorrhoidectomy: results of a double-blind, randomized study. Dis Colon Rectum. 2003;46:1097–102.

97. Alvandipour M, Tavallaei M, Rezaei F, Khodabakhsh H. Postoperative outcomes of intrasphincteric botox injection during hemorrhoidectomy: a double-blind clinical trial. J Res Med Sci. 2021;30(26):53. https://doi.org/10.4103/jrms.JRMS_612_18.

98. Sirikurnpiboon S, Jivapaisarnpong P. Botulinum toxin injection for analgesic effect after Hemorrhoidectomy: a randomized control trial. J Anus Rectum Colon. 2020;4(4):186–92. https://doi.org/10.23922/jarc.2020-027.

99. Yaghoobi Notash A, Sadeghian E, Heshmati A, Sorush A. Effectiveness of local botulinum toxin injection for perianal pain after Hemorrhoidectomy. Middle East J Dig Dis. 2022;14(3):330–4.

100. Patti R, Almasio PL, Arcara M, Sammartano S, Romano P, Fede C, Di Vita G. Botulinum toxin vs. topical glyceryl trinitrate ointment for pain control in patients undergoing hemorrhoidectomy: a randomized trial. Dis Colon Rectum. 2006;49(11):1741–8.

101. Rodriguez-Acevedo O, Elstner KE, Jacombs ASW, Read JW, Martins RT, Arduini F, Wehrhahm M, Craft C, Cosman PH, Dardano AN, Ibrahim N. Preoperative botulinum toxin A enabling defect closure and laparoscopic repair of complex ventral hernia. Surg Endosc. 2018;32(2):831–9.

102. Niu EF, Kozak GM, McAuliffe PB, Amro C, Bascone C, Honig SE, Elsamaloty LH, Hao M, Broach RB, Kovach SJ 3rd, Fischer JP. Preoperative botulinum toxin for Abdominal Wall reconstruction in massive hernia defects-a propensity-matched analysis. Ann Plast Surg. 2023;90(6S Suppl 5):S543–6.
103. Stevens J, Baillie C, Choi B, Chapman A, Kostalas M, Ratnasingham K. The use of botulinum toxin in the acute management of symptomatic complex incisional hernia: a case series. Hernia. 2023;27(3):593–9.

Correction to: Botulinum Toxin Treatment in Aesthetic Medicine

Correction to:
Chapter 13 in: B. Jabbari, *Botulinum Toxin Treatment*,
https://doi.org/10.1007/978-3-031-54471-2_13

In the original version of the chapter "Botulinum Toxin Treatment in Aesthetic Medicine", owing to an oversight, Marie Noland and Marissa Dennis were mentioned as the authors of Chapter 13 in the Preface of the initially published version of this book but were not included in the chapter metadata. This has now been corrected.

The updated version of this chapter can be found at
https://doi.org/10.1007/978-3-031-54471-2_13

B. Jabbari, *Botulinum Toxin Treatment*,
https://doi.org/10.1007/978-3-031-54471-2_20

Index

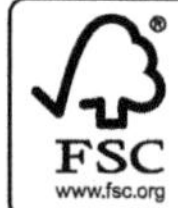

MIX
Papier aus verantwortungsvollen Quellen
Paper from responsible sources
FSC® C105338

If you have any concerns about our products,
you can contact us on
ProductSafety@springernature.com

In case Publisher is established outside the EU,
the EU authorized representative is:
**Springer Nature Customer Service Center GmbH
Europaplatz 3, 69115 Heidelberg, Germany**

Printed by Libri Plureos GmbH
in Hamburg, Germany